AF681857

Bariatric Surgery

A Primer for Your Medical Practice

Bariatric Surgery

A Primer for Your Medical Practice

Edited by

Francis A. Farraye, MD, MSc
Clinical Director, Section of Gastroenterology
Co-Director, Center for Digestive Disorders
Boston Medical Center
Boston, Mass

R. Armour Forse, MD, PhD
Chairman, Department of Surgery
Creighton University Medical Center
Omaha, Neb

SLACK
INCORPORATED

An innovative information, education, and management company
6900 Grove Road • Thorofare, NJ 08086

Copyright © 2006 by SLACK Incorporated

ISBN-10: 1-55642-736-0
ISBN-13: 978-1-55642-736-7

Top Right and Bottom Left Cover Images: Copyright © 2004 Massachusetts Medical Society. All rights reserved.
Top Left and Bottom Right Cover Images: Reproduced, with permission of Dr. Michel Gagner and Springer-Verlag, from Gentileschi P, Kini S, Catarci M, Gagner M. Evidence-based medicine: open and laparoscopic bariatric surgery. *Surg Endosc.* 2002;16:736-744.

All rights reserved. No part of this book may be reproduced, stored in a retrieval system or transmitted in any form or by any means, electronic, mechanical, photocopying, recording or otherwise, without written permission from the publisher, except for brief quotations embodied in critical articles and reviews.

The procedures and practices described in this book should be implemented in a manner consistent with the professional standards set for the circumstances that apply in each specific situation. Every effort has been made to confirm the accuracy of the information presented and to correctly relate generally accepted practices. The author, editor, and publisher cannot accept responsibility for errors or exclusions or for the outcome of the application of the material presented herein. There is no expressed or implied warranty of this book or information imparted by it.

Care has been taken to ensure that drug selection and dosages are in accordance with currently accepted/recommended practice. Due to continuing research, changes in government policy and regulations, and various effects of drug reactions and interactions, it is recommended that the reader carefully review all materials and literature provided for each drug, especially those that are new or not frequently used.

The work SLACK Incorporated publishes is peer reviewed. Prior to publication, recognized leaders in the field, educators, and clinicians provide important feedback on the concepts and content that we publish. We welcome feedback on this work.

Printed in the United States of America.

Library of Congress Cataloging-in-Publication Data

Bariatric surgery : a primer for your medical practice / edited by
Francis A. Farraye, R. Armour Forse.
p. ; cm.
Includes bibliographical references and index.
ISBN-13: 978-1-55642-736-7 (alk. paper)
ISBN-10: 1-55642-736-0 (alk. paper)
1. Obesity--Surgery. 2. Morbid obesity--Surgery. I. Farraye, Francis A. II. Forse, R. Armour.
[DNLM: 1. Obesity--surgery. 2. Bariatrics--methods. WD 210 B252 2005]
RD540.B377 2005
617.4'3--dc22

2005012842

Published by: SLACK Incorporated
6900 Grove Road
Thorofare, NJ 08086 USA
Telephone: 856-848-1000
Fax: 856-853-5991
www.slackbooks.com

Contact SLACK Incorporated for more information about other books in this field or about the availability of our books from distributors outside the United States.

For permission to reprint material in another publication, contact SLACK Incorporated. Authorization to photocopy items for internal, personal, or academic use is granted by SLACK Incorporated provided that the appropriate fee is paid directly to Copyright Clearance Center. Prior to photocopying items, please contact the Copyright Clearance Center at 222 Rosewood Drive, Danvers, MA 01923 USA; phone: 978-750-8400; Web site: www.copyright.com; email: info@copyright.com.

Last digit is print number: 10 9 8 7 6 5 4 3 2 1

Dedication

This book is dedicated to my loving and devoted family: my wife, Renee M. Remily, MD; my children, Jennifer and Alexis; and in particular to my parents who taught me that perseverance and commitment can result in great accomplishments.

Francis A. Farraye

This book is dedicated to the thousands of bariatric patients who taught me the importance of treating the whole patient, and to never giving up; to Dr. Lloyd MacLean, a great surgeon, who taught me to be a bariatric surgeon; to Adrienne O'Brien, a true friend and colleague, whose loyalty, dedication, and love to our practice was felt by all; and to my father whose lessons in life and medicine never seem to get old.

R. Armour Forse

Contents

Acknowledgments

We would like to thank the authors who did an outstanding job. The depth of experience and excellence in the field of bariatric surgery is evident in these very practical and informative chapters. Their efforts elevated this book from an idea to a reality and helped considerably with the editing process. A special note of thanks to our colleagues at the Boston University Medical Center and, in particular, to Dr. Christopher Huang, who worked tirelessly in providing care to our patients with postoperative gastrointestinal problems.

Furthermore, we greatly appreciate the superb efforts of Carie Lambert whose tireless editing resulted in clear and uniform content. On behalf of all the authors, we thank you for your dedication and professionalism. Finally, we would like to thank the staff members at SLACK Incorporated, specifically Carrie Kotlar, who recognized the importance of this topic and produced this publication on an accelerated timeline without sacrificing quality.

About the Editors

Francis A. Farraye, MD, MSc is an Associate Professor of Medicine and Epidemiology at the Boston University School of Medicine in Boston, Mass. He is also the Clinical Director in the Section of Gastroenterology and Co-Director of the Center for Digestive Disorders at Boston Medical Center. After graduating from the State University of New York at Stony Brook, Dr. Farraye earned his medical degree from the Albert Einstein College of Medicine in New York and his master's degree in Epidemiology from the Harvard School of Public Health. He completed an internship and residency in internal medicine, as well as a research and clinical fellowship in gastroenterology at Beth Israel Hospital in Boston.

Dr. Farraye's clinical interests are in the care of patients with inflammatory bowel disease, endoscopy in patients after bariatric surgery, and the management of colon polyps and colorectal cancer. He is studying the significance of adenomas found in patients with ulcerative colitis, management and diagnosis of dysplasia and cancer in patients with inflammatory bowel disease, and predictors of pouchitis after ileal pouch anal anastomosis. In the area of colorectal cancer, he is involved in several ongoing research studies, including modifying behavior in patients with colon polyps, identifying barriers to colorectal cancer screening, and gender differences in the tolerability of colon cancer screening with flexible sigmoidoscopy.

A frequent speaker and invited lecturer on topics including the management of inflammatory bowel disease, colorectal cancer screening, and endoscopy in the bariatric surgery patient, Dr. Farraye has authored or coauthored over 150 original scientific manuscripts, chapters, reviews, and abstracts. His work has been published in the *American Journal of Gastroenterology, Gastroenterology, Alimentary Pharmacology and Therapeutics, Gastrointestinal Endoscopy, Annals of Internal Medicine, JAMA,* and others. In addition, he has developed an interactive teaching DVD on the complications of bariatric surgery and the performance of endoscopy after bariatric surgery.

Dr. Farraye is a Fellow of the American College of Physicians and the American College of Gastroenterology. Nationally, he serves as Chair of the Patient Care Committee, Vice Chair of the Board of Governors, Governor in Massachusetts, and member of the Board of Trustees for the American College of Gastroenterology. He serves as AGA representative on the National Colorectal Cancer Round Table as Co-Chairman of the Standards Committee. He has served as the Chairman of the lower gastrointestinal disorders section of the Annual Scientific Program Committee of the American Society of Gastrointestinal Endoscopy. He is a member of the Chapter Medical Advisory Committee for the New England Crohn's and Colitis Foundation of America (CCFA) and is its immediate past Chairman. The New England CCFA named Dr. Farraye Humanitarian of the Year in 2003.

R. Armour Forse, MD, PhD is the Dr. & Mrs. Arnold W. Lempka Professor and Chair in the Department of Surgery at Creighton University, Omaha, Neb and the Chief of the Surgical Services at Creighton University Medical Center in Omaha, Neb.

Dr. Forse was previously the Laslo N. Tauber Professor of Surgery at Boston University and the Vice Chairman of Surgery at Boston Medical Center. Dr. Forse received his undergraduate, medical, and post-doctorate degrees from McGill University in Montreal, Quebec, Canada. He completed his surgical internship and residency at Royal Victoria Hospital in Montreal, where he also served as chief surgical resident. His research fellowships include experimental surgery at McGill University and surgical metabolism at Columbia University College of Physicians and Surgeons in New York. Dr. Forse was an Assistant Professor of Surgery at McGill University and later an Associate Professor of Surgery at Harvard Medical School, where he co-founded and directed the Center for Minimally Invasive Surgery and directed the Clowes Laboratory of Surgical Metabolism.

Dr. Forse's clinical interests are in the areas of gastrointestinal surgery including bariatric surgery, minimally invasive surgery, trauma, care of the critically ill patient, and nutrition, including obesity. He has been involved with bariatric surgery for over 25 years and has performed thousands of procedures, including jeujuno-ileal bypass, gastroplasty, gastric bypass, laparoscopic gastric bypass, and revision bariatric surgery. His research interests currently include the development of transluminal surgery, the effectiveness of revision surgery, and the effects on nutrients on various diseases. His basic research interests include adipocyte biology as it applies to cell differentiation and proliferation in obesity, abdominal compartment syndrome in obesity, cell signaling in macrophages and Kuppfer cells, and nutrient-disease interactions.

Dr. Forse is a frequent speaker on topics including bariatric surgery, nutritional support, and the treatment of sepsis. He has authored and coauthored over 380 papers, chapters, and abstracts, and has coedited 4 previous medical books. His publications have appeared in *American Journal of Clinical Nutrition, American Journal of Physiology, American Journal of Surgery, Annals of Surgery, Biochemistry Journal, Critical Care Medicine, New England Journal of Medicine,* and *Obesity Research.*

Dr. Forse is a Fellow of the American College of Surgeons, the American College of Critical Care Medicine, and the Royal College of Surgeons in Canada, and he is a member of over 25 surgical societies.

Contributing Authors

Wendy A. Anderson, MS, RD, LDN
Boston Medical Center
Boston, Mass

Caroline M. Apovian, MD
Boston Medical Center
Boston University School of Medicine
Boston, Mass

Laura Foresta, RD, LDN
Boston Medical Center
Boston, Mass

Donald T. Hess, Jr, MD
Boston Medical Center
Boston University School of Medicine
Boston, Mass

Christopher S. Huang, MD
Boston Medical Center
Boston University School of Medicine
Boston, Mass

Nawfal Istfan, MD, PhD
Boston Medical Center
Boston University School of Medicine
Boston, Mass

David M. Lambert, MD
Creighton University Medical Center
Omaha, Neb

Keith P. Lewis, RPh, MD
Boston Medical Center
Boston University School of Medicine
Boston, Mass

Linda Lin, PhD
Emmanuel College
Boston, Mass

Brian C. Lucey, MD
Boston Medical Center
Boston University School of Medicine
Boston, Mass

Marie E. McDonnell, MD
Boston Medical Center
Boston University School of Medicine
Boston, Mass

John R. Pender, MD
East Carolina University
Greenville, NC

Frank Perna, PhD, EdD
Solomon Carter Fuller Center
Boston, Mass

Walter J. Pories, MD
East Carolina University
Greenville, NC

Jennifer Rosenblum, MD
Massachusetts General Hospital
Harvard Medical School
Boston, Mass

Jorge A. Soto, MD
Boston Medical Center
Boston University School of Medicine
Boston, Mass

Heather K. Stein, MD, MPH
Massachusetts General Hospital
Harvard Medical School
Boston, Mass

Ranjan Sudan, MD
Creighton University Medical Center
Omaha, Neb

Jose C. Varghese, MD
Boston Medical Center
Boston University School of Medicine
Boston, Mass

Preface

Obesity has reached epidemic proportions in the United States and other parts of the world. This chronic disease is a factor in many illnesses, resulting in suffering and premature death. Medical investigators and providers are studying and developing new pharmacologic, medical, and surgical treatments for obesity.

Bariatric surgery is, in appropriate and carefully selected patients, an effective treatment for obesity. While the field of bariatric surgery is relatively new—only about 50 years old—it is developing rapidly, offering innovative options for patients who have failed to lose weight by diet, exercise, and pharmacologic methods. Multidisciplinary teams help to assure the care of these individuals, but as the number of patients undergoing weight-loss surgery increases, more clinicians will see bariatric patients in their practices.

The editors and authors developed this text as a complete primer and reference manual for students and residents as well as practicing health care providers who see patients considering bariatric surgery and those who have undergone the surgery. This book reviews problems that the patient faces immediately around the surgery as well as the long-term issues such as adjustments in lifestyle and health care management following weight-loss surgery. The text is authored by authorities who participate in the multidisciplinary care of bariatric patients. Here, they address assessment and selection as well as the patients' treatment before surgery, options for surgical intervention, and postoperative medical management. Access to this information can help providers understand the process of bariatric care and thus better provide for those undergoing or considering these procedures.

Francis A. Farraye, MD, MSc
R. Armour Forse, MD, PhD

Foreword

"Doctor, should I be considering bariatric surgery?" With the increasing number of overweight and obese patients and a rise in media attention, primary care providers are being asked to answer this question more frequently than ever before. *Bariatric Surgery: A Primer for Your Medical Practice* is a timely text that provides the information practitioners need. Although the prevalence of all obesity classification groups is increasing, the steepest rise is occurring in the severely (morbidly) obese category. According to the latest statistics of the Behavioral Risk Factor Surveillance System (BRFSS), the prevalence of self-reported clinically severe obesity (body mass index [BMI] $\geq$40 kg/m^2) quadrupled from about 1 in 200 adult Americans to 1 in 50 over the last 15 years. The prevalence of a BMI $\geq$50 kg/m^2 increased by a factor of 5, from about 1 in 2000 to 1 in 400. Thus, it can be expected that every primary care provider will have a subpopulation of severely obese patients in his or her practice.

What therapies should we offer our overweight and obese patients? Low-calorie diets, increased physical activity, and behavior therapy form the basis for lifestyle management across all body BMI ranges. However, the evidence is limited that these strategies alone, or in combination with very low-calorie diets (VLCDs) or pharmacotherapy, are effective in persons with clinically severe or extreme class III obesity. In contrast to these nonsurgical approaches, bariatric surgery has been demonstrated to be an effective treatment option and should be considered for patients who are severely obese. As a result of the high visibility of bariatric surgery in the media, more patients are asking their physicians whether they are candidates for one of several procedures. Accordingly, primary care providers need to become familiar with the identification, evaluation, and perioperative management of the bariatric surgical patient. Primary practitioners will also be expected to monitor and manage their patients on a long-term basis. This textbook provides the foundation of care for selecting and managing patients who elect to undergo bariatric surgery.

Why is a textbook devoted to bariatric surgery needed? Quite simply, there is no other surgical procedure that more profoundly alters the medical, psychological, and social status of an individual than bariatric surgery. From preoperative evaluation of the patient's risk status, assessment of readiness for change, knowledge about diet, social support and coping ability, to postoperative management of surgical complications and dietary changes, the primary care provider is an extended member of the multidisciplinary team that cares for the bariatric surgical patient. Because very little training in obesity care and bariatric surgery occurs in medical school, residency, and continuing medical education, clinicians must rely on self-directed resources. *Bariatric Surgery: A Primer for Your Medical Practice* is a well-written and informative text that covers all aspects of the surgical process, including deciphering the most commonly performed surgical procedures, evaluating the patient preoperatively, identifying and managing immediate and long-term complications, and providing psychological support. The chapters that review endoscopy and imaging are particularly instructive because they provide guidance regarding appropriate testing and illustrative pictures of the surgically altered anatomy with and without complications. The text also provides a much needed crash course on nutrition and nutritional deficiencies. The combined restrictive-malabsorptive surgical procedures place patients at high risk for development of both macro- and micronutrient deficiencies unless properly counseled and supplemented. Chronic deficiencies in iron, vitamin B_{12}, calcium, and vitamin D are particularly concerning and represent the greatest long-term risk. Fortunately, these deficiencies are predictable and preventable.

Although *Bariatric Surgery: A Primer for Your Medical Practice* is mainly intended for primary health care providers, others including medical students, residents, and subspecialists who care for bariatric patients will be equally informed. I am confident that this book will be a valuable resource to many clinicians in the coming years.

Robert F. Kushner, MD
Professor of Medicine
Northwestern University Feinberg School of Medicine
Chicago, Ill

1 THE OBESITY EPIDEMIC

John R. Pender, MD and Walter J. Pories, MD

Introduction

Each year, more Americans are becoming overweight. Increases in comorbidity and decreases in life span are being seen in our population as a result of this growing epidemic. Once considered an issue of vanity, research in obesity has linked this problem with increased mortality and comorbidities. Obesity is becoming a commonly seen health issue that is endangering the lives of more individuals each year. Obesity is directly related to increased risk of gallbladder disease,[1] musculoskeletal disorders,[1] severe pancreatitis,[2] infertility,[3] urinary incontinence,[4] sleep apnea,[5] cancer,[5] bacterial panniculitis,[6] diverticulitis,[7] and idiopathic intracranial hypertension.[8] An increased risk of cardiovascular disease, hyperlipidemia, hypertension, and diabetes are associated with an increased waist-to-hip girth.[9] The disabilities caused by obesity are psychosocial as well as physiologic; decreased quality of life in the obese population has been well documented, as has an increase in psychological problems. As the prevalence of obesity and related disorders increases, so must the efforts of the health care industry to educate patients on prevention and to establish treatments that save and improve the quality of patients' lives.

In the last few decades, the prevalence of obesity has radically increased. In the United States alone, 300,000 annual deaths are attributed to obesity[10]; researchers ascribe these deaths to direct as well as indirect effects of the condition. The mortality rate of individuals who are overweight is twice that of nonobese individuals.[11] Severe obesity can result in a significant reduction of an individual's life expectancy—by as much as 22%.[12] The ethnicity and gender of a patient with obesity are factors in shorter life expectancy (discussed later). Age is also significant. Compared to their older counterparts, younger adults lose more years of their lives because of obesity. The increasing number of individuals who are classified as overweight has some medical professionals calling the prevalence of morbid obesity an epidemic and has others calling for obesity to be officially recognized as a separate disease process. The United States, in particular, needs to directly address this epidemic.

As research of obesity has increased and improved, so have treatments for the disorder. Medical research has resulted in the development of diets, exercise regimens, pharmacologic advancements, and surgical treatments. Advances in obesity surgery have led to weight loss that is permanent in those who comply with required lifestyle changes. However, as with all diseases, a comprehensive health care plan is necessary to address prevention and thus minimize the number of individuals suffering from and needing treatment for obesity.

Definition of Obesity-Related Terms

Simply, obesity is the state of having too much adipose tissue to be healthy. The standard for a healthy weight is defined by the percentage of body fat that increases an individual's risk of morbidity and mortality. Assessment of human body composition helps in the differentiation of lean muscle weight and adipose tissue weight. The body of a 6-foot-tall, 260-pound football player cannot be compared to that of a 5-foot-tall, 60-year-old desk clerk who also weighs 260 pounds.

Several methods to determine body composition exist, some of which use expensive and time-consuming methods involving the use of radioisotopes, laboratory values, and machines to perform calculations. All have the common purpose of determining what percentage of a subject's total weight is fat and what percentage is lean. Total body water, total body potassium, urinary creatinine excretion, densitometry, neutron-activation analysis, absorptiometry, bioelectrical impedance, total-body electrical conductivity, computerized tomography, magnetic resonance imaging, and anthropometry are all methods for determining the amount of fat in a human body. Some of these are only available in laboratories, and others require only a set of scales and a measuring tape. For the bariatric surgeon, a method that can be applied in clinical practice is the best choice. Unfortunately, as with most tests, simplicity usually means less accuracy.

In 1959, Metropolitan Life Insurance Company (Met Life) developed actuarial tables to determine a client's longevity in relation to weight. Developed by statisticians, these tables demonstrate what weight an individual should be if he or she is a certain height with a certain frame size. Studies since 1959 have classified individuals' weights using these tables as the standard. A patient whose weight is 20% over the ideal body weight (IBW) presented in this table is considered "overweight."[13,14]

The Met Life tables have several inconsistencies.[15] First, the heights on the chart include a person's height with 1-inch-heeled shoes. Not all versions of these tables specify this detail. Second, the tables are specific for adults over 25 years of age and are not appropriate for evaluation of children or young adults (individuals who are less likely to have life insurance). Finally, the Met Life tables present unreasonably low weights for taller individuals (regardless of gender). As average height and weight increase, as they have in the last 25 years, the standards set in the Met Life tables are even more unrealistic.[16] Because of these and other conditions, the Met Life tables are used less frequently as standards for healthy weight.

Today, the body mass index (BMI) is the most commonly used and universally accepted method to classify an individual's state of obesity in relation to that of others. BMI is calculated as the patient's weight in kilograms divided by his or her height in meters squared (kg/m^2). This method is quite simple and easy to use; however, the system has limitations. First, because BMI is calculated by weight and height, it does not take into consideration the composition of the individual's weight. A physically fit athlete with a large amount

Table 1-1

Classification of Weight by NHLBI and WHO[22]

BMI Range	NHLBI Terms	WHO Terms	Classification
<18.5	Underweight	Underweight	—
18.5 to 24.9	Normal	Normal	—
25 to 29.9	Overweight	Preobese	—
30 to 34.9	Mildly obese	Mildly obese	I
35 to 39.9	Moderately obese	Moderately obese	II
≥40	Morbidly obese	Morbidly obese	III
≥50	Super obese	Super obese	III*

* "Super obese" is included in Class III, although it has its own lower BMI limit.

Adapted from World Health Organization. *Obesity: preventing and managing the global epidemic.* Report of a WHO Consultation presented at: the World Health Organization; June 3-5, 1997; Geneva, Switzerland. Publication WHO/NUT/NCD/98.1.

of muscle weight can have the same BMI as that of an individual who is indeed overweight. Second, BMI does not consider the difference in fat cells and their distribution.[17] Clinicians and health officials have attempted to overcome the BMI system's shortcomings by adding modifications, such as measuring the ratio of waist-to-hip circumferences; however, this adds to the complexity of a simple test.[18] Even with its limitations, the method is useful because BMI has been demonstrated to correlate with a patient's risk of obesity-related morbidity and mortality[19] and therefore can assist the physician in assessing the individual's overall health.

The National Heart, Lung, and Blood Institute's (NHLBI) definitions for the division between overweight and obesity are currently the most frequently used weight-classification system. The World Health Organization (WHO) classification system is similar to the NHLBI terminology[20]: both use BMI of 18.5 to 24.9 kg/m^2 ("normal" weight) as a reference category to the 4 weight classes (Table 1-1) and, with the exception of BMI of 25.0 to 29.9, both organizations use the same categories. (For this category, the WHO uses the term "preobese" and the NHLBI uses the term "overweight.") Individuals with a BMI ≥30 are considered "obese."[21,22] A BMI ≥40 corresponds to 100 pounds over IBW, categorizing the patient as "morbidly obese."[14] "Super obese" is used for patients in obesity class III whose BMI is ≥50.

Obesity-Related Surveys

International Surveys

Several recent surveys have compared the prevalence of individuals with obesity today with that of the past. In Europe, the Seven Countries Study included data on the prevalence of obesity in Yugoslavia, Italy, Finland, the Netherlands, and Greece. This study evaluated the connection between obesity and mortality and revealed that obesity and its complications have become an increasing health problem throughout Europe.[23] In the United Kingdom, the National Health and Growth Study has run uninterrupted for over 23 years. This study along with the International Obesity Task Force has identified an alarming increase in the prevalence of obesity, especially in school-age children.[24,25]

In 1997, the WHO held a "Consultation on Obesity" to review information on obesity throughout the world and recommend international action to improve existing programs for obesity prevention and treatment. At this meeting, the WHO recommended the BMI system (see Table 1-1) as the international weight-classification standard. Most importantly, the final report formally declared obesity as a threat to global health, recognizing that more populations than ever before are struggling with the issues related to obesity.[22] Obesity is not a problem unique to the United States; it is a worldwide epidemic.

United States Surveys

Surveys specific to the United States show alarming trends of obesity in Americans. Two US-specific surveys are worth noting: the Behavioral Risk Factor Surveillance System (BRFSS), which is a telephone survey conducted by the Centers for Disease Control and Prevention, and the National Health and Nutrition Examination Survey (NHANES), a statistically representative probability sample. The BRFSS questions a cross-section of noninstitutionalized, civilian adults to determine behaviors that increase risks for the top 10 causes of death in the United States.[26] Between 1986 and 2003, collected data were examined to evaluate national obesity trends. During this 17-year data period, the number of individuals with a BMI ≥40 quadrupled. The prevalence of obesity (BMI ≥30) only increased by a factor of 2, but the prevalence of super obesity (BMI ≥50) increased by a factor of 5.[27] This is impressive, particularly considering the self-reporting bias of telephone surveys.

The National Health Survey Act of 1956 instituted the NHANES. From 1960 to 1962, the National Health Examination Survey (NHES I) was the first survey under the Act to collect data on Americans' health. Following were the NHANES I (1971 to 1975), the NHANES II (1976 to 1980), and the NHANES III (1988 to 1994),[28] each a comprehensive health examination of a noninstitutionalized, civilian population.[29] In 1999, the NHANES became a continuing survey on the amount, distribution, and effects of illness and disability in the United States.

The NHANES I (1971 to 1975) included interviews of approximately 32,000 persons age 1 to 74 years. Of the interviewed sample, 23,808 people received a medical examination at the end of the study.[30] A longitudinal follow-up study was then undertaken: the Epidemiologic Follow-Up Study (NHEFS) investigated the relationships between behavioral, nutritional, and clinical factors of persons aged 25 to 74 years who completed a medical examination for NHANES I (n=14,407).[29] Using this information, the NHEFS has demonstrated the hospital utilization, morbidity, and mortality of the cohort, as well as the changes in risk factors, impairment, and institutionalization.[28]

A second study, during 1976 to 1980, interviewed and examined 20,322 individuals age 6 to 74 years. The NHANES II continued the measurement and monitoring of the nutritional status and health of the US population. The NHANES III sampled 33,994 Americans who were 2 years of age and older from 1988 to 1994. The Hispanic Health and Nutrition Examination Survey (HHANES) was also conducted (1982 to 1984) to obtain health and nutrition information specific to US Hispanics, including Cuban Americans, Puerto Ricans, and Mexican Americans.[31]

An epidemiologic follow-up study has been instituted for each of the subsequent cohorts of all of the NHANES. Current collection teams use a mobile exam unit to collect exam information on every survey subject using standardized measurements.

Data from these studies have been used to determine obesity trends in America since 1960.[28] The 1999-to-2000 survey included height and weight measurements for the 4115 adult men and women in this multistage, stratified survey. Early survey results show that obesity rates in the United States were relatively stable between 1960 and 1980. The more recent NHANES III data indicate an estimated 22% overall prevalence of obesity,[32] with an estimated 8% increase between 1988 and 1994.[28] The NHANES III's estimated prevalence of obesity is almost twice that reported by the BRFSS. In NHANES III, actual height and weight are measured, whereas the BRFSS is a self-reporting survey.[28] The tendency of individuals to over-report height and under-report weight in the self-reporting process can explain this discrepancy. Nonetheless, both surveys reveal an alarming trend in obesity.

Demographics of Americans With Obesity

The prevalence of obesity was relatively constant during the periods of the NHES, the NHANES I, and the NHANES II (1960 to 1980). However, the NHANES data specifically demonstrate significant increases—regardless of gender, ethnicity, or age—in the age-adjusted prevalence in America from the NHANES III (1988 to 1994) to the first phase of the continuous NHANES (1999 to 2000): overweight—55.9% to 64.5%; obesity—22.9% to 30.5%; and morbid obesity—2.9% to 4.7%.[28] By 2002, 30.4% of those interviewed were obese and 65.1% were overweight.[33]

Some demographic subgroups experience obesity more frequently than others. The following sections discuss the increasing prevalence of obesity in Americans according to gender, ethnicity, and age.

Gender

Being overweight is a problem that affects individuals regardless of gender. In general, trends show slightly higher rates of obesity in females (Table 1-2),[33] with increases in prevalence rates following similar patterns. The only exception to this is NHANES data on men age 60 to 74 years, for which the increase since 1960 has been greater than those of female and other male subgroups.[28]

BMI calculations depend completely on an individual's height and weight. For past NHANES, gender-specific values for overweight (BMI ≥27.8 for males, BMI ≥27.3 for females) were used[33]; however, current obesity standards (see Table 1-1) do not include separate tables for males and females.

Ethnicity

Assessing different ethnic groups helps specify which groups have higher rates of obesity and thus are at higher risk for the related morbidities. These rates can be the result of genetics, education, environment, or cultural practices and biases, among other factors. Obesity trends seem to differ by gender for the 3 major ethnic groups, hereby identified as African Americans (referring to non-Hispanic Blacks), Whites (referring to non-Hispanic Whites), and Hispanics (Cuban Americans, Puerto Ricans, and Mexican Americans). Other small ethnic groups were not separately classified in the NHANES.[28]

Past NHANES (I and II) do not include adequate sample sizes of Hispanics in the United States.[31] However, from 1982 to 1984, the HHANES collected data on US Hispanics.[34] This survey was limited in that data were collected from a specific geographic area of

Table 1-2

Trends in Age-Adjusted and Age-Specific Prevalence of Obesity for Adults 20 to 74 Years of Age (1960 to 2000)[28]

Gender	Age† (y)	Prevalence of Obesity (%)				
		NHES I (n=6126)	*NHANES I (n=12,911)*	*NHANES II (n=11,765)*	*NHANES III (n=14,468)*	*NHANES* (n=3,601)*
Combined Data	20 to 74	13.4	14.5	15.0	23.3	30.9
Male	20 to 74	10.7	12.1	12.7	20.6	27.7
	20 to 39	9.8	10.2	9.8	14.9	23.7
	40 to 59	12.6	14.7	15.4	25.4	28.8
	60 to 74	8.4	10.5	13.5	23.8	35.8
Female	20 to 74	15.8	16.6	17.0	25.9	34.0
	20 to 39	9.3	11.2	12.3	20.6	28.4
	40 to 59	18.5	19.7	20.4	30.4	37.8
	60 to 74	26.2	23.4	21.3	28.6	39.6

† Estimated prevalences were age-standardized by the direct method to the 2000 Census population using the age groups in this table.

* Includes data collected through the continuous NHANES from 1999 to 2000.

Adapted from Flegal KM, Carroll MD, Ogden CL, Johnson CL. Prevalence and trends in obesity among US adults, 1999-2000. *JAMA*. 2002;288(14):1723-1727.

the United States[34]; however, because the HHANES information represents 84% of the Mexican-origin population in the United States, comparison between the HHANES and NHANES III can reliably estimate trends in obesity for US Hispanics.[31]

According to reports from 1999 to 2000, 74.7% of Hispanic males were overweight (BMI ≥25), a rate that was higher than those of White and African American males, whose estimated prevalence of overweight were 67.4% and 60.7%, respectively (Table 1-3).[28] These rates do not differ greatly from expanding findings in the 1999 to 2002 NHANES for the same 3 subgroups—73.1%, 69.4%, and 62.9%, respectively.[33] Prevalence of obesity (BMI ≥30) during 1999 to 2000 was not significantly different between the 3 ethnic groups of males—28.9% (Hispanic), 27.3% (White), and 28.1% (African American) (see Table 1-3)[28]; and there were no significant changes in the prevalence of obesity for these 3 groups of men (27.3%, 28.2%, and 27.9%, respectively) between 1999 to 2000 and 2001 to 2002.[33] These show slight increases from data of NHANES III (1988 to 1994): 23.9% (Hispanic males), 21.1% (African Americans), and 20.3% (Whites).[28]

Women of different ethnic subgroups have greater differences on estimated prevalence of overweight, according to these studies. According to 1999 to 2000 NHANES data, African American females had the highest prevalence of overweight (BMI ≥25)—77.3%—when compared with Hispanic (71.9%) and White (57.3%) females. Data from 1999 to 2002 NHANES assessments did not differ greatly: prevalence of obesity remained consistent

Table 1-3

Prevalence of Overweight and Obesity by Gender, Age, and Ethnicity from NHANES Data (1999 to 2000)[28]

		Sample Size (n)				Prevalence (%) of Overweight (BMI ≥25), Obesity (BMI ≥30)			
Gender	*Age*† *(y)*	*All**	*White*	*Black*	*Hispanic*	*All**	*White*	*Black*	*Hispanic*
Combined	≥20	4115	1831	794	1105	64.5, 30.5	62.3, 28.7	69.6, 39.9‡	73.4‡, 34.4
Male	≥20	2043	946	374	538	67.2, 27.5	67.4, 27.3	60.7, 28.1	74.7, 28.9
	20 to 39	666	276	125	184	60.5, 23.7	61.0, 22.0	52.6, 27.4	67.5, 30.4
	40 to 59	595	262	127	157	70.0, 28.8	69.9, 28.5	63.9, 29.9	79.1, 27.0
	≥60	782	408	122	197	74.1, 31.8	74.3, 34.3	69.1, 26.4	79.6, 29.7
Female	≥20	2072	885	420	567	61.9, 33.4	57.3, 30.1	77.3‡, 49.7‡	71.9, 39.7
	20 to 39	640	249	140	180	54.3, 28.4	49.0, 24.4	70.8‡, 46.2‡	61.6, 30.6
	40 to 59	653	249	141	193	66.1, 37.8	61.0, 34.2	81.5‡, 53.2‡	79.3, 48.5
	≥60	779	387	139	194	68.1, 35.0	65.8, 33.3	81.7‡, 50.2‡	77.5, 41.0

† Estimated prevalences were age-standardized by the direct method to the 2000 Census population using the age groups in this table.

* Includes ethnic groups not shown separately.

‡ Significantly different from whites, *P* <.05 (with Bonferroni correction).

Adapted from Flegal KM, Carroll MD, Ogden CL, Johnson CL. Prevalence and trends in obesity among US adults, 1999-2000. *JAMA*. 2002;288(14):1723-1727.

(77.2%, 71.7%, and 57.2% for African American, Hispanic, and White females).[33] Trends for the prevalence of obesity (BMI ≥30) for females were similar—49.7% of African Americans, 39.7% of Hispanics, and 30.1% of Whites were assessed as obese in 2000[28]—and did not significantly change by 2002 (49.0%, 38.4%, and 30.7%, respectively).[33] These percentages do, however, show a significant increase in obesity prevalence from NHANES III (1988 to 1994)—38.2% (African American), 35.3% (Hispanic), and 22.9% (White)—particularly in African American females.[28]

AGE

Obesity is no longer only a concern for adults. More than ever before, infants, children, and adolescents are becoming obese and experiencing comorbidities that can accompany the disease. Prevention, diagnosis, and treatment for obesity differ for different age groups, as shown below. Research is focusing on subgroups according to age: children (0 to 12 years), adolescents (13 to 18 years), adults (19 to 59 years), and seniors (≥60 years). The data presented below are classified in different age groups according to the National Longitudinal Survey of Youth (children 4 to 12 years of age)[35] and the NHANES: preschool children (0 to 5 years, with minimal data coverage before 2 years), children (6 to 19 years), and adults (≥20 years).[28,33,34]

This book focuses on obesity in the adult population; however, in addition to the brief discussion below, Chapter 6 addresses obesity in pediatric and elderly groups.

Children—0 to 19 years of age

According to the NHANES data, the prevalence of overweight has increased in preschool girls: 10.8% of 4- to 5-year-old girls were overweight in 1988 to 1994 compared to 5.8% in 1971 to 1974. Smaller increases from the NHANES I to the NHANES III were also recorded for girls who were 12 to 23 months of age (6.1% to 9.5%) and 2 to 3 years of age (2.0% to 4.8%). Changes for boys of this age were insignificant between the 2 surveys: 7.5% to 7.5% for 12- to 23-month-olds, a decrease of 3.1% to 2.1% for 2- to 3-year olds, and an increase of 4.4% to 5.0% for 4- to 5-year olds. When comparing data specific to children between the ages of 6 months and 5 years, prevalence of overweight was higher in girls than boys, and investigators reported a higher prevalence in Hispanic preschoolers than those classified as African American or White.[36]

The National Longitudinal Survey of Youth studied the prevalence of overweight in 8270 children, ages 4 to 12 years, from 1986 to 1998. Children were interviewed several times during the study period; an in-home interview included the collection of demographic data, height and weight measurement (or parental reporting of the measurement), and calculation of the child's BMI. A child was classified as "overweight" if his or her BMI was >95th percentile on the weight growth curve for his or her gender and age.[35] (The term "obesity" is not used when referring to children or adolescents.)

This study shows significant increases in the prevalence of overweight among Hispanic, African American, and White children. By 1998, rates in Hispanic children had increased to 21.8%, with similar increases in the cohort of African American children (21.5%)—a >120% increase in both groups. Overweight prevalence increased (12.3%) in White children as well (a >50% increase). Demographic differences in the prevalence of childhood overweight by 1998 could be seen as overweight increased fastest among minorities and southerners. Additionally, low-income Hispanic and African American boys had a 27.4% increase of prevalence of overweight during the study period. Also, overweight children in 1998 were heavier than those in 1986.[35]

These trends have been further supported by the NHANES data from 1999 to 2000. "At risk for overweight" was defined as at or above the 85th percentile but less than the 95th percentile of the sex-specific BMI for age. Children above the 95th percentile of the sex-specific BMI-for-age growth chart are defined as "overweight." These percentiles are defined by the 2000 Centers for Disease Control and Prevention Growth Chart. These growth charts are based on national data from 1963 to 1994 and are sex-specific for BMI (Table 1-4).[33]

Table 1-4

Prevalence of At Risk for Overweight and Overweight in Children by Sex, Age, and Ethnic Group: US, 1999 to 2000[*34]

		At Risk for Overweight and Overweight (BMI for Age ≥85th Percentile)—Prevalence, % (SE)				Overweight (BMI for Age ≥95th Percentile)—Prevalence, % (SE)			
Gender	*Age (y)*	*All*	*White*	*Black*	*Hispanic*	*All*	*White*	*Black*	*Hispanic*
Combined	6 to 19	31.0 (1.1)	28.2 (1.6) †‡	35.4 (0.9)‡§	39.9 (1.3)†§	16.0 (0.8)	13.6 (1.1)†‡	20.5 (0.8)§	22.2 (1.1)§
	2 to 5	22.6 (1.5)	20.8 (2.0)	23.2 (2.3)	26.3 (2.7)	10.3 (1.2)	8.6 (1.5)	8.8 (1.5)	13.1 (2.0)
	6 to 11	31.2 (1.8)	28.6 (2.6)‡	33.7 (1.6)	38.9 (2.2)§	15.8 (1.1)	13.5 (1.5)†‡	19.8 (1.4)§	21.8 (1.7)§
	12 to 19	30.9 (1.0)	27.9 (1.5)†‡	36.8 (1.3)§	40.7 (1.6)§	16.1 (0.8)	13.7 (1.1)†‡	21.1 (1.2)§	22.5 (1.3)§
Boys	6 to 19	31.8 (1.4)	29.2 (2.4)‡	31.0 (1.3)‡	42.8 (1.6)†§	16.8 (0.8)	14.3 (1.1)‡	17.9 (1.0)‡	22.5 (1.3)†§
	2 to 5	23.0 (2.3)	21.7 (3.2)	20.9 (2.5)	27.6 (3.1)	9.9 (1.6)	8.2 (1.9)	8.0 (1.8)	14.1 (2.1)
	6 to 11	32.5 (2.3)	29.3 (3.8)‡	29.7 (2.2)‡	43.9 (3.0)†§	16.9 (1.3)	14.0 (1.5)‡	17.0 (1.5)‡	26.5 (2.2)†§
	12 to 19	31.2 (1.5)	29.2 (2.3)‡	32.1 (2.1)‡	41.9 (1.8)†§	16.7 (0.9)	14.6 (1.3)‡	18.7 (1.7)	24.7 (1.9)§
Girls	6 to 19	30.3 (1.3)	27.0 (1.7)†‡	40.1 (1.4)§	36.6 (1.8)§	15.1 (1.1)	12.9 (1.6)†‡	23.2 (1.1)§	18.5 (1.4)§
	2 to 5	22.3 (1.8)	20.0 (2.3)	25.6 (3.0)	25.0 (3.8)	10.7 (1.5)	9.1 (2.0)	9.6 (1.8)	12.2 (3.4)
	6 to 11	29.9 (2.1)	27.7 (2.8)	37.9 (2.8)	33.8 (2.6)	14.7 (1.6)	13.1 (2.3)†	22.8 (2.5)§	17.1 (2.0)
	12 to 19	30.5 (1.3)	26.5 (2.0)†‡	41.9 (1.7)§	39.3 (2.3)§	15.4 (1.2)	12.7 (1.8)†	23.6 (1.8)§	19.9 (1.9)

* BMI was rounded to the nearest tenth. Pregnant girls were excluded. "All" category included ethnic groups not shown separately.

† Significantly different from blacks at $P < .05$, with Bonferroni adjustment.

‡ Significantly different from Hispanics at $P < .05$, with Bonferroni adjustment.

§ Significantly different from whites at $P < .05$, with Bonferroni adjustment.

Adapted from Kuczmarski RJ. Flegal KM, Campbell SM. Johnson CL. Increasing prevalence of overweight among US adults: the National Health and Nutrition Examination Surveys, 1960 to 1991. *JAMA*. 1994;272(3):205-211.

NHANES 1999 to 2002 data revealed that 22.6% of children 2 to 5 years of age were at risk for overweight or were overweight (BMI ≥85), and 10.3% of preschoolers (2 to 5 years of age) were overweight (BMI ≥95).[33] Among preschool-age children, Hispanic boys had the highest prevalence of being at risk for or being overweight (27.6%) compared to African American (20.9%) and White (21.7%) boys ages 2 to 5 years. Regarding overweight prevalence, Hispanic preschool boys again had higher rates. Prevalence of risk and overweight in preschool girls did not differ significantly by ethnicity; however, the gender-specific rates of girls and boys with BMI ≥85 (22.3% and 23.0%, respectively) and BMI ≥95 (10.7% and 9.9%, respectively) were similar.[33]

Prevalence of overweight in school-age children was similar. Nearly one-third (31.0%) of children ages 6 to 19 years were at risk for or were overweight, and 16.0% were classified as overweight. Hispanic boys also had the highest rate of being at risk for or being overweight (42.8%) compared to White (29.2%) and African American (31.0%) boys. Hispanic boys of this age group also had the highest rate of being overweight (25.5%). The prevalence of overweight of African American and Hispanic girls (23.2% and 18.5%, respectively) was significantly higher than those among White girls (12.9%).[33]

Reports separating NHANES data for adolescents revealed the prevalence of overweight among 12 to 19 year olds as 15.5% in 1999 to 2000 compared to a prevalence of 10.5% in the NHANES III.[37]

Adults

Greater body weight is associated with a higher relative risk of death. This was confirmed by a study of approximately a million subjects in the American Cancer Society's Cancer Prevention Study I.[38] Evidence suggests that the relative risk associated with greater BMI declines with age, such that a younger adult (19 to 24 years of age) with a BMI >25 will have a higher relative risk of death from any cause than will an older patient with obesity. Additionally, the younger an individual is when his or her BMI surpasses 25, the greater that individual's relative risk of death is by any cause.[39]

The longer an individual has had diabetes and/or hypertension, the less likely this person is to see these comorbidities reversed by weight loss. Specifically, a younger individual with obesity has a higher risk of death by cardiovascular disease than does an older individual with a similar BMI.

Combining Gender, Ethnicity, and Age

Separating prevalence of overweight (BMI ≥25) according to NHANES (1999 to 2000) data by gender, ethnicity, and age exposes the most dangerous trends for African American females who are 40 to 59 years of age (81.5%) and ≥60 years of age (81.7%) and for Hispanic males who are 40 to 59 years of age (79.1%) and ≥60 years of age (79.6%).[28] Separated data for the prevalence of obesity (BMI ≥30) shows that almost half of African American females are obese, with the highest rates existing in those who are 40 to 59 years of age (53.2%) (see Table 1-3).[28]

Effects of Obesity

The Cost of Obesity

The cost of obesity-related disease, second only to that of tobacco-related costs, consumes close to 6% of American health care dollars per year.[40] The direct cost of obesity totals $70 million, with the combined direct and indirect cost of obesity being estimated at $117 billion.[41] This estimated financial burden from obesity is based on the estimated proportion of the diseases and prevalence of the diseases.[42] The problem is not unique to the United States: Europe's obesity-related health care costs are one-third of those in the United States.[42]

Mortality of Patients With Obesity

Researchers estimate that, every year, more than 300,000 deaths in the United States are attributable to obesity,[10] which is now the second leading cause of preventable death in the nation.[21] The NHANES data shows a significant number of years of life lost (YLL) when comparing the life expectancy of the overweight to that of the nonobese. Estimated years lost between gender and ethnicity groups were also significant in individuals whose BMIs are ≥45. Maximum YLL for White males was 13, while White women lost approximately 8 years. Young African American men and women lost even more years; the maximum for African American males was 20 YLL and for African American females was 5 YLL. For African American individuals over 60 years of age, however, the YLL was not significant for those with BMI between 30 and 45.[12]

Research on the effects of obesity that specifically addresses other ethnic groups—specifically Hispanics—is limited. General research, however, would indicate that obesity decreases the life expectancy of any individual, regardless of gender or ethnicity.

Comorbidities of Patients With Obesity

Numerous comorbid conditions are present in patients with obesity and morbid obesity, most of which are indirectly caused by or are intensified by an individual's overweight state. The comorbidities are one serious consideration when a patient and his or her surgeon discuss the option of bariatric surgery (Chapter 3). Research shows and physician experience supports that weight loss can decrease or even cure comorbidities seen in relation to obesity.[43] These complications are briefly discussed below.

Type 2 Diabetes Mellitus

The most serious comorbidity is type 2 diabetes mellitus. One-third of patients with obesity meet the criteria of the American Diabetic Association for type 2 diabetes, and another third have impaired glucose tolerance or pre-diabetes. The most worrisome part of this problem is that morbidly obese children are now being seen in increasing number with diabetic glucose tolerance curves.

Metabolic Syndrome

Syndrome X is the combination of metabolic risk factors in one individual that combines central obesity with increased resistance to insulin, hyperinsulinemia, dyslipidemia, essential hypertension, non-insulin–dependent diabetes, and an increased risk of cardiovascular disease.[9,44] The severity of this syndrome is associated with the distribution of fat (concentrated mostly on the hips versus the abdomen).[45] Abdominal distribution fat cells correlate with higher glucose and insulin levels.[45] Investigators estimate that 20 to 25% of Americans suffer from Syndrome X.[46] This metabolic syndrome is well documented[44] but not completely understood. The condition is not diagnosed by a standard test but must be recognized and diagnosed by health care professionals who recognize the combination of comorbid conditions. Also called "insulin-resistance syndrome," Syndrome X is closely associated with insulin resistance, which can be genetically inherited.[46]

Respiratory Disease

Intermittent obstruction of the pharynx results in episodes of apnea during sleep. This occurs frequently in the obese because of reduced tone in the pharyngeal muscles and redundant soft tissue. Obstructive Sleep Apnea (OSA), the most frequently seen form of sleep apnea in obese patients, results in daytime drowsiness, morning headaches, and cognitive dysfunction (Chapter 5). Obesity Hypoventilation Syndrome is associated with hypercarbia and hypoxemia while awake. This syndrome is the result of decreased lung volumes. This can also cause right heart failure as well. Surgery for obesity is associated with significant improvements in lung volumes, arterial blood gases, and sleep apnea.[47]

Gastroesophageal Reflux Disease

There is an increase in the prevalence of gastroesophageal reflux disease (GERD) in the obese. It is estimated that between 37% and 72% of patients with obesity suffer from GERD. Increased abdominal pressure is believed to overcome the lower esophageal resting pressure, resulting in reflux.[48,49]

Hypertension

Investigators have developed several theories to explain the increased prevalence of high blood pressure in the obese. Sodium reabsorption and increased catecholamine sensitivity, because of the metabolic syndrome of central obesity, can cause hypertension. Other theories are based on increased abdominal pressure and its effects on the renin-angiotensin-aldosterone system. In addition, sodium retention, increased blood pressure, and proteinuria are seen in the severely obese.[9,50]

Idiopathic Intracranial Hypertension

Headaches, visual disturbances, pulsatile tinnitis, cranial nerve dysfunction, and increased cerebrospinal fluid (CSF) pressure affect the patient with idiopathic intracranial hypertension. Also called pseudotumor cerebri (PTC), this syndrome is most commonly seen in obese females. In a study of 8 patients with PTC before obesity surgery, 100% of the patients had resolution of their symptoms and a decrease in their CSF pressures after the surgical treatment.[8,51]

Hormone Imbalance and Cancer

Infertility, irregular menses, and hirsutism are commonly seen in the female with obesity. Elevated levels of estradiol and dehydroepiandrosterone sulfate (also known as DHEAS sulfate) and increases in sex-hormone–binding globulin have been measured preoperatively in patients with obesity.[3] These increases occur in the obese because androgens are converted into estrogens in the fat tissue, which directly correlates with the degree of adiposity in women. Men tend to have normal levels of testosterone. Reports of higher mortality rates from breast, ovarian, endometrial, colon, and prostate cancers have also been reported.[3,5]

Psychosocial Health

"Disdain for the obese is one of the last widely permitted prejudices in the United States."[52] Patients with obesity report an overwhelming discrimination and prejudice towards themselves because of their weight.[53] Although there is no single personality type to characterize the individual suffering from obesity, these patients do demonstrate higher levels of Axis I disorders.[54,55] Specifically, these patients have higher rates of depression, eating disorders, and anxiety disorders.[55-57] However, this patient population does not demonstrate greater level of psychopathology than those that are not obese.[54] (This topic is discussed at length in Chapter 12.)

Quality of life (QOL) is compromised in this patient population. Disparagement of the body self-image and recurrent health problems in the obese population lead to several measures of coping that impede their QOL. They are often compliant with the social stereotypes applied to themselves. They avoid situations in which being obese could be a problem (ie, relationships). These coping measures lead to difficulty with many social situations, including employment, marriage, and sexual relations. Weight loss has been demonstrated to improve these psychological aspects of obesity; however, dieting can produce untoward psychological effects. Participants in diet programs demonstrate adverse reactions to the program (eg, depression, nervousness, irritability, and weakness).[56]

Pregnancy and Delivery-Related Issues

Research links obesity with increased risks of pregnancy complications,[41,58] fetal morbidities, preterm birth, and increased frequency of induced delivery and cesarean section.[58] A woman's prepregnancy BMI is a proven predictor of her baby's birthweight, and lower Apgar scores are more frequent in mothers with obesity. The deliveries of mothers experiencing prepregnancy obesity cost as much as 5 times more and their infants are 3.5 times more likely to require admission to the neonatal intensive care unit than those of mothers who are not obese before pregnancy.[58]

Other Comorbid Conditions

Increased abdominal pressure resulting from obesity can cause other comorbid conditions, including pressure on the urinary tract, which results in urgency and incontinence.[4] Poor venous return from the lower extremities secondary to increased abdominal pressure causes venous stasis ulcer in the obese.[59] Musculoskeletal problems plague the morbidly obese with an estimated 50% rate of some degree of disability, including sharp limitations of activity, with dependence on canes and wheelchairs in a significant number. They suffer from pain in weight-bearing joints and from ruptured or compressed vertebral discs. Obesity is a contraindication for repair of most of these orthopedic issues. Weight loss has proven an effective way to decrease, and even cure, these comorbidities.

Increased rates of diabetes, wound infections, subcutaneous injections of insulin, ventral hernia, and poor blood flow to the pannus have all been blamed on the development of pannicular abscess.[6] Obviously, losing weight will reduce or remove the pannus and the risk of this serious and sometimes fatal complication of obesity.

Obesity has also been demonstrated as an important prognostic indicator in most severe diseases. For example, obesity is proven as an important prognostic factor in acute pancreatitis. Increased retroperitoneal fat was suggested to be the reason for the increase in severity of pancreatitis in the obese.[2] Diverticular disease has also been demonstrated to require surgery and is more common in young obese patients.[7]

Conclusion

The increasing prevalence of overweight and obesity is disturbing. Obesity is a risk factor for many chronic diseases including diabetes, hypertension, heart disease, stroke, hypercholesterolemia, some cancers, and degenerative joint disease. The rise in the prevalence of diabetes has increased with the prevalence of obesity, illustrating the link between these morbid conditions.[60] Obesity also increases pregnancy complications and can cause serious problems in newborns of mothers with obesity. The rate of children suffering from overweight is steadily increasing; therefore, the comorbidities of obesity are being seen at earlier ages and are causing longer-term health issues in the obese population.

Regardless of the method of weight loss, these comorbid conditions can be reduced. Because of this, some medical professionals and researchers are petitioning for obesity to be recognized as an independent disease process. Doing so would definitely mobilize resources to help combat this increasing problem.

There is a consensus that the recent increase in the prevalence of obesity in the United States is due to changes in environmental conditions.[61] Over the period of the increase, several factors in the environment have changed. However, no definitive conclusions can be made about specific environmental factors and their relative contributions to this epidemic. The underlying explanation for overweight is an imbalance in the energy equation. Energy consumed is in excess to that expended. However, the determinants of this imbalance are poorly understood.[62] Throughout the world, health organizations are developing task forces to define the problem and develop a plan of prevention. However, diet programs and pharmacotherapy so far have demonstrated dismal success rates in weight reduction. Further, in the few that succeed, at least 15% to 30% return to pre-diet weight with cessation of the weight loss method.[63] Bariatric surgery is presently the only definitive cure for obesity.

The 1991 NIH Consensus Conference on the Surgery of Obesity underscored the importance of this threshold with its declaration that diets, exercise, behavioral modification, and drugs are not effective in the morbidly obese.[64] Based on that conclusion and a review of the therapies available at that time, the panelists concluded that weight-loss surgery may be the next step for people who remain severely obese after they try nonsurgical approaches or for individuals who have an obesity-related disease. A candidate for bariatric surgery has at least one of the following:

- A BMI >40
- A BMI >35 with a life-threatening comorbid condition (eg, diabetes, severe sleep apnea, or heart disease)
- Obesity-related physical problems that interfere with employment, walking, or family function.

The panelists also recommended age limits to >18 years of age and recommended 2 operations, the vertical banded gastroplasty and the gastric bypass as the preferred procedures.

These guidelines proved to be invaluable; however, the qualifications for bariatric surgery candidates are changing. Bariatric surgery has evolved with additional operations and the introduction of laparoscopic techniques, and surgical treatment may, in the near future, have a place in the treatment of children and adolescents with morbid obesity.[1] (The problem of overweight in children and adolescents is discussed in Chapter 6.)

The world epidemic of obesity is resulting in increased morbidity and mortality in affected individuals. This epidemic is costing governments large amounts of money, time, and manpower. Despite a campaign of obesity awareness and prevention in 2000,[33] the prevalence of overweight and obesity has increased and continues to do so. The goal of any task force to combat obesity should be to prevent weight gain in the normal weight population, reduce weight in the overweight population and encourage them to maintain a lower body weight. Whatever the solution, it will surely contain a combination of education, diet, exercise, pharmacotherapy, and surgery. Therefore, continued research in these areas is very important in the fight against the obesity epidemic.

References

1. Van Itallie TB. Obesity: adverse effects on health and longevity. *Am J Clin Nutr.* 1979;32(suppl 12):2723-2733.
2. Funnell IC, Bornman PC, Weakley SP, Terblanche J, Marks IN. Obesity: an important prognostic factor in acute pancreatitis. *Br J Surg.* 1993;80(4):484-486.
3. Deitel M, To TB, Stone E, Sutherland DJ, Wilk EJ. Sex hormonal changes accompanying loss of massive excess weight. *Gastroenterol Clin North Am.* 1987;16(3):511-515.
4. Bump RC, Sugerman HJ, Fantl JA, McClish DK. Obesity and lower urinary tract function in women: effect of surgically induced weight loss. *Am J Obstet Gynecol.* 1992;167(2):392-397.
5. Garfinkel L. Overweight and cancer. *Ann Intern Med.* 1985;103(6, pt 2):1034-1036.
6. Nauta RJ. A radical approach to bacterial panniculitis of the abdominal wall in the morbidly obese. *Surgery.* 1990;107(2):134-139.
7. Schauer PR, Ramos R, Ghiatas AA, Sirinek KR. Virulent diverticular disease in young obese men. *Am J Surg.* 1992;164(5):443-446.
8. Sugerman HJ, Felton WL 3rd, Salvant JB Jr, Sismanis A, Kellum JM. Effects of surgically induced weight loss on idiopathic intracranial hypertension on morbid obesity. *Neurology.* 1995;45(9):1655-1659.
9. Gillum RF. The association of body fat distribution with hypertension, hypertensive heart disease, coronary heart disease, diabetes and cardiovascular risk factors in men and women aged 18-79 years. *J Chronic Dis.* 1987;40(5):421-428.
10. Allison DB, Fontaine KR, Manson JE, Stevens J, VanItallie TB. Annual deaths attributable to obesity in the United States. *JAMA.* 1999;282(16):1530-1538.
11. NIH Conference. Gastrointestinal surgery for severe obesity. Consensus Development Conference Panel. *Ann Intern Med.* 1991;115(12):956-961.
12. Fontaine KR, Redden DT, Wang C, Westfall AO, Allison DB. Years of life lost due to obesity. *JAMA.* 2003;289(2):187-193.
13. Metropolitan Life Insurance Company. 1983 Metropolitan height and weight tables. *Stat Bull Metrop Life Insur Co.* 1983;64:2-9.
14. Williamson DF. Descriptive epidemiology of body weight and weight change in U.S. adults. *Ann Intern Med.* 1993;119(7, pt 2):646-649.

15. Harrison GG. Height-weight tables. *Ann Intern Med.* 1985;103(6, pt 2):989-994.
16. Halls SB. About the "Metropolitan Life" height and weight charts. Health calculators and charts. Available at: http://www.halls.md/ideal-weight/met.htm. Accessed March 31, 2005.
17. Lukaski HC. Methods for the assessment of human body composition: traditional and new. *Am J Clin Nutr.* 1987;46(4):537-556.
18. Snijder MB, Dekker JM, Visser M, et al. Associations of hip and thigh circumferences independent of waist circumference with the incidence of type 2 diabetes: the Hoorn Study. *Am J Clin Nutr.* 2003;77(5):1192–1197.
19. Calle EE, Thun MJ, Petrelli JM, Rodriguez C, Heath CW Jr. Body-mass index and mortality in a prospective cohort of U.S. adults. *N Engl J Med.* 1999;341(15):1097–1105.
20. *The Practical Guide: Identification, Evaluation, and Treatment of Overweight and Obesity in Adults.* Bethesda, MD: National Institutes of Health; National Heart, Lung, and Blood Institutes; and North American Association for the Study of Obesity; 2000. NIH publication 00-4084. Available at: http://www.nhlbi.nih.gov/guidelines/obesity/prctgd_c.pdf. Accessed April 1, 2005.
21. Clinical guidelines on the identification, evaluation, and treatment of overweight and obesity in adults—the evidence report. National Institutes of Health. *Obes Res.* 1998;6(suppl 2):51S-209S.
22. World Health Organization. Obesity: preventing and managing the global epidemic. Report of a WHO Consultation presented at: the World Health Organization; June 3-5, 1997; Geneva, Switzerland. Publication WHO/NUT/NCD/98.1.
23. Kluthe R, Schubert A. Obesity in Europe. *Ann Intern Med.* 1985;103(6, pt 2):1037-1042.
24. Rona RJ. The National Study of Health and Growth (NSHG): 23 years on the road. *Int J Epidemiol.* 1995;24(suppl 1):S69-S74.
25. Lobstein T, Rigby N, Leach R. EU Platform on Diet, Physical Activity and Health. EU Platform Briefing Paper. International Association for the Study of Obesity: London, UK; March 15, 2005.
26. Mokdad AH, Serdula MK, Dietz WH, Bowman BA, Marks JS, Koplan JP. The continuing epidemic of obesity in the United States. *JAMA.* 2000;284(13):1650-1651.
27. Sturm R. Increases in clinically severe obesity in the United States, 1986-2000. *Arch Intern Med.* 2003;163(18):2146-2148.
28. Flegal KM, Carroll MD, Ogden CL, Johnson CL. Prevalence and trends in obesity among US adults, 1999-2000. *JAMA.* 2002;288(14):1723-1727.
29. Cox CS, Mussolino ME, Rothwell ST, et al. Plan and operation of the NHANES I Epidemiologic Follow-Up Study 1992. Washington, DC: US DHHS, Centers for Disease Control and Prevention, National Center for Health Statistics; 1997. DHHS publication no: PHS 98-131. Available at: http://www.cdc.gov/nchs/data/nhanes/nhefs/sr01_035.pdf. Accessed March 31, 2005.
30. National Health and Nutrition Examination Survey. NHANES I Data Files Documentation Codebook, 1971-75. National Center for Health Statistics. DHHS Centers for Disease Control and Prevention website. Available at: http://www.cdc.gov/nchs/about/major/nhanes/nhanesi.htm. Accessed April 1, 2005.
31. Hispanic Health and Nutrition Examination Survey (HHANES) public-use data files. National Center for Health Statistics. DHHS Centers for Disease Control and Prevention website. Available at: http://www.cdc.gov/nchs/products/elec_prods/subject/hhanes.htm. Accessed April 2, 2005.
32. Flegal KM, Carroll MD, Kuczmarski RJ, Johnson CL. Overweight and obesity in the United States: prevalence and trends, 1960-1994. *Int J Obes Relat Metab Disord.* 1998;22(1):39-47.
33. Hedley AA, Ogden CL, Johnson CL, Carroll MD, Curtain LR, Flegal KM. Prevalence of overweight and obesity among US children, adolescents, and adults, 1999-2002. *JAMA.* 2004;291(23):2847-2850.
34. Kuczmarski RJ. Flegal KM, Campbell SM. Johnson CL. Increasing prevalence of overweight among US adults: the National Health and Nutrition Examination Surveys, 1960 to 1991. *JAMA.* 1994;272(3):205-211.
35. Strauss RS, Pollack HA. Epidemic increase in childhood overweight, 1986-1998. *JAMA.* 2001;286(22):2845-2848.
36. Ogden CL, Troiano RP, Briefel RR, Kuczmarski RJ, Flegal KM, Johnson CL. Prevalence of overweight among preschool children in the United States, 1971 through 1994. *Pediatrics.* 1997;99(4):E1. Available at: http://pediatrics.aappublications.org/cgi/reprint/99/4/e1. Accessed April 4, 2005.

37. Ogden CL, Flegal KM, Carroll MD, Johnson CL. Prevalence and trends in overweight among US children and adolescents, 1999-2000. *JAMA*. 2002;288(14):1728-1732.

38. Lew EA. Mortality and weight: insured lives and the American Cancer Society Studies. *Ann Intern Med.* 1985;103(6, pt 2): 1024-1029.

39. Stevens J, Cai J, Pamuk ER, Williamson DF, Thun MJ, Wood JL. The effect of age on the association between body-mass index and mortality. *N Engl J Med.* 1998;338(1):1-7.

40. Martin LF, White S, Lindstrom W Jr. Cost-benefit analysis for the treatment of severe obesity. *World J Surg.* 1998;22(9):1008-1017.

41. The Surgeon General's call to action to prevent and decrease overweight and obesity: 2001. Rockville, MD: US Department of Health and Human Services, Public Health Service, Office of the Surgeon General; 2001. Available at: http://www.surgeongeneral.gov/topics/obesity/. Accessed March 31, 2005.

42. Colditz GA. Economic cost of obesity and inactivity. *Med Sci Sports Exerc.* 1999;31(suppl 11):S663-S667.

43. Raum WJ. Postoperative medical management of bariatric patients. In: Martin LF, Ed. *Obesity Surgery.* New York, NY: McGraw-Hill; 2004:133-159.

44. Björntorp P. Abdominal obesity and the metabolic syndrome. *Ann Intern Med.* 1992;24(6):465-468.

45. Kissebah AH, Vydelingum N, Murray R, et al. Relation of body fat distribution to metabolic complications of obesity. *J Clin Endocrinol Metab.* 1982;54(2):254-260.

46. Metabolic syndrome. American Heart Association Web site. Available at: http://www.americanheart.org/presenter.jhtml?identifier=534. Accessed April 5, 2005.

47. Sugerman HJ, Fairman RP, Sood RK, Engle K, Wolfe L, Kellum JM. Long-term effects of gastric surgery for treating respiratory insufficiency of obesity. *Am J Clin Nutr.* 1992;55(suppl 2):597S-601S.

48. Kahrilas PJ. Gastroesophageal reflux disease. *JAMA.* 1996;276(12):983-988.

49. Kim CH, Sarr MG. Severe reflux esophagitis after vertical banded gastroplasty for treatment of morbid obesity. *Mayo Clin Proc.* 1992;67(1):33-35.

50. Bloomfield GL, Blocher CR, Fakhry IF, Sica DA, Sugerman HJ. Elevated intra-abdominal pressure increases plasma renin activity and aldosterone levels. *J Trauma Inj Infect Crit Care.* 1997;42(6):997-1004.

51. Sugerman HJ, Felton WL 3rd, Sismanis A, Kellum JM, De Maria EJ, Sugerman EL. Gastric surgery for pseudotumor cerebri associated with severe obesity. *Ann Surg.* 1999;229(5):634-640.

52. Buchwald H, Ikramuddin S. Laparoscopic adjustable gastric banding in bariatric surgery: an overview of the LAP-BAND. Introduction. *Am J Surg.* 2002;184(6B):1S-3S.

53. Rand, CS, Macgregor AM. Morbidly obese patients' perceptions of social discrimination before and after surgery for obesity. *South Med J.* 1990 Dec;83(12):1390-1395.

54. Stunkard AJ, Wadden TA. Psychological aspects of severe obesity. *Am J Clin Nutr.* 1992;55(suppl 2):524S-532S.

55. Herpertz S, Kielmann R, Wolf AM, Langkafel M, Senf W, Hebebrand J. Does obesity surgery improve psychosocial functioning? A systematic review. *Int J Obes Relat Metab Disord.* 2003;27(11):1300-1314.

56. Sarlio-Lähteenkorva S, Stunkard A, Rissanen A. Psychosocial factors and quality of life in obesity. *Int J Obes Relat Metab Disord.* 1995;19(suppl 6):S1-S5.

57. Onyike CU, Crum RM, Lee HB, Lyketsos CG, Eaton WW. Is obesity associated with major depression? Results from the Third National Health and Nutrition Examination Survey. *Am J Epidemiol.* 2003;158(12):1139-1147.

58. Galtier-Dereure F, Boegner C, Bringer J. Obesity and pregnancy: complications and cost. *Am J Clin Nutr.* 2000;71(5):1242S-1248S.

59. Sugerman HJ, Sugerman EL, Wolfe L, Kellum JM Jr, Schweitzer MA, DeMaria EJ. Risks and benefits of gastric bypass in morbidly obese patients with severe venous stasis disease. *Ann Surg.* 2001;234(1):41-46.

60. Harris MI, Flegal KM, Cowie CC, et al. Prevalence of diabetes, impaired fasting glucose, and impaired glucose tolerance in U.S. adults: The Third National Health and Nutrition Examination Survey, 1988-1994. *Diabetes Care.* 1998;21(4):518-524.

61. Jeffery RW, Utter J. The changing environment and population obesity in the United States. *Obes Res.* 2003; 11(suppl):12S-22S.

62. Methods for voluntary weight loss and control. NIH Technology Assessment Conference Panel. Consensus Development Conference. *Ann Intern Med.* 1993;119(7 pt 2):764-770.

63. Ayyad C, Anderson T. Long-term efficacy of dietary treatment of obesity: a systematic review of studies published between 1931 and 1999. *Obes Rev.* 2000;1(2):113-119.

64. Gastrointestinal surgery for severe obesity. NIH consensus statement online. 1991 Mar 25-27;9(1):1-20. Available at: http://consensus.nih.gov/cons/084/084_statement.htm#2_What_Ar. Accessed April 4, 2005.

2

Medical Treatment of Obesity

Jennifer Rosenblum, MD and Heather K. Stein, MD, MPH

Introduction

Treatment of an individual with obesity requires assessment of the patient's current medical status as well as development of a management plan for weight reduction. Assessment of an individual includes determining his or her degree of obesity, identifying potentially reversible factors contributing to the obesity, and evaluating medical complications that are related to the patient's weight. A management plan of the patient's obesity incorporates treating obesity-related comorbidities and creating an appropriate weight-reduction-and-maintenance plan. This chapter will review the assessment and treatment of a patient with obesity and provide guidelines for using behavioral and pharmacologic therapy for weight management.

Assessment

Severity of Obesity—The Body Mass Index

Assessment of the patient with obesity begins with understanding the degree of his or her obesity. This provides a global conceptualization of the patient's risk of obesity-related comorbidities and helps direct the treatment strategies. The body mass index (BMI)—a measure of an individual's weight in relation to his or her height—can be considered a "vital sign" and provides the health care provider with a standard for classifying the

Table 2-1
Classification of Weight by Body Mass Index and Associated Disease Risk

Description	BMI (kg/m^2)	Obesity Class	Disease Risk
Underweight	<18.5	—	—
Normal	18.5-24.9	—	—
Overweight	25-29.9	—	Increased
Mild obesity	30-34.9	I	High
Moderate obesity	35-39.9	II	Very high
Morbid obesity	≥40	III	Extremely high
Super obesity	≥50	—	—

Adapted from *The Practical Guide: Identification, Evaluation, and Treatment of Overweight and Obesity in Adults.*[1]

patient's obesity status. BMI is calculated as a ratio of weight (measured in kilograms) to height (measured in meters squared).

$$\text{BMI (kg/m}^2\text{)} = \frac{\text{Weight (kg)}}{(\text{Height in Meters})^2}$$

If pounds and inches are used to measure weight and height, the following formula can be used:

$$\text{BMI (kg/m}^2\text{)} = \frac{\text{Weight in Pounds}}{(\text{Height in Inches})^2} \times 703$$

BMI helps to stratify patients into different classes of obesity, which in turn are associated with varying degree of disease risk (Table 2-1). The BMI as a classification system has limitations (Chapter 1); for example, it often overestimates body fat in muscular individuals and underestimates body fat in those who have lost muscle mass by as much as 2 to 3 points. However, it is currently the measure of obesity with the greatest utility in clinical care. Calculating BMI is the initial step in assessing a patient's obesity.

The History and Physical Examination

The next step in assessing an individual with obesity is a comprehensive history and a physical examination, which facilitate a greater understanding of a patient's obesity and the impact it has on the patient's overall health status. This, in turn, helps direct the health care provider in choosing the most appropriate treatment regimen. The following is a review of the history and physical examination with particular attention to details specific to the evaluation of obesity.

The History

History of Present Illness

The clinical assessment begins with questions about the patient's current experience with his or her weight. It is helpful to understand the patient's motivation for pursuing the medical visit related to weight management. This opportunity to explore the patient's past weight-loss attempts will help the physician recommend appropriate medical therapy. It is also important to do a brief nutritional assessment of the patient's appetite and eating habits. Practically, this information will help guide the decision-making process for the patient's treatment. It is possible that, as the study of obesity advances, this information will reflect different patterns of obesity, each of which might respond to a different therapy. Table 2-2 reviews the history of present illness in detail.

Past Medical History

Review of the patient's past medical history begins with an examination of possible medical causes for a patient's obesity. The most common reversible cause of obesity is drug-induced weight gain, which will be discussed in an upcoming section. Medical causes of obesity are rare but can include endocrine diseases such as hypothyroidism, hyperprolactinemia, Cushing's syndrome, and neurologic diseases arising from traumatic brain injury.

A patient's past medical history also focuses on the medical complications or comorbidities of the patient's obesity. Over 50 medical problems have been linked to obesity as weight-related complications. Some—such as sleep apnea, type 2 diabetes mellitus, and coronary artery disease (CAD)—have a greater impact on the patient's overall health than do others. The provider should consider this hierarchy when gauging the urgency of treating the patient's obesity. The information in Table 2-3 provides a model through which the medical complications of obesity can be considered and reviewed.

Past Surgical History

The surgical history is an important factor in any patient's history but is particularly relevant in those who are being considered for bariatric surgery. The surgical history will help the patient's physician determine which bariatric procedure, if indicated, should be recommended to the patient (Chapter 3). For example, a patient who has had multiple previous abdominal surgeries may have developed adhesions; therefore, an open approach might be preferred because laparoscopy could be difficult or impossible to perform.

Table 2-2

Features of the History of Present Illness

1. History of patient's weight
   - ❖ Age of onset of obesity
   - ❖ Highest and lowest lifetime weights
   - ❖ Highest and lowest recent weights
   - ❖ Patterns of weight change
     - Slow, steady increase in weight versus recent, rapid onset
     - Change related to medical condition
     - Change related to a life event
   - ❖ Identifiable triggers of weight gain
2. Past history of weight-loss attempts
   - ❖ Prior attempts with diets
     - Commercial
     - Medically supervised
     - Liquid or protein-sparing modified fast
   - ❖ Prior use of prescribed medications
   - ❖ Prior use of over-the-counter medications or natural supplements
3. Brief nutritional assessment
   - ❖ Role of appetite in patient's eating habits
   - ❖ Review of current eating habits
     - Large portions
     - Poor food choices
     - Constant grazing or snacking
     - Binge eating
     - Fast-food consumption
   - ❖ Review of patient's physical activity

Medications

A review of the patient's current and past medications provides further insight into his or her current medical-treatment regimen. It is important to note if the patient is taking medications that are known to induce weight gain. If so, the patient might benefit from an adjustment or change of medication to reduce the impact on his or her weight. Table 2-4 includes a list of medications known to cause weight gain.

Social History

Evaluation of social history gives the health care provider an opportunity to screen the patient for cigarette, alcohol, and drug use. Cigarette smoking increases the risk of cardiovascular disease and thromboembolism, beyond the increased risk in this population that is attributable to their weight. Although smoking cessation may result in weight gain in some patients, all patients who are currently smoking should be educated about this heightened risk and strongly encouraged to stop. Alcohol contains "empty" or nutrient-void calories that can contribute to a patient's weight gain; therefore, it is important to report how much alcohol the patient consumes. Furthermore, the provider should inquire about the patient's substance-abuse history, as active substance abuse would be a contraindication to bariatric surgery. Patients currently abusing drugs and/or alcohol can be treated and reconsidered for surgery after a period of sobriety.

Table 2-3
Medical Complications of Obesity

Metabolic	Hypertension (HTN) Type 2 diabetes mellitus Dyslipidemia Gallstones Pancreatitis	Central sleep apnea Hypercoagulability (platelet dysfunction) Polycystic ovary syndrome (PCOS) Nonalcoholic fatty liver disease
Anatomic	Gastroesophageal reflux disease (GERD) Asthma Obstructive sleep apnea Deep vein thrombosis Pulmonary embolism Osteoarthritis Knee pain	Back pain Hip pain Stress incontinence Hernia Venous stasis Decubitus ulcers Fungal skin infections
Degenerative	Atherosclerosis Coronary artery disease (CAD) Congestive heart failure (CHF) Cirrhosis related to nonalcoholic steatohepatitis Degenerative joint disease	End-organ disease in diabetes such as retinopathy and renal failure Vertebral disc disease Peripheral vascular disease
Neoplastic	Breast carcinoma Endometrial carcinoma Cervical cancer Prostate carcinoma	Gallbladder carcinoma Renal cell carcinoma Pancreatic adenocarcinoma Esophagus adenocarcinoma
Psychological	Depression Anxiety	Binge-eating disorder Bulimia nervosa

Adapted from Kaplan LM.[2]

Environmental components also have a significant impact on a patient's obesity. Some patients may not be able to afford healthy food or may live in a location in which healthy food is not easily accessed. Information about a patient's marital status, living situation, children, employment history, and education level helps the provider assess the patient's socioeconomic status and the contribution it might be making to the patient's obesity. It is also important to consider potential cultural factors that may contribute to an individual's food choices and eating patterns.

Family History

The patient's family history of obesity provides insight into the role of genetics contributing to the patient's weight. It is generally thought that people who are obese at a young age or who have many obese family members have a stronger genetic component to their weight regulation. It is also relevant to note family histories of certain comorbidities of

Table 2-4

Medications That Cause Weight Gain

Antipsychotics

risperidone (Risperdal)	fluphenazine (Prolixin)
aripiprazole (Abilify)	ziprasidone (Geodon)
thiothixene (Navane)	thioridazine (Mellaril)
olanzapine (Zyprexa)	chlorpromazine (Thorazine)
haloperidol (Haldol)	clozapine (Clozaril)
perphenazine (Trilafon)	molindone (Moban)
quetiapine (Seroquel)	mesoridazine (Serentil)
loxapine (Loxitane)	

Selective Serotonin Reuptake Inhibitors

citalopram (Celexa)	fluvoxamine (Luvox)
escitalopram (Lexapro)	paroxetine (Paxil)
fluoxetine (Prozac)	sertraline (Zoloft)

Tricyclic Antidepressants

amitriptyline (Elavil)	imipramine (Tofranil)
clomipramine (Anafranil)	nortriptyline (Pamelor)
desipramine (Norpramin)	protriptyline (Vivactil)
doxepin (Sinequan)	

Monoamine Oxidase Inhibitors

phenelzine (Nardil)	tranylcypromine (Parnate)

Other Antidepressants/Mood Stabilizers

mirtazapine (Remeron)	lithium (Lithobid)
venlafaxine (Effexor)	

Steroid Hormones

corticosteroids: prednisone, prednisolone, methylprednisolone	depo-medroxyprogesterone acetate (Depo-Provera)
	megestrol acetate (Megace)

Antiepileptic Drugs

carbamazepine (Tegretol)	gabapentin (Neurontin)
divalproex sodium (Depakote)	

Antidiabetic Medications

insulin	thiazolidinediones—rosiglitazone (Avandia), pioglitazone (Actos)
sulfonylureas—eg, glyburide (Diabeta, Micronase), glipizide (Glucotrol)	

Please note: All drug names in parentheses are trademarked names.

obesity, such as type 2 diabetes, CAD, and malignancies; this information will help further stratify the patient's risk for these diseases.

Psychiatric History

A brief history of the patient's mental health must be performed to disclose any psychiatric issues that may be contributing to a patient's obesity and to determine if further psychiatric assessment and treatment are needed. Questions should assess any mood disorders—including anxiety and depression—that might affect a patient's eating habits by stimulating a desire to eat as an emotional response or "emotional eating." Additionally, it is important to ask questions to determine if the patient has an eating disorder, such as binge-eating disorder or bulimia nervosa (Chapter 12). If the patient has a comorbid psychiatric condition, his or her obesity cannot be treated unless the underlying psychiatric issue is also addressed. This may complicate the treatment of obesity, because some medications used to treat the psychiatric condition (eg, antidepressants or antipsychotics) can contribute to the patient's already existing obesity with additional weight gain.

Review of Systems

A thorough review of systems will elucidate any signs of obesity-related comorbidities and illustrate obesity's impact on the patient's quality of life. This evaluation enables the provider to screen for symptoms of sleep apnea, including snoring, witnessed apnea, daytime somnolence, choking or gasping for air, and morning headaches. The patient's mobility status is also pertinent, as patients with limited mobility may not lose weight as easily as do those who move better and exercise regularly. Considering the extent of the patient's disabilities is necessary in the creation of an appropriate treatment plan.

If not addressed during the patient's past medical history, the system review allows for evaluation of the patient's health-maintenance status. Patients with obesity are not screened as frequently with mammograms, clinical breast exams, Pap smears,[3] and colonoscopy[4]; however, they are at greater risk for cervical, colon, and postmenopausal breast cancers.[46,47] All patients should be strongly encouraged to obtain these cancer-screening tests if they are of the appropriate age and are not yet tested.

The Physical Exam

During the physical exam, the health care provider should note physical features that suggest causes of or comorbidities resulting from obesity. Table 2-5 highlights features of a clinical exam that are relevant to a patient's obesity and current medical status.

Laboratory Tests

A panel of laboratory tests completes the patient's physical examination and the provider's evaluation of possible causes and comorbidities from a patient's obesity. Table 2-6 is a recommended list of laboratory tests.

If suggested by findings in the history and physical examination, a 24-hour urine-free cortisol level can be sent as an initial evaluation for Cushing's syndrome. If this yields a positive result, or if it is negative but there is still a strong clinical suspicion of the disease, further evaluation can be done with an overnight 1-mg dexamethasone-suppression test.

Other Studies

Based on the patient's medical history, other studies should be considered to evaluate the impact of the patient's obesity and medical comorbidities on his or her health. Examples include stress test, echocardiogram, sleep study, pulmonary-function test, upper gastrointestinal (UGI) series or endoscopy, and cancer screening tests such as mammogram, Pap smear, and colonoscopy.

Table 2-5

Physical Examination Findings

General

Mood
Overall capacity for movement
Somnolence

Head, Eyes, Ears, Nose, Throat (HEENT)

Anatomy of tonsils and uvula that may increase risk of obstructive sleep apnea (OSA)
Round face suggestive of Cushing's syndrome
Scleral icterus suggestive of possible end-stage liver disease from nonalcoholic steatohepatitis
Retinopathy suggestive of diabetic eye disease

Neck

Neck circumference >16 cm (female) and >17 cm (male), associated with a substantially greater risk of OSA
Thyroid exam
Dorsal cervical fat pad ("buffalo hump")
Supraclavicular fat pad suggestive of Cushing's syndrome
Increased jugular venous distension from pulmonary HTN and right heart failure secondary to OSA

Pulmonary Exam

Wheezing possibly from GERD or asthma
Rales indicating CHF

Cardiac Exam

Murmurs or gallops suggesting structural or functional changes in the heart resulting from CAD and myocardial infarctions, heart failure, or valvular disease

Abdomen

Measurement of waist circumference: >35 in (female) and >40 in (male) as a criteria for the diagnosis of metabolic syndrome
Thick violaceous striae suggestive of Cushing's syndrome
Ascites suggestive of possible end-stage liver disease from nonalcoholic steatohepatitis
Umbilical and ventral hernias

Extremities

Leg edema
Chronic venous stasis changes
Tenderness, erythema, and asymmetric edema suggestive of deep venous thrombosis

Skin

Fungal infections
Furuncles/folliculitis
Cellulitis or ulcers
Hirsutism suggestive of PCOS and Cushing's syndrome
Ecchymoses suggestive of Cushing's syndrome

Table 2-6
Laboratory Evaluation

CBC	Lipid profile*	PTH*	Vitamin B12
Electrolytes	HbA1c	Vitamin D	Iron studies
Liver function	Insulin*	TSH	PT/INR†/PTT
Renal function	Urine microalbumin/Cr ratio (if HTN or diabetes)		Urinalysis

* Lab should be obtained after the patient has fasted

† INR=international normalized ratio

Management of Obesity

The management of the patient with obesity incorporates a two-pronged approach: providing care for obesity-related comorbidities and treating the obesity itself. The care of comorbidities is beyond the scope of this chapter; however, it is important to closely monitor comorbidities, as their status may change during weight loss or gain.

The first step in managing obesity includes identifying and addressing modifiable factors that are currently contributing to a patient's weight. The next step is to decide which treatment strategies are appropriate for the patient to achieve weight reduction. Available treatment options include diet and exercise therapy, behavior modification, pharmacotherapy, and weight-loss surgery. The assessment of an individual's BMI and weight-related comorbidities should together guide the provider's approach to treatment (Table 2-7).

Energy and Metabolism

The basal metabolic rate or basal energy expenditure (BEE) is the energy needed by an individual to maintain basic body functions during a 24-hour period of complete inactivity. For adults, BEE is estimated by calculating the Harris-Benedict equation, which accounts for age, height, weight, and gender. It does not account for the increased energy requirement of lean muscle mass and, therefore, may underestimate caloric needs in very muscular individuals or overestimate needs in the severely obese. The estimate also does not include the calories needed to sustain daily activities. The calculation is different for males and females.

For males:

$$\text{BEE (kcal/day)} = 66.5 + [13.75 \times \text{weight (kg)}] + [5.0 \times \text{height (cm)}] - [6.78 \times \text{age (yr)}]$$

For females:

$$\text{BEE (kcal/day)} = 655 + [9.56 \times \text{weight (kg)}] + [1.85 \times \text{height (cm)}] - [4.68 \times \text{age (yr)}]$$

Table 2-7
Guide to Selecting Treatment Strategy

Treatment	BMI (kg/m²) 25.0-26.9	27.0-29.9	30.0-34.9	35.0-39.9	≥40.0
Dietary Modification	+	+	+	+	+
Exercise	+	+	+	+	+
Behavioral Modification	+	+	+	+	+
Pharmacotherapy		*	+	+	+
Surgery				x	+

* With comorbidities

x With significant comorbidities, including diabetes mellitus, coronary artery disease, and severe obstructive sleep apnea

Adapted from *The Practical Guide: Identification, Evaluation, and Treatment of Overweight and Obesity in Adults.*[1]

Table 2-8
Physical Activity Level

Level of Activity	Description of Activity	PAL Factor
Sedentary	Little or no exercise	1.2
Low active	Light exercise/sports 1-3 d/wk	1.375
Moderately active	Moderate exercise/sports 3-5 d/wk	1.55
Very active	Hard exercise/sports 6-7 d/wk	1.725
Extra active	Very hard daily exercise/sports and physical job, or 2 times per day training	1.9

The total energy expenditure (TEE) is the number of calories needed to sustain an individual's basic body functions and activities in a 24-hour period. TEE can be estimated by multiplying the BEE by physical activity level (PAL) factor, as specified in Table 2-8: TEE ≈ BEE x PAL. TEE estimates the caloric requirement to maintain current body weight. Reducing the caloric intake by 500 to 1000 kcal/day below the TEE should result in a healthy weight loss of 1 to 2 pounds per week. This caloric reduction occurs through a combination of dietary modification and exercise.

Dietary Therapy

The majority of patients with obesity require dietary modification to achieve weight reduction. Many individuals may have a history of repetitive dieting with subsequent weight regain; therefore, nutritional counseling should emphasize making healthy food choices that can be maintained long-term. It is also important to set realistic weight-loss goals. The general guideline should be to achieve a daily deficit of 500 to 1000 kcal and thus lose 1 to 2 lb per week. A weight reduction of 5% to 10% of initial body weight should be the patient's initial target weight-loss goal, as this can result in significant health benefits. Once this weight loss has been achieved and maintained, an additional 10% weight-loss goal can be set, if clinically indicated. While a 5% to 10% reduction in body weight can improve health risks, it will not satisfy many patients, who may feel discouraged or disappointed if they cannot lose more weight. Setting realistic weight-loss goals early on and providing education about health benefits are key components of nutritional counseling.

Low-calorie diets (LCD) are designed so the individual can achieve a caloric deficit while maintaining a balance of carbohydrates, fat, and protein. Diets should be planned per individual so the design includes a reduction of 500 to 1000 kcal/day compared to usual intake, which translates into 1000 to 1500 kcal/day for most females and 1200 to 1800 kcal/day for most males. The distribution of carbohydrates, fat, and protein should be adjusted according to the individual's medical comorbidities. For example, a patient with diabetes or polycystic ovarian syndrome (PCOS) may be counseled to reduce carbohydrate intake, while an individual with heart disease may be counseled to reduce dietary-fat content. Recent studies suggest that low-carbohydrate diets produce greater short-term weight loss than do low-fat diets[5,6]; however, these studies show no significant differences between the 2 approaches in long-term weight loss.[7] Many clinicians believe that the best diet for an individual is one that can be maintained long-term.

A very low-calorie diet (VLCD) provides fewer than 800 kcal/day. These diets require close medical monitoring, given their risks of dehydration, nutrient deficiencies, renal electrolyte abnormalities, and cardiac arrhythmias. VLCDs often use meal replacements in the form of liquids or snack bars to provide part or all of the caloric needs. The protein-sparing modified fast is a type of VLCD that sometimes uses lean meat and fish as well as supplements to provide micronutrients. Although these hypocaloric diets can result in successful short-term weight loss, this weight loss is not usually sustained. Clinical trials show no difference between VLCDs and LCDs in terms of total weight loss after 1 year.[8] VLCDs are appropriate for most individuals who needs to achieve rapid, short-term weight loss, such as patients who needs to lose weight prior to transplant surgery.

Exercise Therapy

Physical activity is a key component of weight loss and weight maintenance. It also provides health benefits independent of weight loss, including reduction in blood pressure, increase in insulin sensitivity, and improvement in lipid profiles. Exercise facilitates weight reduction by increasing TEE, which, in combination with a calorie-deficit diet, helps achieve a negative energy balance. Activity may play a greater role in weight maintenance and prevention of regain than in actual weight loss.[9] In fact, many patients may not notice any weight loss upon initiation of an exercise regimen; however, they often achieve a reduction in fat mass and an increase in muscle mass, which may be noted by greater energy levels and loose-fitting clothing.

The initiation of an exercise plan must be realistic and achievable for that patient, with the aim to gradually increase activity duration and intensity. Although the exercise prescription should be individualized for each patient, an average target goal for exercise includes 30 to 60 minutes of moderate activity on all or most days of the week. A general guideline is 300 minutes per week of moderate activity, which should increase energy expenditure by 1000 kcal per week. Examples of moderate activity include brisk walking at a pace of 4 mph, shoveling snow or climbing stairs for 15 minutes, gardening for 30 to 45 minutes, swimming or water aerobics for 20 to 30 minutes, or playing basketball or dancing for 30 minutes. Ideally, an exercise program should combine both aerobic activity and strength training. Varying the type of activity can help prevent boredom and burnout and can maximize muscle response.

Patients with severe obesity may be limited in their ability to perform many exercises because of physical limitations such as joint pain and stiffness, lower extremity edema, or significant dyspnea on exertion. The clinician must decide whether cardiopulmonary testing is indicated prior to the patient beginning an exercise program. Furthermore, a consultation with a physical therapist is often helpful to provide the patient with proper instruction on performing activities safely. These individuals can start with simple exercises, such as stretching, light arm weights, and slow-paced walking.

It is important to emphasize to the patient that exercise is a key component of any healthy weight program, whether weight loss is achieved through dietary modification, pharmacotherapy, or surgery. Engaging in a regular exercise regimen will help him or her maintain weight loss and provide additional health benefits in the long-term.

Behavior Modification

It is helpful for patients with obesity to identify, understand, and overcome obstacles that prevent them from successfully following a weight-management plan. Barriers can include issues related to maintaining healthy eating or developing an active lifestyle that includes regular exercise. Each patient has individualized eating and lifestyle behaviors that need to be addressed; some may be more difficult to modify than others.

Eating behaviors that can lead to detrimental weight problems include skipping meals, grazing throughout the day, and eating while watching TV, out of boredom, or late at night. With irregular eating patterns, people consume more calories, generally from unhealthy foods, and subsequently gain weight. By modifying these behaviors, patients can be more mindful of their eating and develop habits that result in lower caloric intake and weight loss.

Addressing unhealthy lifestyle behaviors usually focuses on efforts to incorporate more activity into daily living. As a society, we are becoming less and less active, as our environment caters to convenience and jobs become more sedentary. One lifestyle change commonly needed by patients with obesity is more activity, which enables them to expend more energy and thus lose weight. For some patients, this requires commitment to a regular exercise program, as discussed in the previous section. Behavior modification should address potential barriers to instituting such a program: eg, some patients with obesity may be uncomfortable exercising in a public gym or swimming pool, and others may feel like they cannot commit to a full exercise program so they do not exercise at all. Addressing issues and overcoming obstacles can help the patient to participate in regular exercise more readily.

Some patients are overwhelmed by the recommended dietary and lifestyle behavioral modifications. These patients should be educated that even small behavioral changes can result in positive outcomes. It is important that the provider help these patients set

Table 2-9

Points about Behavioral Modification

- Be mindful of the patient's and health care provider's attitudes and beliefs about obesity and patients with obesity.
- Assess the patient's motivation and readiness to change, and counsel accordingly.
- Establish a partnership with the patient.
- Set realistic weight loss goals:
  - Focus on health outcomes in addition to pounds lost.
  - Set smaller goals to be achieved between visits.
- Follow-up regularly with the patient.
- Have the patient use food and exercise diaries.
- Elucidate environmental stimuli that may be detrimental to weight-loss effort and encourage the patient to change them.
- Encourage rewards for the patient when goals are met, large or small.
- Focus on successes.

Adapted from *The Practical Guide: Identification, Evaluation, and Treatment of Overweight and Obesity in Adults.*[1]

short-term goals that can be realistically accomplished. They can then gradually build up toward their larger, long-term goals, which will result in sustained weight loss and improvement in health. Table 2-9 offers some general guidelines for the development of a patient-specific behavioral-modification program that should accompany all coordinated weight-loss efforts.

Some unhealthy behaviors result from underlying psychological disorders, such as anxiety, depression, binge-eating disorder, or night-eating syndrome. If the health care provider suspects such a disorder after assessing the patient, he or she should enlist the assistance of a mental health professional. A patient with both obesity and an underlying psychological disorder cannot be fully treated for the obesity until the psychiatric disorder is addressed.

PHARMACOTHERAPY

Medications are often helpful in the treatment of obesity, especially when they are used in combination with diet and exercise therapy to augment weight-loss efforts. Some controversy surrounds the use of anti-obesity drugs because of concerns about safety, potential for abuse, and long-term efficacy. Drug therapy for obesity most often results in only modest weight loss, with success generally considered a 5% to 15% reduction in total body weight. Medications should be considered in the treatment of obesity for patients with BMI >30 or BMI >27 and comorbidities.

The number of medications that are FDA approved to treat obesity is quite small. Current pharmacotherapy for obesity primarily includes medications that decrease appetite and increase satiety and energy expenditure, such as phentermine and sibutramine. Another medication that is commonly prescribed is a lipase inhibitor called orlistat. A small group of medications that are not FDA-approved for obesity treatment have undergone study in clinical trials and have been used "off-label" because of their noted side effect of weight loss. These medications are discussed later in this section.

Medications Approved for Weight Loss

Phentermine

Phentermine (Adipex-P: Teva Phamaceuticals, Sellersville, Pa; Fastin: King Pharmaceuticals, Bristol, Tenn; Ionamin: Celltech Pharmaceuticals Inc, Rochester, NY) is one of the most commonly prescribed anti-obesity drugs. A sympathomimetic amine, phentermine stimulates the release of norepinephrine and results in appetite suppression, increased satiety, and increased energy expenditure. It has been available since the 1960s and is generally well tolerated, effective, and among the least expensive of the medications approved for the treatment of obesity. Short-term trials have shown phentermine to be effective for modest weight loss: 5% to 15% of initial body weight.[10]

When used in combination with fenfluramine, it resulted in significant weight loss; therefore, the combination, called "Phen-Fen," was commonly prescribed for weight loss in the early and mid 1990s. However, in 1997, both fenfluramine and dexfenfluramine were withdrawn from the market because patients taking these medications had an increased incidence of pulmonary hypertension (HTN) and valvular abnormalities. Further studies have suggested that these abnormalities were likely increased with the combination therapy, compared to monotherapy, and that the adverse effects were directly related to dose and duration of use. It has also been suggested that the natural history after discontinuation was likely regression as opposed to progression of abnormalities.[11-13] Although it is generally thought that the cardiopulmonary effects seen with the use of "Phen-Fen" were due to fenfluramine and not phentermine, phentermine cannot be totally excluded as the cause. Therefore, patients should be cautioned to discontinue phentermine if they experience dyspnea, angina, syncope, or decreased exercise tolerance. However, overall, phentermine is generally well tolerated, with possible side effects including dry mouth, insomnia, nervousness and agitation, palpitations, and constipation.

Phentermine can cause elevations in heart rate and blood pressure, so patients should be monitored monthly while taking this medication. It can be prescribed as 15 to 37.5 mg/day taken 30 to 60 minutes before breakfast. It is approved for short-term—3- to 4-month—treatment; however, many obesity experts prescribe it long-term with continued monitoring for patients in whom the regimen is effective and well tolerated. Phentermine is contraindicated in patients with poorly controlled HTN, unstable cardiovascular disease, glaucoma, hyperthyroidism, agitation, or recent use of monoamine oxidase (MAO) inhibitors.

Sibutramine

Sibutramine (Meridia: Abbott Laboratories, Abbott Park, Ill) is indicated for the long-term treatment of obesity; studies show it to be effective for weight loss for up to 1 year or longer. It inhibits the reuptake of norepinephrine and serotonin and, to a lesser degree, dopamine. The increase of norepinephrine and serotonin in neuronal synapses is thought to result in increased satiety and, therefore, reduced caloric intake. This drug also appears to increase resting energy expenditure.

A recent systematic review of sibutramine for obese adults—healthy as well as those with type 2 diabetes, HTN, or hyperlipidemia—concluded that sibutramine plus lifestyle modification are more effective in promoting weight loss than are placebo plus lifestyle modification at 3, 6, and 12 months. Moreover, adults taking sibutramine for 1 year were 19% to 34% more likely to achieve 5% weight loss and 12% to 31% more likely to achieve 10% weight loss—an average of 10 pounds per subject—than were those taking placebo. Those taking sibutramine for 2 years maintained more weight loss than did those receiving placebo (an average 9-pound difference; range 5 to 12 pounds).[14] Therefore, sibutramine is generally effective for both moderate weight loss as well as weight maintenance. However, as with older pharmacological approaches, most individuals regain weight once they stop this medication.

The long-term risk/benefit ratio of sibutramine is not yet determined. Because studies associate sibutramine with increased heart rate and blood pressure,[8] patients taking this medication should be monitored frequently; however, there are no indications that it can cause more serious cardiopulmonary abnormalities. Sibutramine is contraindicated in patients with uncontrolled HTN, congestive heart failure (CHF), CAD, known arrhythmias, and stroke. At the same time, use of sibutramine is linked with minor improvements in high-density lipoprotein cholesterol and triglyceride levels and glycemic control among diabetics.[8] Generally, providers expect obesity-related comorbidities to improve as weight loss occurs; however, there is no direct evidence that sibutramine prevents or reduces obesity-associated morbidity or mortality.[8]

Common side effects include dry mouth, constipation, insomnia, and headache. Less common adverse effects include nausea, diarrhea, dizziness, palpitations, chest pain, restlessness, and anxiety. Because of its effect on serotonin reuptake, use in combination with other serotonin-altering medications can result in the rare but serious serotonin syndrome. Therefore, sibutramine should be avoided in combination with MAO inhibitors, select serotonin reuptake inhibitors, lithium, dextromethorphan, sumatriptan, and dihydroergotamine.

Sibutramine should be started at a dose of 10 mg/day. If the patient does not lose 4 pounds in 4 weeks and does not experience adverse reactions, the physician can increase the patient's dose to 15 mg/day. Patients who are hypersensitive to medication can begin with or adjust to a lower dose of 5 mg/day. This medication should be taken at the same time each day and can be taken before or after a meal.

While only FDA approved for adult use for 1 year, sibutramine has been found to be safe and effective in adults for up to 2 years. It is not yet approved for adolescent use; however, a randomized control trial by Berkowitz and colleagues showed that sibutramine, in combination with behavioral modification, induced significantly more weight loss in adolescents with overweight than in the placebo-treated group.[15]

Less Commonly Used Anorexiants

In addition to phentermine, other available nonamphetamine DEA-Schedule-IV anorexiants include mazindol and diethylpropion. Mazindol—an isoindole compound—and diethylpropion (Tenuate: AH Robbins Co Inc)—a sympathomimetic amine—are both approved for short-term treatment of obesity but may have adverse effects similar to those of amphetamines, including tachycardia, HTN, and dysrhythmias. They have low abuse potential and less stimulant activity than do amphetamines; however, these medications do not result in sustained weight loss beyond 6 months, and patients tend to build rapid tolerance to their anorectic effects.[16]

Other less common medications that are available for short-term treatment of obesity include the DEA Schedule II amphetamines, such as dextroamphetamine, and the Schedule-III sympathomimetic amines: benzphetamine and phendimetrazine. Dextroamphetamine (Dexedrine: Celltech Pharmaceuticals Inc, Rochester, NY) suppresses appetite and increases metabolic rate but has the potential for abuse as well as adverse cardiovascular effects, including tachycardia and HTN.[17] Most obesity experts agree that these drugs are inappropriate for obesity treatment given the availability of newer anorexiants (DEA Schedule IV) with negligible addiction or abuse potential.[18]

Orlistat

Orlistat (Xenical: Hoffmann-La Roche Inc, Nutley, NJ) was approved by the FDA in 1999 for use in obesity treatment. It blocks the absorption of dietary fat by inhibiting gastrointestinal (GI) and pancreatic lipases, causing partially or undigested dietary fat to be excreted in the patient's stool. At the treatment dose of orlistat, approximately 30% of ingested fat absorption is inhibited and eliminated. Pharmacokinetic studies show that approximately 97% of orlistat is excreted in the feces, and less than 2% is excreted renally.[19]

In 1999, Davidson et al published the results of a 2-year randomized trial in which patients who followed a hypocaloric diet and took 120 mg of orlistat 3 times a day had greater weight loss after 1 year than did placebo-dosed patients (8.76 kg versus 5.81 kg; $p < 0.001$). Additionally, patients who continued the orlistat regimen for a second year regained less weight on a maintenance diet than did patients who took a lower dose of orlistat or the placebo.[20] Since the publication of this study, additional clinical trials and literature reviews have supported orlistat's role in both weight loss[21,22] and weight maintenance.[23]

Orlistat also has beneficial effects on obesity-related comorbidities, including glucose intolerance and diabetes. In the "XENical in the Prevention of Diabetes in Obese Subjects" (XENDOS) study, subjects with BMI ≥30 and normal or impaired glucose tolerance participated in lifestyle counseling and took either orlistat or a placebo. After 4 years, patients taking orlistat lost more weight and fewer developed diabetes.[24] Similar results were obtained in a study of patients with diabetes who also experienced more weight loss and improved glycemic control on orlistat.[25] Other studies of orlistat have also noted improvements in cardiovascular risk factors and lipid parameters including total cholesterol,[19,24-26] low-density lipoprotein cholesterol,[19,24-26] triglycerides,[22,25] systolic blood pressure,[24] and diastolic blood pressure.[19,22,24] Orlistat therapy may also improve clinical and pathological findings associated with nonalcoholic steatohepatitis.[27]

The recommended treatment dose of orlistat is 120 mg taken 3 times a day during or up to 1 hour after each meal. Patients start with 1 dose per day and increase frequency of dosage gradually if no side effects are experienced. Patients should be monitored monthly at first and then every 2 to 3 months, based on their tolerance of the medication, as many patients do experience side effects. Gastrointestinal side effects are the most common, including fatty or oily stools, fecal urgency, flatus with discharge, oily spotting,[19] abdominal cramps, intestinal flatus,[28] increased defecation, and oily evacuation.[29] In the XENDOS study, most GI events were characterized as mild to moderate and occurred early in treatment,[24] suggesting that the symptom frequency decreases as the duration of treatment increases. For management of these potential side effects, one study noted a decrease in the incidence in GI events when orlistat was taken with psyllium.[28]

Additional side effects for which patients must be followed include hypoglycemia in patients with type 2 diabetes, particularly those taking insulin or sulfonylureas, according to 2 separate studies. These studies illustrate the need for adjustment of diabetic medications as weight is lost and metabolic parameters improve.[19] Also, patients taking orlistat are at risk for deficiency of fat-soluble vitamins, including A, D, E, and K; therefore, patients should take a daily multivitamin at a different time than they take orlistat.[29] Close monitoring for continued vitamin deficiencies is vital, as patients may require supplementation beyond that provided by the multivitamin. Furthermore, orlistat should be used with extreme caution in a patient who is taking coumadin, because a vitamin-K deficiency can increase the risk of bleeding in this patient. If a patient does combine the 2 medications, the physician must closely monitor the patient's international normalized ratio (INR), and the patient must take the drugs regularly so his physician (and not the patient independently) can adjust the coumadin dose as needed.

Medications That May Cause Weight Loss

Metformin

Metformin (Glucophage: Bristol-Myers Squibb, New York, NY) is FDA-approved for treatment of type 2 diabetes but is currently used "off-label" for weight loss by some obesity-medicine experts. This medication improves glycemic control and increases insulin sensitivity in diabetic patients. Theoretically, by decreasing hyperinsulinemia and insulin resistance, metformin decreases lipogenesis and increases lipolysis, thus promoting weight loss. In short- and long-term studies, it was shown to result in decreased food consumption and weight loss in adults with obesity and type 2 diabetes.[30] By extension, metformin is also being used as treatment for women with PCOS.

Because of documented weight-loss success in individuals with type 2 diabetes and PCOS, metformin is now being studied as treatment for obese individuals without these comorbidities. One randomized trial demonstrated that metformin, compared to placebo, and a hypocaloric diet led to a greater reduction in subjects' body weight, BMI, and visceral adipose tissue in women with abdominal obesity, with and without PCOS.[31] The Diabetes Prevention Program study compared lifestyle-intervention results to those of metformin and of placebo on the progression to diabetes among patients with glucose intolerance. This study revealed that patients taking metformin maintained an approximate 2-kg weight loss after 4 years, a result that was not as effective as lifestyle intervention but was significantly greater than sustained weight loss with placebo.[32] Another clinical trial—comparing 6-month results in subjects with obesity who are taking sibutramine, orlistat, or metformin—demonstrated similar weight reduction for metformin and orlistat (9.9% and 9.1%, respectively), with greater weight reduction seen with sibutramine (13.6%). All 3 medications led to improvement in insulin resistance, lipid profile, and blood pressure.[33]

Data also suggests that metformin can be effective in the treatment of obese adolescents. A randomized trial of metformin in 24 hyperinsulinemic, nondiabetic adolescents with obesity demonstrated greater weight loss, decreased body fat, and enhanced insulin sensitivity with metformin (850 mg twice a day) after 8 weeks.[34] Another study of 29 adolescents with obesity, hyperinsulinemia, and family history of type 2 diabetes showed a small reduction of BMI in those treated with metformin (500 mg twice a day) for 6 months, whereas those given placebo had an increase in BMI.[35]

Most published studies of metformin for obesity treatment are small and relatively short-term; however, preliminary results are promising, especially for use in adolescents where pharmacologic-treatment options are more limited than they are for adults. Clearly, larger long-term studies are needed to demonstrate a sustained effect of metformin on weight loss as well as to determine the optimal dose of treatment. Patients using the drug for obesity at this time should understand and agree to the "off-label" circumstances and should be followed closely for any possible adverse effects.

Topiramate

Topiramate (Topamax: Ortho-McNeil Pharmaceutical Inc, Raritan, NJ) was approved as a treatment for epilepsy and recently has been used as a mood stabilizer. One of the side effects noted in clinical studies of the medication was weight loss. To examine this finding in patients without epilepsy, Bray et al conducted a randomized, double-blind, placebo-controlled trial over 6 months with four doses of topiramate in patients with obesity. Lower doses of 64 mg/day and 96 mg/day were better tolerated, and patients lost 5.0% and 4.8% of their baseline weight, respectively. At higher doses of 192 mg/day and 384 mg/day, patients lost 6.3% of their baseline body weight, but the doses were not as well tolerated.[36] Similar findings were obtained in subsequent, longer-term studies that note topiramate's effect on weight loss[37] and weight maintenance.[38] Some study subjects did experience side effects. In the study by Bray et al, most patients developed adverse reactions—mild to moderate reactions that were dose related—within the first 8 weeks of treatment, but they generally resolved on their own. The most common side effects were paresthesias, memory problems, fatigue, somnolence, anorexia, dizziness, and difficulty concentrating. Adverse effects of depression, upper respiratory infections, renal stones, and acute angle glaucoma have also been reported.[29,36]

Based on these findings, some obesity specialists have started to prescribe low-dose topiramate for treatment of obesity. Clinical observation has shown the drug to be particularly effective for treatment of psychotropic-induced weight gain. Patients who take topiramate for obesity treatment need to understand that it is an "off-label" use of the medication. They should be started on a low dose—25 mg twice a day—and titrated up slowly, increasing by 25 to 50 mg/week to reach a goal dose of 50 to 100 mg twice a day. Patients should be monitored during the titration period for any side effects. If side effects are experienced at one dose, it is reasonable to try the medication at a lower dose prior to discontinuing it all together.

Zonisamide

Zonisamide (Zonegran: Elan Corporation, Dublin, Ireland) is an antiepileptic medication with serotonergic and dopaminergic effects. As with topiramate, studies of zonisamide on epileptic activity have noted weight loss as an adverse effect, which resulted in a further study of the drug for obesity treatment alone. In a randomized, double-blinded trial, patients taking zonisamide lost an average of 5.9 kg over 16 weeks, while those taking placebo lost 0.9 kg. The only adverse effect that was significantly more common in the treatment group was fatigue. When the study was extended in a single-blinded fashion over another 16 weeks, those patients taking zonisamide lost 9.2 kg total, while those taking placebo lost 1.5 kg.[39] The study had limitations including small sample size and a short follow-up. Furthermore, the 5 male subjects all received zonisamide, so it is difficult to extrapolate the efficacy of this therapy to men. Nevertheless, the study does reflect that patients taking zonisamide with a hypocaloric diet lost more weight than did those taking placebo.[40]

Because only one study has investigated zonisamide and it is not FDA approved as obesity treatment, its use for obesity is "off-label"; patients taking the drug for obesity should be instructed on this and monitored closely. Additionally, the patient and the prescribing physician must be aware of its adverse effects: in addition to fatigue (noted above), dizziness, cognitive impairment, and somnolence have been reported in trials of this medication when used to treat epilepsy. A history of kidney stones is a contraindication to therapy with zonisamide, as the medication is known to cause them.

Bupropion

Bupropion (Wellbutrin and Zyban: GlaxoSmithKline, Middlesex, UK) is approved for the treatment of depression and smoking cessation. It works as a noradrenaline and dopamine reuptake inhibitor and does not affect the serotonin system. In studies evaluating the effect of bupropion on the treatment of depression, weight stabilization or loss was noted instead of the weight gain, which is typical of other classes of antidepressants.

As a result, further studies were performed to examine the role of bupropion as a medication to facilitate weight loss.[41] In one study of females who were overweight or had obesity, those taking bupropion experienced greater weight loss after 8 weeks (4.9% total body weight) loss than did those taking placebo (1.3% total body weight loss).[42] These results were supported by the findings of Anderson et al: among males and females with obesity, those taking 300 mg/day, 400 mg/day, and a placebo lost 7.2%, 10.1% and 5.0% of their initial body weight, respectively, after 24 weeks. At 48 weeks, those taking 300 mg/day and 400 mg/day of bupropion maintained a weight loss of 7.5% and 8.6%, respectively.[43] Similar results were obtained in a study of patients with obesity and depression.[44] In all studies, bupropion was well tolerated, with dry mouth, anxiety, and insomnia being most commonly reported as side effects.[42-44]

Although approved for depression and smoking cessation, bupropion used for obesity treatment is an "off-label" use. Patients taking this medication for obesity must understand the circumstances under which it is being prescribed and should be closely followed clinically for any adverse effects.

Choosing a Medication

It is appropriate to consider pharmacological treatment for obesity if a patient has a BMI ≥30 or a BMI ≥27 with medical comorbidities. Table 2-10 includes the medications discussed that are approved for the treatment of obesity. Table 2-11 describes medications that may cause weight loss and are sometimes used "off-label" by obesity specialists as part of a treatment plan. The choice of medication should be based on information obtained during the assessment of the patient's weight history and comorbidities. For example, if a patient reports having an insatiable appetite, treatment with an anorexiant such as phentermine or sibutramine would be most appropriate if there are no medical contraindications. Orlistat is not the best pharmacotherapy for a patient with irritable bowel syndrome because of its GI side effects. If a patient has PCOS or impaired glucose tolerance, early consideration of a trial of metformin would be appropriate.

Prior to starting pharmacotherapy, patients must be educated that the medication is not a "magic bullet." Rather, it is adjunctive therapy designed to augment their other weight-loss efforts, which must include healthy eating, exercise, and behavior modification. This concept should be reinforced during interim visits with regular assessment of the medication's tolerability and effect.

Surgery

Despite the best combination of dietary, exercise, behavioral, and pharmacologic therapies, some patients ultimately need surgery to treat their obesity. These patients may be inclined to believe that they "failed" and that their inability to lose weight with medical therapies reflects poorly on them and their characters. It is important that these patients understand that obesity results from complex interactions of medical, genetic, develop-

Table 2-10

Medications Approved for Treatment of Obesity

Drug	Dose	Adverse Effects	Contraindications	AWP*
Phentermine	15-37.5 mg QD orally	Dry mouth, insomnia, nervousness, agitation, palpitations, constipation, elevations in heart rate and blood pressure	Poorly controlled HTN, active CAD, glaucoma, hyperthyroidism, agitation or use of MAO inhibitors within 14 days	$30.46 (30 mg/d)
Sibutramine	5-15 mg QD orally	Dry mouth, constipation, insomnia, headache, nausea, diarrhea, dizziness, palpitations, chest pain, restlessness, anxiety, elevations in heart rate and blood pressure	Uncontrolled HTN, CHF, CAD, known arrhythmias, stroke	$99.65 (10 mg/d)
Orlistat	120 mg TID orally (before, during, or ≥1 h after meals)	GI side effects including fatty or oily stools, fecal urgency, flatus with discharge, oily spotting, abdominal cramps, and intestinal flatus; malabsorption of vitamins A, D, E, and K	Use with extreme caution in patients taking coumadin and follow the INR closely	$163.81 (360 mg/d)

*Based on average cost of 30-day supply for the most common dose using 2004 average wholesale price.[45]

Table 2-11

Medications that May Cause Weight Loss

Drug	Common Use	Dose	Adverse Effects	Contraindications	AWP*
Metformin	Diabetes mellitus, PCOS	1000-2500 mg orally on BID or TID schedule	Diarrhea, nausea/vomiting, flatulence, abdominal pain, lactic acidosis	CHF, acidosis (lactic, metabolic, diabetic ketoacidosis); caution if impaired liver or renal function, hypersensitivity to metformin	$21.00 (850 mg BID)
Topiramate	Epilepsy, migraine prophylaxis	Start 25 mg orally BID; titrate up in 25-mg increments to maximum of 100 mg BID	Memory and concentration problems, paresthesias, and fatigue	Hypersensitivity to topairamate, impaired liver or renal function, cognitive or behavioral disorders; paresthesias	$306.90 (200 mg QD)
Zonisamide	Epilepsy	400-600 mg total orally on QD or BID schedule	Fatigue, somnolence, cognitive impairment, dizziness	Hypersensitivity to zonisamide or sulfonamides, renal stones	$265.00 (400 mg QD)
Bupropion	Depression, smoking cessation	150 mg orally extended release BID	Dry mouth, anxiety, insomnia	Seizure disorders, MAO-inhibitor use, current eating disorder, hypersensitivity to bupropion	$82.88 (150 mg BID)

*Based on average cost of 30-day supply for the most common dose using 2004 average wholesale price.[4]

mental, hormonal, psychological, environmental, and behavioral factors that are not completely understood. Some of these interactions result in obesity that is recalcitrant to medical therapy and requires surgical intervention. Choice of bariatric surgical procedures and management of the bariatric surgical patient are discussed in Chapter 3.

References

1. *The Practical Guide: Identification, Evaluation, and Treatment of Overweight and Obesity in Adults.* Bethesda, MD: National Institutes of Health; National Heart, Lung, and Blood Institutes; and North American Association for the Study of Obesity; 2000. NIH publication 00-4084.
2. Kaplan LM. Body weight regulation and obesity. *J Gastrointest Surg.* 2003;7(4):443-451.
3. Fontaine KR, Heo M, Allison DB. Body weight and cancer screening among women. *J Womens Health Gend Based Med.* 2001;10(5):463-470.
4. Rosen AB, Schneider EC. Colorectal cancer screening disparities related to obesity and gender. *J Gen Intern Med.* 2004;19(4):332-338.
5. Samaha FF, Iqbal N, Seshadri P, et al. A low-carbohydrate as compare with a low-fat diet in severe obesity. *N Engl J Med.* 2003;348(21):2074-2081.
6. Aude YW, Agatston AS, Lopez-Jimenez F, et al. The national cholesterol education program diet vs a diet lower in carbohydrates and higher in protein and monounsaturated fat. *Arch Intern Med.* 2004;164:2141-2146.
7. Foster GD, Wyatt HR, Hill JO, et al. A randomized trial of a low-carbohydrate diet for obesity. *N Engl J Med.* 2003;348(21):2082-2090.
8. Wadden TA, Foster GD, Letizia KA. One-year behavioral treatment of obesity: comparison of moderate and severe caloric restriction and the effects of weight maintenance therapy. *J Consult Clin Psychol.* 1994;62:165-171.
9. Pate RR, Pratt M, Blair SN, et al. Physical activity and public health. A recommendation from the Centers for Disease Control and Prevention and the American College of Sports Medicine. *JAMA.* 1995;273:402-407.
10. Munro JF, MacCuish AC, Wilson EM, Duncan LJ. Comparison of continuous and intermittent anorectic therapy in obesity. *Br Med J.* 1968;1:352-354.
11. Weissman NJ. Appetite suppressants and valvular heart disease. *Am J Med Sci.* 2001;321:285-291.
12. St John Sutton M. Silver lining to the cloud over anorexogen-related cardiac valvulopathy? *Ann Intern Med.* 2001;134:335-337.
13. Jick H. Heart valve disorders and appetite-suppressant drugs. *JAMA.* 2000;283:1738-1740.
14. Arterburn DE, Crane PK, Veenstra DL. The efficacy and safety of sibutramine for weight loss: a systematic review. *Arch Intern Med.* 2004;164:994-1003.
15. Berkowitz RI, Wadden TA, Tershakovec AM, Cronquist JL. Behavior therapy and sibutramine for the treatment of adolescent obesity: a randomized controlled trial. *JAMA.* 2003;289:1805-1812.
16. Seaton DA, Duncan LJ, Rose K, Scott AM. Diethyl-propion in the treatment of "refractory" obesity. *Br Med J.* 1961;5231:1009-1111.
17. Bays H, Dujovne C. Phamacotherapy of obesity: currently marketed and upcoming agents. *Am J Cardiovasc Drugs.* 2002(4);2:245-253.
18. Glazer G. Long-term pharmacotherapy of obesity 2000: a review of efficacy and safety. *Arch Intern Med.* 2001;161:1814-1824.
19. Curran MP, Scott LJ. Orlistat: a review of its use in the management of patients with obesity. *Drugs.* 2004;64(24):2845-2864.
20. Davidson MH, Hauptman J, DiGirolamo M, et al. Weight control and risk factor reduction in obese subjects treated for 2 years with orlistat: a randomized controlled trial. *JAMA.* 1999;281(3):235-242.
21. Weigle DS. Pharmacological therapy of obesity: past, present, and future. *J Clin Endocrinol Metab.* 2003;88(6):2462-2469.
22. Padwal R, Li SK, Lau DCW. Long-term pharmacotherapy for overweight and obesity: a systematic review and meta-analysis of randomized controlled trials. *Int J Obes Relat Metab Disord.* 2003;27(12):1437-1446.

23. Hill JO, Hauptman J, Anderson JW, et al. Orlistat, a lipase inhibitor, for weight maintenance after conventional dieting: a 1-y study. *Am J Clin Nutr.* 1999;69(6):1108-1116.

24. Torgerson JS, Hauptman J, Boldrin MN, Sjostrom L. XENical in the prevention of diabetes in obese subjects (XENDOS) study: a randomized study of orlistat as an adjunct to lifestyle changes for the prevention of type 2 diabetes in obese patients. *Diabetes Care.* 2004;27(1):155-161.

25. Hollander PA, Elbein SC, Hirsch IB, et al. Role of orlistat in the treatment of obese patients with type 2 diabetes. A 1-year randomized double-blind study. *Diabetes Care.* 1998;21(8):1288-1294.

26. Lindgarde F. The effect of orlistat on body weight and coronary heart disease risk profile in obese patients: the Swedish Multimorbidity Study. *J Intern Med.* 2000;248(3):245-254.

27. Harrison SA, Fincke C, Helinski D, Torgerson S, Hayashi P. A pilot study of orlistat treatment in obese, non-alcoholic steatohepatitis patients. *Aliment Pharmacol Ther.* 2004;20(6):623-628.

28. Cavaliere H, Floriano I, Medeiros-Neto G. Gastrointestinal side effects of orlistat may be prevented by concomitant prescription of natural fibers (psyllium mucilloid). *Int J Obes Relat Metab Disord.* 2001;25(7):1095-1099.

29. Waitman JA, Arrone LJ. Pharmacotherapy of obesity. *Obes Manage.* 2005;1(1):15-19.

30. Lee A, Morley JE. Metformin decreases food consumption and induces weight loss in subjects with obesity with type II non-insulin-dependent diabetes. *Obes Res.* 1998;6:47-53.

31. Pasquali R, Gambineri A, Biscotti D, et al. Effect of long-term treatment with metformin added to hypocaloric diet on body composition, fat distribution, and androgen and insulin levels in abdominally obese women with and without the polycystic ovary syndrome. *J Clin Endocrin Metab* 2000;85:2767-2774.

32. Knowler WC, Barrett-Connor E, Fowler SE, et al. Reduction in the incidence of type 2 diabetes with lifestyle intervention or metformin. *N Engl J Med.* 2002;346(6):393-403.

33. Gokcel A, Gumurdulu Y, Karakose H, et al. Evaluation of the safety and efficacy of sibutramine, orlistat and metformin in the treatment of obesity. *Diabetes Obes Metab.* 2002;4:49-55.

34. Kay JP, Alemzadeh R, Langley G, D'Angelo L, Smith P, Holshouser S. Beneficial effects of metformin in normoglycemic morbidly obese adolescents. *Metabolism.* 2001;50:1457-1461.

35. Freemark M, Bursey D. The effects of metformin on body mass index and glucose tolerance in obese adolescents with fasting hyperinsulinemia and a family history of type 2 diabetes. *Pediatrics.* 2001;107:E55.

36. Bray GA, Hollander P, Klein S, et al. A 6-month randomized, placebo-controlled, dose-ranging trial of topiramate for weight loss in obesity. *Obes Res.* 2003;11(6):722-733.

37. Wilding J, Van Gaal L, Rissanen A, Vercruysse R, Fitchet M: OBES-002 Study Group. A randomized double-blind placebo-controlled study of the long-term efficacy and safety of topiramate in the treatment of obese subjects. *Int J Obes Relat Metab Disord.* 2004;28(11):1399-1410.

38. Astrup A, Caterson I, Zelissen P, et al. Topiramate: long-term maintenance of weight loss induced by a low-calorie diet in obese subjects. *Obes Res.* 2004;12(10):1658-1669.

39. Gadde KM, Franciscy DM, Wagner HR 2nd, Krishnan KR. Zonisamide for weight loss in obese adults: a randomized controlled trial. *JAMA.* 2003;289(14):1820-1825.

40. Kim CS. Zonisamide effective for weight loss in women. *J Fam Pract.* 2003;52(8):600-601.

41. Appolinario JC, Bueno JR, Coutinho W. Psychotropic drugs in the treatment of obesity: what promise? *CNS Drugs.* 2004;18(10):629-651.

42. Gadde KM, Parker, BC, Maner LG, et al. Bupropion for weight loss: an investigation of efficacy and tolerability in overweight and obese women. *Obes Res.* 2001;9(9):544-551.

43. Anderson JW, Greenway FL, Fujioka K, Gadde KM, McKenney J, O'Neil PM. Bupropion SR enhances weight loss: a 48-week double-blind, placebo-controlled trial. *Obes Res.* 2002;10(7):633-641.

44. Jain AK, Kaplan RA, Gadde KM, et al. Bupropion SR vs. placebo for weight loss in obese patients with depressive symptoms. *Obes Res.* 2002;10(10):1049-1056.

45. PDR Staff. *2004 Red Book: Pharmacy's Fundamental Reference.* 108th ed. South Montbale, NJ: Thomson Healthcare; 2004.

46. Pan SY, Johnson KC, Ugnat A-M, et al. Association of obeisty and cancer risk in Canada. *Am J Epidemiol.* 2004;159(3):259-268.

47. Lacey JV Jr, Swanson CA, Brinton LA, et al. Obesity as a potential risk factor for adenocarcinomas and squamous cell carcinomas of the uterine cervix. *Cancer.* 2003;98(4):814-821.

3

Choice of Bariatric Procedures

David M. Lambert, MD; Ranjan Sudan, MD; and R. Armour Forse, MD, PhD

Introduction

Surgery for morbid obesity has been used in a small minority of patients since the 1950s to alleviate both the morbid obesity and associated comorbid conditions.[1] More recently, and especially with the use of advanced laparoscopic techniques, the number of bariatric procedures has risen: from 16,000 cases per year in the early 1990s to over 100,000 cases in 2003.[2] Significant decreases in excess body weight (EBW) are possible through obesity surgery, and, more importantly, comorbidities—such as HTN, type 2 diabetes mellitus, gastroesophageal reflux disease (GERD), arthritis, respiratory problems, urinary incontinence, depression, headaches, hyperlipidemia, and hormonal disturbances (polycystic ovary disease and dysmenorrhea)—can be effectively treated and often cured.[3] As a result of these improvements in health, not only is the morbidity and utilization of health care decreased, but life expectancy is also increased.[4,5]

History

Early Ideas

After the end of World War II, food rationing ended and common food items became cheap and plentiful. Through the following years, lifestyles changed: people began eating larger portions and making poorer choices in what they ate, and they became more sedentary. These changes led to physicians seeing patients who were significantly overweight. These patients began to develop medical problems directly related to their excessive weight.[6]

As surgeons realized that the most obese patients were refractory to available diets and drug therapies, they began devising surgical procedures to provide weight loss to these patients.[6] From past experiences, surgeons knew that patients undergoing resection of significant amounts of small bowel lost large amounts of weight.

The evolution of obesity surgery has been through 3 main classifications of techniques: malabsorptive—bypassing intestinal length so calories are not absorbed; restrictive—restricting the amount of food that can be ingested and bringing a sensation of satiety earlier; and combined—using both malabsorptive and restrictive components together to bring about weight loss. Other methods have also been devised that do not fit into these categories. The following is a discussion of the history of the development of bariatric surgery with operations grouped by technique.

Malabsorptive Procedures

Jejunoileal Bypass

In 1954, Kremen, Linner, and Nelson, of The University of Minnesota, published the report of what is now called the jejunoileal bypass (JIB).[7,8] This procedure and those similar to it are called malabsorptive procedures. The surgeon bypasses a variable length of the patient's small intestine, thereby decreasing the surface area available for absorption of calories as well as nutrients. The first JIB was conducted earlier that year and has been reported as the first such surgery of its kind (personal communication, April 2005).[8]

Around this same time, Dr. Victor Henriksson, in Sweden, performed a similar procedure; however, he resected the excluded portion of the small intestine and thus eliminated the option of reversing the procedure.[7] Throughout the 1950s and 1960s, several different groups performed variations of these operations for the treatment of obesity.[6,7,9] Because of nutritional and electrolyte disturbances (some severe) in patients undergoing JIBs, almost all cases required reversal. Other complications seen in these patients were gallstone and kidney-stone formation and diarrhea. Occasionally, bacterial overgrowth in the bypassed segment led to bacterial translocation and occasionally acute liver failure.[6] This liver failure often progressed to death in these patients and led to abandonment of this procedure in essentially all centers.

Incidentally, a partial ileal bypass—a much less severe version of the JIB—is used by some surgeons with excellent results in patients with familial hypercholesterolemia who cannot tolerate lipid-lowering drugs. Patients have obtained normal lipid levels, and reversal of atherosclerosis has even been documented.[6,10]

Restrictive Procedures

As purely malabsorptive procedures were associated with the risk of serious and life-threatening complications, surgeons used a number of purely restrictive procedures. These procedures were designed to limit the amount of food taken in orally by the patient. They have no affect on absorption and earlier procedures did not involve surgery on the intestine.

Jaw Wiring

The first truly restrictive procedure was wiring a patient's jaw closed. This obviously limited what foods were ingested, but when the wires were removed, patients steadily regained weight to preprocedure weights as the diet was increased.

Intragastric Devices

Another interesting restrictive idea involves an intragastric balloon (the Garren-Edwards gastric bubble or the BioEnterics Intragastric Balloon, BioEnterics: Santa Barbara, Calif). This device was placed in the stomach endoscopically and filled with fluid to occupy space and therefore limit the amount of food ingested. Use of this device incurred a moderate amount of weight loss; however, other procedures proved to be far more effective in weight loss, both in terms of quantity and sustained duration.[11,12]

Gastroplasty

Mason and Printen described the first surgical restrictive procedure for weight loss in 1971: the horizontal gastroplasty.[7] The principle of gastroplasty was to divide the patient's stomach into two interconnected compartments. One below the esophagogastric junction was to be small, limiting food intake and causing a sense of early satiety. This procedure, however, did not result in significant sustained weight loss. Modifications of this procedure by Gomez and colleagues also failed to produce the degree of weight loss or sustained weight loss.[7,13]

Eventually, through various modifications, Mason discovered that better results were obtained when (1) the created stomach pouch was very small, (2) the pouch was oriented along the lesser curve, and (3) the pouch stoma was small and reinforced with nondistensible material. This new procedure, named the vertical banded gastroplasty (VBG), improved the weight-loss results from the original gastroplasty[6,7] and is still a surgical option today.

Gastric Banding

The next evolution of restrictive procedures was by means of a band placed on the stomach without cutting or crushing the stomach. These bands also created two interconnected gastric compartments. The first bands used for obesity surgery were developed in the late 1970s and early 1980s; they were not adjustable and had limited success.[7] Kuzmak developed the first adjustable gastric band in 1986,[14] and variations of it are used today.

Combined Procedures

Gastric Bypass

Because of limited success with the gastroplasty and other restrictive operations, Mason looked to procedures combining the restrictive and malabsorptive components. By doing this, the degree of severe malabsorption and its related complications could be decreased. In the late 1960s, Mason and Ito first described the gastric bypass.[13] This is predominately a restrictive procedure with a lesser amount of malabsorption and was the first of the combined malabsorptive/restrictive procedures. It bypasses a smaller portion of the proximal small intestine, thus incorporating less malabsorption, and includes the restriction of food intake by making a small gastric pouch through which food can pass.

In the next few decades, the gastric bypass procedure underwent multiple modifications by various surgeons and, in its modified state, has become the standard by which other bariatric procedures are judged.[13] The Roux-en-Y gastric bypass (RYGB), as it is now called, derives its name from the way in which the gastrointestinal (GI) tract is reconstructed, as originally described by Cesar Roux, a Swiss surgeon.[7]

Biliopancreatic Diversion and Duodenal Switch

The biliopancreatic diversion (BPD) was described by Dr. Nicola Scopinaro and is primarily a malabsorptive procedure with a gastric-restrictive component.[7,13,15] A distal gastric resection is performed to reduce the stomach capacity to 250 cc. The small bowel is bypassed to create a 50-cc common channel and an alimentary limb of 250 cm. The biliopancreatic limb carries bile and pancreatic enzymes to the point where the alimentary limb transitions into the common channel. This avoids many of the problems associated with the blind limb of the JIB.

Further modifications of the BPD by Legace et al and by Hess and Hess resulted in the following changes and a new technique: the biliopancreatic diversion with duodenal switch (BPD/DS).[7,13] The partial gastrectomy was changed to a resection of the greater curvature ("sleeve gastrectomy") with sparing of the pylorus and anastomosis of the alimentary limb to the cuff of the proximal duodenum. This minimized the ulcerogenicity of the operation and reduced dumping symptoms.

Laparoscopic Procedures

With the increasing use of laparoscopic techniques, bariatric surgeons began to develop laparoscopic versions of the weight-loss procedures. The laparoscopic RYGB was initially reported by Wittgrove, Clark, and Tremblay in 1994,[16] with modifications by de la Torre and Scott[17] and by Higa and colleagues.[18] The VBG was performed laparoscopically first in the mid-1990s.[19,20] The gastric band was placed laparoscopically first in the early 1990s by Broadbent et al[21] and Catona et al,[22] and the first report of laparoscopic adjustable-gastric–band (LAGB) placement was by Forsell et al.[23] LAGB has become the standard of the totally restrictive procedures.[13] The BPD/DS was initially performed laparoscopically by Ren and associates and reported in 2000.[24] Robotic technology has been applied to virtually every bariatric procedure as well.[25-27]

Experimental Procedures/Evolving Technologies

Hypothalamic Stimulation

Other novel methods for surgical weight loss have been tried as well. In 1974, Quaade and his colleagues used stereotaxic stimulation and electrocoagulation of sites in the lateral hypothalamus. This led to decreased caloric intake and a decrease in body weight, but the results were temporary.[7]

Gastric Stimulation

More recently, Cigaina[28] used electrical stimulation of the gastric antrum to induce gastroparesis and weight loss. Initial results show weight loss associated with a decreased appetite and early satiety in some patients. Further studies are in progress throughout the world.[29,30]

Options

Various options exist in bariatric surgery. The procedures can be classified by their altered absorption of nutrients (malabsorptive procedures), limitation of intake (restric-

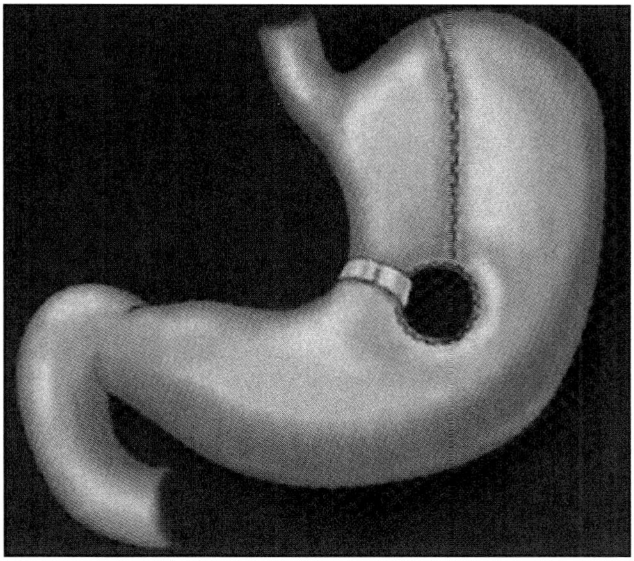

Figure 3-1. Diagram of VBG. (Reprinted, with permission of Dr. Michel Gagner and Springer-Verlag, from Gentileschi P, Kini S, Catarci M, Gagner M. Evidence-based medicine: open and laparoscopic bariatric surgery. *Surg Endosc.* 2002;16:736-744.) *For a full-color version, see page CA-I of the Color Atlas.*

tive procedures), or a combination of both. For the reasons detailed above, the purely malabsorptive procedures are not routinely performed today.

In general, the choice of procedure depends on the experiences and preferences of the surgeon and the patient. The surgeon's responsibility lies in knowing which procedures he or she can perform safely and effectively. The patients, when given a choice, choose the procedure that best suits their needs, based on risks and benefits as well as their own values. An algorithm has been proposed to aid in these choices and takes into account body mass index (BMI), age, gender, race, body habitus, and comorbidities.[31] However, the choice is best made after full discussion between the surgeon and patient.

The following is a more detailed description of the most commonly performed procedures for morbid obesity at this time.

Restrictive Procedures

Vertical Banded Gastroplasty

VBG is a purely restrictive procedure for the treatment of morbid obesity; there is no small-intestinal bypass and hence no malabsorptive component. A small pouch of 50 cc is created in the upper part of the stomach with an area of narrowing to restrict the flow of food into the distal stomach (Figure 3-1). The pouch is usually stapled, cut, and divided from the remainder of the fundus of the stomach. A piece of polypropylene mesh is placed around the stoma to lessen the chances of expansion of the stoma. If the pouch is not separated from the stomach (and to a lesser extent even when the stomach is completely divided) and the staple-line opens and forms a gastrogastric fistula, then the restriction is lessened, reversing the results of the surgery and causing weight regain (Chapter 7). The operation can also fail if the patient makes poor food choices, such as high-carbohydrate, calorie-dense foods (Chapter 8).

Risks seen with this procedure include bleeding, infection, leak/perforation, anastomotic stenosis, and internal hernia/small-bowel obstruction. There is also a risk of ulceration and stenosis at the stoma or dilation of the stoma (leading to weight regain).

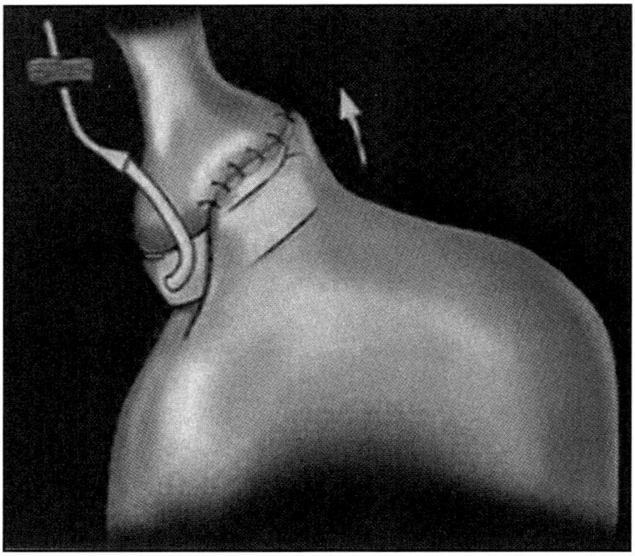

Figure 3-2. Diagram of LAGB. (Reproduced, with permission of Dr. Michel Gagner and Springer-Verlag, from Gentileschi P, Kini S, Catarci M, Gagner M. Evidence-based medicine: open and laparoscopic bariatric surgery. *Surg Endosc.* 2002;16:736-744.) *For a full-color version, see page CA-I of the Color Atlas.*

Patients can have a foreign-body reaction to the mesh material. Metabolic deficiencies are rare after purely restrictive procedures. (Postoperative complications are discussed in detail in Chapter 7.)

Weight loss after the open procedure is 40% to 77% of EBW at 4 years[33] and after the laparoscopic procedure is 61% to 75% long-term.[34] Hospital stay after laparoscopic VBG is generally short: between 1 and 5 days.[34] Mortality with this procedure is low: 0% to 1.1%.[34]

Laparoscopic Adjustable Gastric Banding

LAGB is also a purely restrictive procedure for weight loss. A silicone device consisting of a band with an inflatable balloon is placed around the upper portion of the stomach (Figure 3-2). The band is connected to a subcutaneous injection port by tubing. Sutures are placed in the stomach wall to form a tunnel around the band to help hold it in place. The band compartmentalizes the proximal stomach, creating a small gastric pouch (about 30-cc capacity), and its outlet into the remainder of the stomach is adjusted by either injecting or removing fluid from the access port.

To allow for healing and to encourage scar tissue that will hold the device in place, the balloon is not inflated upon placement. Once the patient has recovered from surgery, the balloon is inflated slowly over time. The patient should lose weight slowly after adjustment (inflation) of the band: about 1 lb per week. When weight loss plateaus, the balloon is inflated more. Weight loss is the guide for adjusting the balloon. The band provides restriction, and the small pouch allows the feeling of satiety sooner than is normal for the patient. This procedure requires absolute commitment of the patient to close follow-up and adjustment of the band when required. Prudent selection of patients for this procedure will likely maximize results. The benefits of this procedure are that there are no anastomoses with the potential for leaks, and the procedure is completely and easily reversible, as there has been no reconstruction. Additionally, hospital stay is short—1 to 3 days, and reoperative rate is relatively low (2% to 8.9%).[34]

Risks seen with this procedure include bleeding, infection, and leak/perforation. The stomach distal to the band can herniate through the band ("slipped" band), leading to an obstruction. This is a foreign body and will continue to be associated with the inherent problems that go along with that: device failure (band leak, tube leak), device infection, and erosion of the device into the stomach. Metabolic deficiencies are rare after purely restrictive procedures.

Experience with the LAGB in Europe and Australia is fairly extensive, and results have been good, as have short-term results in the United States.[35] Percentage losses of EBW at 1, 2, and 3 years have been reported to be 43%, 58%, and 55%, respectively, in a European study of 500 patients.[36] The early trial for FDA approval of the LapBand device (INAMED Corp.; Santa Barbara, Calif) demonstrated EBW loss of 35% at 1 year and 36% at 3 years.[36] Other studies have shown weight loss in the range of 40% to 70%[34] and 44% to 68%[33] at 4 years, though this was in a small number of patients.

There is still a need for demonstration through long-term studies of the long-term efficacy and durability of weight loss. The mortality rate of patients undergoing this procedure is very low, with most studies reporting no deaths.[32,36,37]

Combined Procedures

Roux-en-Y Gastric Bypass

RYGB is considered the "gold standard" operation for morbid obesity and accounts for approximately 70% of bariatric procedures.[34,38] Studies directly comparing the effectiveness (weight loss) between RYGB and VBG, the previously preferred procedure, continue to show greater weight loss after RYGB.[32,36]

This procedure has 3 basic steps. First, the surgeon creates a small (approximately 15 to 30 cc) gastric pouch that accounts for the restrictive component. Then, the surgeon makes a separate limb (the biliopancreatic limb) that extends approximately 50 cm from the ligament of Treitz to conduct biliary and pancreatic secretions until they are mixed with chyme at the distal anastomosis. Finally, the GI tract is rearranged to bring a 75 to 150–cm length of jejunum (the alimentary limb) up to the gastric pouch to carry food from the gastric pouch to the distal anastomosis. Figure 3-3 shows this reconstruction. The delay in mixing of chyme and digestive enzymes accounts for the malabsorptive component. The RYGB can also be fashioned so that there is a much larger amount of bypassed small intestine—the distal RYGB—making the distal anastomosis 150 cm proximal to the ileocecal valve. This procedure has been used by some surgeons, predominately in patients classified as "super obese" (BMI ≥50 kg/m^2). These operations can be carried out in either an open or a laparoscopic approach.

Risks seen with this procedure include bleeding, infection, incisional hernia, leak, anastomotic stenosis or ulceration, nutrient and calorie malnutrition, and internal hernia/small-bowel obstruction.

Loss of EBW is high with this operation: 50% to 68% at 10 years for open operations[13,39] and 60% to 68% at 1 year for laparoscopic procedures.[37,40] Long-term data are accumulating for the laparoscopic procedures, which appear to provide equal weight loss with identical complication profiles but improved rates of wound infections and incisional hernias.[36,37,40-42] Hospital stay also appears to be shorter with the laparoscopic technique in several studies: 1.6 to 4 days for laparoscopic versus 4 to 8 days for open.[13,34,40] Mortality is low with either the open or laparoscopic approach: 0% to 1.5% in multiple studies.[34,43]

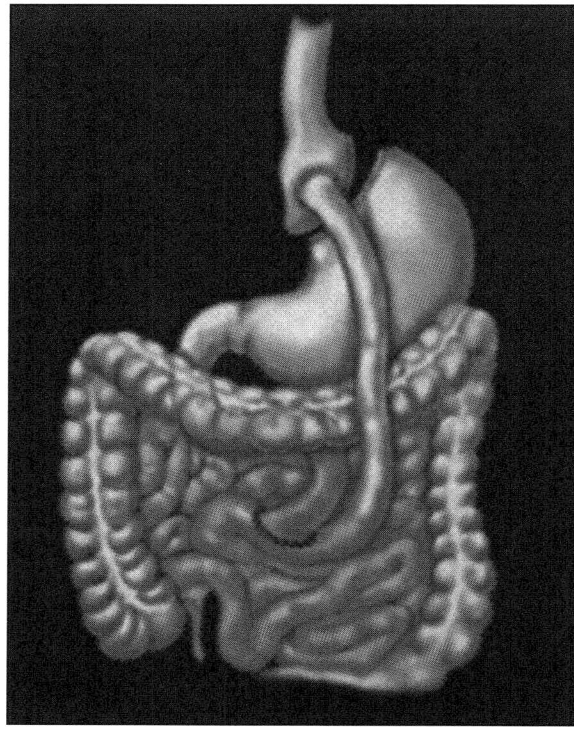

Figure 3-3. Diagram of RYGB. (Reproduced, with permission of Dr. Michel Gagner and Springer-Verlag, from Gentileschi P, Kini S, Catarci M, Gagner M. Evidence-based medicine: open and laparoscopic bariatric surgery. *Surg Endosc.* 2002;16:736-744.) *For a full-color version, see page CA-II of the Color Atlas.*

Biliopancreatic Diversion and Duodenal Switch

The BPD and BPD/DS are procedures that incorporate both restrictive and malabsorptive components (Figure 3-4). BPD is predominately a malabsorptive procedure, with approximately 50 to 100 cm of terminal ileum (the common channel) in which the mixing of the digestive enzymes and chyme for digestion and absorption can occur. Approximately 150 to 200 cm of ileum are used for the enteric limb to carry chyme from the remaining stomach to the distal anastomosis and the common channel. There is a small restrictive component given by a partial gastrectomy (either distal gastrectomy or a "sleeve" gastrectomy), which leaves a gastric pouch with a capacity of about 150 to 250 cc. The alimentary limb can be anastomosed either to the proximal stomach after distal gastrectomy—the BPD—or to the duodenal stump, preserving the pylorus—the BPD/DS. The BPD/DS reduces dumping symptoms (epigastric pain, nausea, palpitations, sweating, dizziness, and occasionally syncope) and other side effects seen with BPD (diarrhea, ulcers, protein malnutrition).[44,45] The gallbladder and appendix are also usually removed. This procedure is most often conducted via an open approach but can be completed laparoscopically, although technically it is the most demanding laparoscopic procedure to perform.

Patients are able to eat more (volume and variety) after the BPD and BPD/DS than after the RYGB. Because of a larger stomach pouch, however, greater malabsorption helps maintain weight loss. These patients have more frequent and foul-smelling stool and flatus.[45]

Risks seen with this procedure include bleeding, infection, incisional hernia, leak, anastomotic stenosis, nutrient and calorie malnutrition, and internal hernia/small-bowel obstruction. There is also a risk of hypocalcemia and hypovitaminosis D, which can

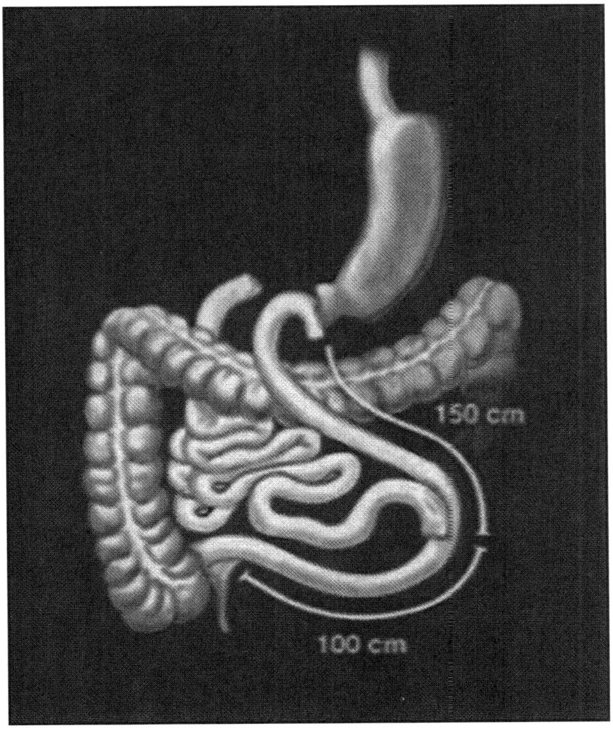

Figure 3-4. Diagram of BPD/DS. (Reproduced, with permission of Dr. Michel Gagner and Springer-Verlag, from Gentileschi P, Kini S, Catarci M, Gagner M. Evidence-based medicine: open and laparoscopic bariatric surgery. *Surg Endosc.* 2002;16:736-744.) *For a full-color version, see page CA-II of the Color Atlas.*

potentially lead to osteoporosis. It is important to monitor calcium and vitamin-D levels routinely to prevent these problems. Elevated parathormone levels can also be seen with low calcium levels.

Long-term weight loss after BPD and BPD/DS are excellent, according to multiple studies.[32,37,46] Patients lose an average of 70% to 80% of EBW in the long term.[45]

Mortality related to open techniques is low: less than 2%.[32,47] Side effects after this procedure are similar to those of other surgical procedures, including leaks, stenoses, and nutritional deficiencies.

Emerging Technologies

Gastric Stimulation

Gastric pacing is a new experimental modality for weight loss, and the mechanism of action is not fully understood. The device consists of a generator and bipolar lead. The lead is attached to the anterior wall of the stomach using laparoscopic techniques, and the generator is implanted under the skin in the left upper quadrant of the abdominal wall. The generator provides an electrical stimulus to the stomach producing retrograde impulses in the stomach and thereby inducing some gastroparesis and early satiety. An excellent review is given in the article by Shikora.[30]

Risks seen with this procedure include bleeding, infection, and device malfunction or failure. Abdominal pain, nausea, and vomiting have also been reported.

Early results of this procedure in humans showed weight loss in the 20% range, with relapses if the device was not functioning (such as when the battery failed). Risks associated with this procedure (eg, bleeding, infection, injury to intra-abdominal organs, and hernias) are minimal and are the same as those commonly associated with any surgical procedure. There is also the potential for device-related issues, such as failure, lead displacement, and erosion.

Current Operative Indications/Approach

"Overweight" is defined by a BMI ≥25, "obesity" as a BMI ≥30, and "morbid obesity" as a BMI ≥40, with "super-obese" defined as a BMI ≥50.[7] A BMI ≥40 represents approximately 100 lbs over ideal body weight (IBW).[2] (BMI is calculated by the division of the individual's weight in kilograms by his or her height in meters squared.) The current indication for considering bariatric surgery is an adult patient who is morbidly obese, per this definition, or someone with a BMI of 35 to 40 with serious comorbid conditions.[48] (For more information about obesity-related definitions and statistics, see Chapter 1.)

Patients should be well informed about the effects of morbid obesity on overall health and educated about the risks and benefits of weight-loss surgery. Patients must understand the potential nutritional risks involved (deficiencies related to the specific procedures) and also must be able to participate in long-term follow-up. It is important that the surgeon work with a highly skilled bariatric team: a group of specialists who can address the different aspects of weight-loss surgery and assist in educating the patient in risks, benefits, and responsibilities. Working with the members of the bariatric team—a bariatric nurse, a medical specialist, a dietician, and a psychologist, in addition to the bariatric surgeon—will ensure that the patient is accurately assessed for surgery and is prepared for the outcomes. Including the patient's primary-care physician may also improve the patient's long-term care after surgery (Chapter 9).

Other considerations for obesity surgery include the patient's psychologic history. Each patient routinely undergoes psychological evaluation prior to surgery to fully evaluate concerns and ensure that the patient is a good candidate for bariatric surgery. If the patient has had problems with alcohol or substance abuse in the past, the disorder should be under control. Patients should be free of significant psychiatric disorders, particularly suicidal ideation or attempts. (See Chapter 12 for discussion of bariatric-related psychological issues and assessment.)

Weight-loss surgery in children and adolescents is an area of controversy at this time. (See Chapter 6 for further discussion.)

Indications for surgery are given in Table 3-1.

Risks

As with any surgical procedure, there are risks associated with weight-loss surgery. It is important for patients to understand these risks so each can give informed consent before proceeding with obesity surgery. It is incumbent on the physician to ensure that the patient and family members are familiar with these risks and their relative incidence. These risks are best classified as short-term and long-term risks. Risks categorized as postoperative complications are discussed in detail in Chapter 7.

Short Term

Risks normally associated with any operative procedure are minimal after bariatric surgery.

Table 3-1
Operative Indications for Bariatric Surgery

- BMI ≥40
- BMI ≥35 with serious comorbid conditions
- Acceptable operative candidate
- Motivated to adhere to the postoperative lifestyle changes
- Well informed regarding risks of surgery
- Able to participate in long-term follow-up
- No substance abuse issues
- No (or under control) significant psychiatric conditions

Bleeding

The risk of significant bleeding is ≤1%, regardless of the operation chosen.[33,34]

Deep Venous Thrombosis and Pulmonary Embolism

The risk of deep venous thrombosis after bariatric surgery is reported to be ≤3% in open cases (primarily in RYGB and VBG) and ≤2% in laparoscopic cases (RYGB, VBG, and LAGB).[33,34] The risk of pulmonary embolism is <1%.[33] Therefore, thrombosis prophylaxis (such as sequential compression devices and low-dose unfractionated heparin or low-molecular–weight heparin) must be instituted. Placement of a vena cava filter in patients with even higher risks (eg, severe pulmonary hypertension, previous deep venous thrombosis, immobility, protein C and S deficiencies) should be considered.

Wound-Related Risks

The risk of wound-related complications, such as infections and hernias, is ever present after any surgery; however, their incidence is reduced after laparoscopic surgery in many studies. While wound infections have been reported in up to 5% of open RYGB and VBG,[13,33] they are reported in <2% of laparoscopic cases (laparoscopic RYGB and LAGB).[33,34,40] Patients are routinely given perioperative antibiotics to decrease the risk of postoperative infection.

Incisional hernias are reported to occur in up to 23.9% of open RYGB and 5.12% of VBG; however, their incidence is <4% of laparoscopic RYGB and laparoscopic VBG.[13,33,34]

Leaks

Perhaps the most concerning of the possible complications of bariatric surgery is GI leak. Symptoms commonly seen with leaks include fever, tachycardia, low urine output, leukocytosis, and shoulder pain. Patients with postoperative leaks may have surprisingly few signs in the face of significant sepsis; because of this, it is important to maintain a high index of suspicion. While the incidence of surgically related leaks is low, the consequences can be devastating. Leaks have been reported in <5% of cases regardless of technique: the incidence of gastric perforation after LAGB and laparoscopic VBG and RYGB is <1%.[33,34] Several options are available to check for leaks at the anastomoses during surgery: insufflation with air, instillation of methylene blue dye, and endoscopy. Regardless of the test chosen, leaks must be sought out intraoperatively to prevent a return to the operating room. Frequently, a water-soluble–contrast upper-gastrointestinal (UGI) study is performed postoperatively as well (Chapter 11).

Gastroesophageal Reflux Disease

GERD is a condition that commonly affects patients with obesity; the majority of RYGB patients respond with a rapid decrease in their symptoms because both acid and bile exposure to the distal esophagus is significantly reduced. RYGB, by drastically reducing the stomach's size and thus separating a majority of the stomach's acid-producing cells from the esophagus, is a very effective surgical treatment for GERD in morbidly obese patients. In contrast, purely restrictive procedures can sometimes be associated with the development of reflux symptoms: in <2% of patients after VBG and variably after LAGB (<1% to 25%-30%).[49-52]

A problem rarely seen after LAGB is dilation of the esophagus related to partial obstruction. If the band is too tight, the patient can experience some reflux symptoms and partial obstruction. Over time, the esophagus can dilate and, if not remedied by deflation or removal of the band, the esophagus can become nonfunctional. The development of reflux symptoms postoperatively in these patients should be investigated.

Pulmonary

Obesity is associated with sleep apnea and Pickwickian syndrome, and patients with these disorders are at risk for pulmonary complications after surgery. Prevention of atelectasis and pneumonia is centered on deep breathing and incentive spirometry, as well as early ambulation. Patients with sleep apnea are closely monitored because they may have more problems with sedation from narcotics, and subsequent hypoxemia can be fatal. Patients with sleep apnea who are using continuous positive-airway–pressure (CPAP) devices are encouraged to continue CPAP postoperatively until they have lost significant amounts of weight and have been reevaluated to ensure that their sleep apnea has resolved.

Cardiac

Metabolic syndrome is a constellation of diseases that increase a patient's risk of developing heart disease, stroke, and diabetes. The diseases include obesity, HTN, dyslipidemia, and glucose intolerance, all of which can increase the postoperative risks in patients undergoing weight-loss surgery. These patients should be evaluated as are any patients undergoing major operative procedures. Cardiac risk is very low, and selected cardiac work-up in high-risk patients is recommended preoperatively.

Diabetes Mellitus

The effect of weight-loss surgery on type 2 diabetes is remarkable. Blood sugars frequently normalize rapidly after surgery—well before significant weight loss occurs—and these patients need reduced doses or elimination of medications to avoid hypoglycemia. This is discussed in detail in Chapter 9.

Dehydration and Fluids

Patients are unable to take in large amounts of fluid postoperatively and can easily become dehydrated. Symptoms include lightheadedness, nausea, malaise, loss of consciousness, and diaphoresis. Patients are encouraged to record fluid intake and consume fluids in small amounts once diet allows to prevent dehydration. Fluid replacement is addressed in Chapter 7.

Long Term

Long-term risks generally occur several weeks to years after surgery and include internal hernias, small-bowel obstructions, anastomotic problems (stenosis and ulceration), device problems (LAGB), and nutritional deficiencies.

Internal Hernias, Bowel Obstructions

Internal hernias and small-bowel obstructions are reported to occur in less than 3.5% of patients after open or laparoscopic RYGB[33,34,42] and in 0.01% to 0.03% of patients after VBG or LAGB.[33] Symptoms seen in the setting of obstruction or internal hernia include abdominal pain, nausea, and vomiting. The presence and persistence of these symptoms should lead to early work-up. This can be difficult, as inappropriate eating (diet and/or behavior) can produce similar symptoms.

Anastomotic Problems

Stenosis of the gastrojejunal anastomosis leading to dysphagia and vomiting occurs in 1.6% to 6.3% of patients after RYGB (laparoscopic or open), <2% of patients after VBG (laparoscopic or open), and 1.97% after LAGB.[33,34] This can often be treated with endoscopic dilatation with good results (Chapter 10). Ulceration in the area of the anastomosis or gastric constriction occurs in 4.1% of patients after RYGB but in <0.2% of patients after VBG or LAGB.[33]

Some potential problems associated with the LAGB and VBG are due to a foreign body—the gastric band—being present near the GI tract. Erosion of the band into the lumen of the stomach has been reported in 0.59% of LAGB cases and 0.26% of VBG cases.[33] Infection of the device has been reported in 0.36% of cases after LAGB and 0.05% of cases after VBG.[33]

Nutritional Deficiencies

Nutritional deficiencies are possible after any of the procedures described above; however, they are rare after purely restrictive procedures (VBG and LAGB). The reason for this is that the GI tract is left intact (except for making a small pouch in the upper portion of the stomach), and there is no malabsorptive component of this weight-loss method. Some abnormalities may be seen in patients with intractable vomiting, ie, hypokalemic, hypochloremic metabolic alkalosis. This responds to rehydration and control of emesis.

Nutritional deficiencies occur more frequently after weight-loss surgery involving bypass of small intestine. The most commonly experienced deficiencies after BPD are iron, anemia, calcium, fat-soluble vitamins (predominately vitamin D), and protein. Kalfarentos et al[53] compared patients undergoing BPD or RYGB and noted a 15.2% incidence of low ferritin in BPD patients, as compared to 37.7% after RYGB. These investigators also showed no difference in hemoglobin, iron, folate, or albumin between the 2 groups (although 1 RYGB patient and 2 BPD patients had albumin levels below 3 g/dl and required hospitalization and parenteral nutrition).

Hypocalcemia and vitamin-D deficiencies after BPD and BPD/DS have been described in several reports[41,44,54,55] and can be explained by the fat malabsorption due to the procedure. Elevated parathormone and alkaline phosphatase suggest bone resorption; however, evidence of increased bone resorption was seen in only 3% of patients in a study by Slater and colleagues.[54]

Because segments of the small intestine are bypassed with the BPD and BPD/DS, it is important to monitor for deficiency of fat-soluble vitamins (A, D, E, and K). Clinical indications of these deficiencies include rashes and night-vision disturbances with vitamin-A deficiency; neurologic disturbances—particularly cerebellar signs—with vitamin-E deficiency; abnormal bleeding and easy bruising with vitamin-K deficiency; and osteoporosis and pathologic bone fracture with vitamin-D deficiency. Serum assays for these vitamins are available and should be checked annually or as indicated.

While a few cases of progressive liver dysfunction in postoperative bariatric patients have been reported,[56] the extensive problems that were experienced by patients after JIB have not been seen consistently after other procedures. Cases of progressive hepatic dysfunction with cirrhosis have been reported after distal RYGB and BPD[46,57]; however, improvement in liver morphology has also been seen with BPD.[44]

Nutritional risks following RYGB differ from those after other weight-loss surgeries because the procedure bypasses the stomach and small intestine differently than do BPD and BPD/DS. The nutrients often seen to be deficient with RYGB are iron (20% to 49%), vitamin B12 (26% to 70%), and folate (9% to 35%). Deficiencies of any of these nutrients can cause anemia, which is seen in 18% to 54% of patients.[39] Iron is absorbed mostly in the duodenum; therefore, bypass of this area can lead to iron-deficiency anemia. Vitamin-B12 deficiency is also a possible cause of anemia after RYGB. This is most likely related to inadequate mixing of food-bound vitamin B12 and intrinsic factor. The cause of folate deficiency is unknown, but inadequate intake is felt to be the most likely cause. Calcium deficiency can also be seen after RYGB.

Regardless of the operative procedure chosen, postoperative vitamin and mineral supplementation with life-long follow-up and surveillance for deficiencies is required. It is important that patients understand the importance of this and commit to participating in this follow-up (Chapter 8).

Results

Results of the varying surgical procedures fall into 2 groups: (1) weight loss, which is discussed above, and (2) resolution of comorbidities. Resolution of comorbidities is uniform, regardless of procedure.

Sleep Apnea

Sleep apnea resolves in 46% to 67% of cases across all procedures.[58,59] However, 1 study, albeit a small study, cautioned that patients may be at risk for recurrence, even without weight regain.[60] Studies for specific procedures also note resolution of sleep apnea, specifically after LAGB (94% resolution),[61] BPD (91.7% resolution),[61] and RYGB (up to 92% resolution).[62,63]

Hypertension

HTN also resolves in a majority of patients and improves in most of the remaining patients. It was reported to resolve in 71.4% of patients after BPD[64] and 43% to 66% of patients after RYGB,[62,63,65-67] with documentation of persistent improvement 5 to 7 years postoperatively.[68] However, the benefit may not always be sustained.[69] HTN is also associated with advancing age and has been seen to recur as patients aged after bariatric surgery.

Diabetes Mellitus

Diabetes is consistently and dramatically improved by weight-loss surgery. Research shows resolution in 81.8% after BPD.[64] Studies involving RYGB showed similar rates of resolution of diabetes and normalization of fasting blood glucose with long-term follow-up (9 or more years).[62,63,65-68,70] These changes were seen as early as 4 months after surgery, before the majority of excess weight had been lost.[71]

Other Comorbidities

Bariatric surgery also brings about improvement in other comorbidities including GERD.[61] RYGB has been compared to Nissen fundoplication for its effectiveness in treating GERD in patients with morbid obesity.

Dyslipidemia also improves with weight loss: surgery and the weight loss not only decrease cholesterol, triglycerides, and low-density lipids, but also increase high-density lipids,[63,68] leading some to surmise that the risk of coronary artery disease also decreases.[66] Multiple studies evaluating the effects of partial ileal bypass have shown reversal of atherosclerosis postoperatively.[10]

Venous stasis resolved in 95% of patients[72] and asthma in 50%.[63] Studies also report decreased incidences of arthritis, infertility, and even pseudotumor cerebri[62,73] after bariatric surgery.

Patients notice significant improvement in psychological and social areas as well. Depression improves in approximately 25% of patients.[61,74] Patients also report improvement in self-confidence and social life[45] and in sexual function.[45,75] Studies specifically investigating marital stability after weight-loss surgery, however, show little change: "unconflicted" marriages—ones that are harmonious before surgery—tend to continue in stability, and bariatric surgery does not decrease problems in "conflicted" marriages.[7] Psychological issues are discussed in great detail in Chapter 12.

Expectations

Dietary

In the immediate postoperative period, patients will, in general, be restricted to small portions (about 1 oz at a time) of liquids. It is important for postoperative patients to consume liquids frequently to avoid dehydration. Inattention to the amount of liquids taken in can rapidly lead to dehydration and its attendant sequelae. Patients are allowed to advanced their diets to pureed foods and then to soft foods gradually. The amount of time it takes to advance to regular food varies from institution to institution and even from surgeon to surgeon.[76]

Patients are encouraged to eat slowly and chew their food well to avoid eating too rapidly and to allow the feeling of satiety to occur. Food should be eaten in small volumes. Liquids are not to be consumed with solid foods because of the limited space available in the stomach; rather liquids should be taken at least 30 minutes before or after meals. Proteins should be the preferred foodstuff over fats and carbohydrates, and it is recommended that patients take in at least 60 g of protein daily. Vitamin and mineral supplements are recommended for virtually all patients to avoid deficiencies. BPD and BPD/DS patients should take water-soluble analogs of fat-soluble vitamins. Parenteral B12 and iron may also be needed.

Bariatric-surgery patients will have significant lifestyle alterations in the form of dietary modifications. Those patients who have restrictive procedures (VBG, LAGB, or RYGB) will have the greatest changes to make. Because of the extremely small size of the gastric pouch, these patients must eat very small portions. In the event of dietary "indiscretions," patients will experience abdominal pain, nausea, and vomiting. Patients who have had a RYGB must also minimize the amounts of concentrated sugars/carbohydrates that they eat. Because these patients have a gastrojejunal anastomosis between the gastric pouch and the enteric limb, they are at risk for the dumping syndrome when carbohydrates rapidly enter the small intestine. The symptoms of dumping are tachycardia, diaphoresis, tremulousness, abdominal cramping, nausea, diarrhea, and generalized malaise after eating sugars. The diagnosis is easily made based on symptoms in relation to dietary intake. While the BPD/DS patients may not experience dumping symptoms with carbohydrates, their weight loss will be suboptimal if they consume simple sugars. Chapter 8 discusses postoperative nutritional requirements in detail.

Laboratory Follow-up

It is imperative that physicians check vitamin and mineral levels in those patients who have had any malabsorptive procedure (RYGB, BPD, and BPD/DS). Patients who have had RYGB are at risk for anemia because of alterations in intrinsic factor availability and decreased absorption of vitamin B12 and folate. Patients who have had BPD or BPD/DS are at risk for deficiencies in vitamins A and D and, to a lesser extent, E and K, as well as iron. Other parameters to monitor include serum protein, albumin, pre-albumin, iron studies, and serum calcium. It should also be noted that nutritional and vitamin deficiencies have been noted in patients with purely restrictive procedures, despite the lack of rearrangement of the GI tract.[77]

Psychological

Because of the psychological and social changes seen after bariatric surgery (Chapter 12), patients need resources for support. Support groups are important because they allow patients to understand the changes in and implications to their lives as seen through the experiences of others. Patients may also need counseling resources. While most patients will have improvement in mood and social functioning, others do not cope as well with the drastic changes in body image and interactions with others. There have been patients who have committed suicide after weight-loss surgery, and patients should be appropriately monitored.

Summary

Bariatric surgery, while medically a safe option overall, is associated with risks—both short and long term. There are several options for surgical treatment of obesity, each with its own risks and benefits. Before pursuing any of these options, patients should be well educated about what to expect from weight-loss surgery, including preoperative and post-operative care as well as long-term follow-up. Surgery for morbid obesity is an extremely effective treatment and remains the most effective option for the appropriate patient.

References

1. Brody F. Minimally invasive surgery for morbid obesity. *Cleve Clin J Med.* 2004;71(4):289,293,296-298.
2. Steinbrook R. Surgery for severe obesity. *N Engl J Med.* 2004;350(11):1075-1079.
3. Raum WJ. Postoperative medical management of bariatric patients. In: Martin LF, Ed. *Obesity Surgery.* New York, NY: McGraw-Hill; 2004:133-159.
4. Christou NV, Sampalis JS, Lieberman M, et al. Surgery decreases long-term mortality, morbidity, and health care use in morbidly obese patients. *Ann Surg.* 2004;240(3):416-423.
5. Flum DR, Dellinger EP. Impact of gastric bypass operation on survival: a population-based analysis. *J Am Coll Surg.* 2004;199:543-551.
6. Martin LF. The evolution of surgery for morbid obesity. In: Martin LF, Ed. *Obesity Surgery.* New York, NY: McGraw-Hill; 2004:15-47.
7. Buchwald H, Buchwald JN. Evolution of operative procedures for the management of morbid obesity 1950-2000. *Obes Surg.* 2002;12:705-717.
8. Kremen AJ, Linner JH, Nelson CH. An experimental evaluation of the nutritional importance of proximal and distal small intestine. *Ann Surg.* 1954;140(3):439-448.
9. Payne JH, DeWind LT. Surgical treatment of obesity. *Am J Surg.* 1969;118:141-147.
10. Buchwald H, Varco RL, Matts JP, et al. Effect of partial ileal bypass surgery on mortality and morbidity from coronary heart disease in patients with hypercholesterolemia. Report of the Program on the Surgical Control of the Hyperlipidemias (POSCH). *N Engl J Med.* 1990;323:946-955.
11. Kirby DF, Wade JB, Mills PR, et al. A prospective assessment of the Garren-Edwards Gastric Bubble and bariatric surgery in the treatment of morbid obesity. *Am Surg.* 1990;56(10):575-580.
12. Doldi SB, Micheletto G, Perrini MN, Rapetti R. Intragastric balloon: another option for treatment of obesity and morbid obesity. *Hepatogastroenterology.* 2004;51(55):294-297.
13. Jones KB Jr. Bariatric surgery—where do we go from here? *Int Surg.* 2004;89:51-57.
14. Kuzmak L. Silicone gastric banding: a simple and effective operation for morbid obesity. *Contemp Surg.* 1986;28:13-18.
15. Scopinaro N, Gianetta E, Civalleri D, Bonalumi U, Bachi V. Bilio-pancreatic bypass for obesity: II. Initial experience in man. *Brit J Surg.* 1979;66:618-620.
16. Wittgrove AC, Clark GW, Tremblay LJ. Laparoscopic gastric bypass, Roux-en-Y: preliminary report of five cases. *Obes Surg.* 1994;4:353-357.
17. de la Torre RA, Scott JS. Laparoscopic Roux-en-Y gastric bypass: a totally intra-abdominal approach—technique and preliminary report. *Obes Surg.* 1999;9:492-498.
18. Higa KD, Boone KB, Ho T, Davies OG. Laparoscopic Roux-en-Y gastric bypass for morbid obesity: technique and preliminary results of our first 400 patients. *Arch Surg.* 2000;135(9):1029-1033.
19. Hess DW, Hess DS. Laparoscopic vertical banded gastroplasty with complete transection of the staple-line. *Obes Surg.* 1994;4:44-46.
20. Chua TY, Mediola RM. Laparoscopic vertical banded gastroplasty: the Milwaukee experience. *Obes Surg.* 1995;5:77-80.

21. Broadbent R, Tracey M, Harrington P. Laparoscopic gastric banding: a preliminary report. *Obes Surg.* 1993;3:63-67.

22. Catona A, Gossenberg M, LaManna A, Mussini G. Laparoscopic gastric banding: preliminary series. *Obes Surg.* 1993;3:207-209.

23. Forsell P, Hallberg D, Hellers G. Gastric banding for morbid obesity: initial experience with a new adjustable band. *Obes Surg.* 1993;3:369-374.

24. Ren CJ, Patterson E, Gagner M. Early results of laparoscopic biliopancreatic diversion with duodenal switch: a case series of 40 consecutive patients. *Obes Surg.* 2000;10(6):514-523.

25. Jacobsen G, Elli F, Horgan S. Robotic surgery update. *Surg Endosc.* 2004;18:1186-1191.

26. Muhlmann G, Klaus A, Kirchmayr W, et al. DaVinci robotic-assisted laparoscopic bariatric surgery: is it justified in a routine setting? *Obes Surg.* 2003;13(6):848-854.

27. Talamini MA, Chapman S, Horgan S, Melvin WS, The Academic Robotics Group. A prospective analysis of 211 robotic-assisted surgical procedures. *Surg Endosc.* 2003;17(10):1521-1524.

28. Cigaina V. Gastric pacing as therapy for morbid obesity: preliminary results. *Obes Surg.* 2002;12(suppl 1):12-16.

29. De Luca M, Segato G, Busetto L, et al. Progress in implantable gastric stimulation: summary of results of the European multi-center study. *Obes Surg.* 2004;14(suppl 1):S33-S39.

30. Shikora SA. Implantable gastric stimulation for weight loss. *J Gastrointest Surg.* 2004;8:408-412.

31. Buchwald H. A bariatric surgery algorithm. *Obes Surg.* 2002;12(6):733-746.

32. Gentileschi P, Kini S, Catarci M, Gagner M. Evidence-based medicine: open and laparoscopic bariatric surgery. *Surg Endosc.* 2002;16:736-744.

33. Chapman AE, Kiroff G, Game P, et al. Laparoscopic adjustable gastric banding in the treatment of obesity: a systematic literature review. *Surgery.* 2004;135(3):326-351.

34. Schauer PR, Ikramuddin S. Laparoscopic surgery for morbid obesity. *Surg Clin North Am.* 2001;81(5):1145-1179.

35. Ren CJ, Weiner M, Allen JW. Favorable early results of gastric banding for morbid obesity: the American experience. *Surg Endosc.* 2004;18:543-546.

36. Melvin WS. Roux-en-Y gastric bypass is the operation of choice for bariatric surgery. *J Gastrointest Surg.* 2004;8(4):398-405.

37. Rabkin RA, Rabkin JM, Metcalf B, Lazo M, Rossi M, Lehman-Becker LB. Nutritional markers following duodenal switch for morbid obesity. *Obes Surg.* 2004;14(1):84-90.

38. Pories WJ, Roth JS. Gastric bypass. In: Martin LF, Ed. *Obesity Surgery.* New York, NY: McGraw-Hill; 2004:213-225.

39. Brolin RE. Gastric bypass. *Surg Clin North Am.* 2001;81(5):1077-1095.

40. Nguyen NT, Goldman C, Rosenquist CJ, et al. Laparoscopic versus open gastric bypass: a randomized study of outcomes, quality of life, and costs. *Ann Surg.* 2001;234(3):279-289.

41. Lujan JA, Frutos MD, Hernandez Q, et al. Laparoscopic versus open gastric bypass in the treatment of morbid obesity: a randomized prospective study. *Ann Surg.* 2004;239(4):433-437.

42. Smith SC, Edwards CB, Goodman GN, Halverson RC, Simper SC. Open vs laparoscopic Roux-en-Y gastric bypass: comparison of operative morbidity and mortality. *Obes Surg.* 2004;14:73-76.

43. Dresel A, Kuhn JA, McCarty TM. Laparoscopic Roux-en-Y gastric bypass in morbidly obese and super morbidly obese patients. *Am J Surg.* 2004;187:230-232.

44. Marceau P, Hould FS, Lebel S, Marceau S, Biron S. Malabsorptive obesity surgery. *Surg Clin North Am.* 2001;81(5):1113-1127.

45. Marceau P, Hould FS, Simard S, et al. Biliopancreatic diversion with duodenal switch. *World J Surg.* 1998;22:947-954.

46. Baltasar A, del Rio J, Escriva C, Arlandis F, Martinez R, Serra C. Preliminary results of the duodenal switch. *Obes Surg.* 1997;7(6):500-504.

47. Lagace M, Marceau P, Marceau S, et al. Biliopancreatic diversion with a new type of gastrectomy: some previous conclusions revisited. *Obes Surg.* 1995;5:411-418.

48. NIH Consensus Statement Online. Gastrointestinal surgery for severe obesity. 1991 Mar 25-27;9(1):1-20. Available at: http://consensus.nih.gov/cons/084/084_statement.htm. Accessed December 31, 2004.

49. Schauer P, Hamad G, Ikramuddin S. Surgical management of gastroesophageal reflux disease in obese patients. *Semin Laparosc Surg.* 2001;8(4):256-264.

50. Dixon JB, O'Brien PE. Gastroesophageal reflux in obesity: the effect of lap-band placement. *Obes Surg.* 1999;9(6):527-531.

51. Ovrebo KK, Hatlebakk JG, Viste A, Bassoe HH, Svanes K. Gastroesophageal reflux in morbidly obese patients treated with gastric banding or vertical banded gastroplasty. *Ann Surg.* 1998;228(1):51-58.

52. Lundell L, Ruth M, Olbe L. Vertical banded gastroplasty or gastric banding for morbid obesity: effects on gastro-oesophageal reflux. *Eur J Surg.* 1997;163(7):525-531.

53. Kalfarentos F, Papadoulas S, Skroubis G, Kehagias I, Loukidi A, Mead N. Prospective evaluation of biliopancreatic diversion with Roux-en-Y gastric bypass in the super obese. *J Gastrointest Surg.* 2004;8(4):479-488.

54. Slater GH, Ren CJ, Seigel N, et al. Serum fat-soluble vitamin deficiency and abnormal calcium metabolism after malabsorptive bariatric surgery. *J Gastrointest Surg.* 2004;8(1):48-55.

55. Gould J, Garren M, Starling J. Bariatric surgery. *WMJ.* 2004;103(2):27-28.

56. Baltasar A, Serra C, Perez N, Bou R, Bengochea M. Clinical hepatic impairment after the duodenal switch. *Obes Surg.* 2004;14:77-83.

57. Grimm IS, Schindler W, Haluszka O. Steatohepatitis and fatal hepatic failure after biliopancreatic diversion. *Am J Gastroenterol.* 1992;87:775-779.

58. Valencia-Flores M, Orea A, Herrera M, et al. Effect of bariatric surgery on obstructive sleep apnea and hypopnea syndrome, electrocardiogram, and pulmonary arterial pressure. *Obes Surg.* 2004;14(6):755-762.

59. Pories WJ, MacDonald KG Jr, Morgan EJ, et al. Surgical treatment of obesity and its effect on diabetes: 10-y follow-up. *Am J Clin Nutr.* 1992;55(2 suppl):582S-585S.

60. Pillar G, Peled R, Lavie P. Recurrence of sleep apnea without concomitant weight increase 7.5 years after weight reduction surgery. *Chest.* 1994;106(6):1702-1704.

61. O'Brien PE, Dixon JB. Lap-band: outcomes and results. *J Laparoendosc Adv Surg Tech A.* 2003;13(4):265-270.

62. Pories WJ, Swanson MS, MacDonald KG, et al. Who would have thought it? An operation proves to be the most effective therapy for adult-onset diabetes mellitus. *Ann Surg.* 1995;222(3):339-350.

63. Dhabuwala A, Cannan RJ, Stubbs RS. Improvement in co-morbidities following weight loss from gastric bypass surgery. *Obes Surg.* 2000;10(5)428-435.

64. Dolan K, Hatzifotis M, Newbury L, Lowe N, Fielding G. A clinical and nutritional comparison of biliopancreatic diversion with and without duodenal switch. *Ann Surg.* 2004;240:51-56.

65. Sugerman HJ, Wolfe LG, Sica DA, Clore JN. Diabetes and hypertension in severe obesity and effects of gastric bypass-induced weight loss. *Ann Surg.* 2003;237(6):751-756.

66. Cowan GS Jr, Buffington CK. Significant changes in blood pressure, glucose, and lipids with gastric bypass surgery. *World J Surg.* 1998;22(9):987-992.

67. Reinhold RB. Late results of gastric bypass surgery for morbid obesity. *J Am Coll Nutr.* 1994:13(4):326-331.

68. Gleysteen JJ, Barboriak JJ, Sasse EA. Sustained coronary-risk-factor reduction after gastric bypass for morbid obesity. *Am J Clin Nutr.* 1990;51(5):774-778.

69. Sjostrom L, Lindroos AK, Peltonen M, et al. Lifestyle, diabetes, and cardiovascular risk factors 10 years after bariatric surgery. *N Engl J Med.* 2004;351(26):2683-2693.

70. MacDonald KG Jr, Long SD, Swanson MS, et al. The gastric bypass operation reduces the progression and mortality of non-insulin-dependent diabetes mellitus. *J Gastrointest Surg.* 1997;1(3):213-220.

71. Pories WJ, Caro JF, Flickinger EG, Meelheim HD, Swanson MS. The control of diabetes mellitus (NIDDM) in the morbidly obese with the Greenville Gastric Bypass. *Ann Surg.* 1987;206(3):316-323.

72. Sugerman HJ, Sugerman EL, Wolfe L, Kellum JM Jr, Schweitzer MA, DeMaria EJ. Risks and benefits of gastric bypass in morbidly obese patients with severe venous stasis disease. *Ann Surg.* 2001:234(1):41-46.

73. Sugerman HJ, Felton WL III, Sismanis A, Kellum JM, DeMaria EJ, Sugerman EL. Gastric surgery for pseudotumor cerebri associated with severe obesity. *Ann Surg.* 1999;229(5):634-640.

74. Holzwarth R, Huber D, Majkrzak A, Tareen B. Outcome of gastric bypass patients. *Obes Surg.* 2002;12(2):261-264.

75. Stunkard AJ, Stinnett JL, Smoller JW. Psychological and social aspects of the surgical treatment of obesity. *Am J Psychiatry*. 1986;143(4):417-429.

76. Marcason W. What are the dietary guidelines following bariatric surgery? *J Am Diet Assoc*. 2004;104(3):487-488.

77. Benotti P, Martin LF. Preoperative evaluation and preparation of bariatric surgery candidates. In: Martin LF, Ed. *Obesity Surgery*. New York, NY: McGraw-Hill; 2004:95-109.

Recommended Readings

DeMaria EJ. Laparoscopic adjustable silicone gastric banding. *Surg Clin North Am*. 2001;81(5):1129-1144.

Doherty C. Vertical banded gastroplasty. *Surg Clin North Am*. 2001;81(5):1097-1112.

Martin LF, ed. *Obesity Surgery*. New York, NY: McGraw-Hill; 2004.

4

Preoperative Evaluation of the Patient Undergoing Bariatric Surgery

Nawfal Istfan, MD, PhD and Wendy A. Anderson, MS, RD, LDN

Introduction

As the number of individuals seeking bariatric surgery continues to increase,[1,2] so does the need for primary-care providers (PCPs) to better understand the principles for the preoperative evaluation of bariatric-surgery patients. The surgical treatment of obesity is based on the alteration of the patient's normal gastrointestinal anatomy, with significant physical and psychological consequences; therefore, patients must be screened properly to ensure appropriate selection. Primary-care physicians often refer their patients with morbid obesity for bariatric surgery before fully evaluating the overall impact of the treatment. Coupled with increasing interest by the media, this lack of caution will lead to poorly selected and unprepared patients undergoing potentially dangerous surgery with permanent consequences.

The pre-bariatric–surgery evaluation helps ensure that the patient with obesity and intractable obesity-related comorbid conditions is more likely to achieve significant medical improvement if the individual undergoes a risky surgical procedure. Evaluation helps to identify patients in need of intensive medical and psychological preparation for the surgery and those needing help postoperatively to cope with the consequences of altered gastrointestinal anatomy. This chapter outlines basic principles of preoperative evaluation for bariatric surgery, which determine: (1) if weight-loss surgery is a reasonable medical decision; (2) if the patient is prepared to undertake the necessary lifestyle changes; and (3) if the multidisciplinary bariatric team can reduce the surgical risk and prevent future nutritional and metabolic deficiencies. Table 4-1 outlines 7 basic questions for this process. The following sections address these issues to help the PCP evaluate the eligibility of patients with morbid obesity for bariatric surgery and identify high-risk patients.

Table 4-1

Basic Questions in the Assessment of Patients With Morbid Obesity to Determine Candidacy for Bariatric Surgery

- Is there a reversible primary cause for the patient's obesity?
- What are the medical benefits of weight-loss surgery for this patient?
- Is surgery the only option for this patient?
- What are the risks and the potential for surgical-risk reduction?
- Are there any contraindications or predictors of poor outcome?
- Is the patient prepared to undergo surgery and make necessary lifestyle changes?
- Does the patient have any pre-existing nutritional insufficiency issues?

Identifiable Causes of Obesity

The main objective of the preoperative evaluation is to exclude patients with treatable causes of obesity from further consideration of unnecessary bariatric surgery. While obesity is easily identified as a common phenotypic manifestation, its behavioral and metabolic classifications remain poorly understood. Despite recent advances in the understanding of the molecular biology of fat cells, our current knowledge of the genetics of obesity does not allow etiologic classification in the majority of patients. However, there are several well-known clinical conditions in which obesity is a secondary manifestation of primary and identifiable disease. In preparing to diagnose and treat the primary obesity disease, it is essential that every effort be made to identify secondary obesity syndromes prior to committing patients with obesity to bariatric surgery.

Thyroid and Adrenal Syndromes

Clinical and biochemical markers for hypothyroidism and adrenal disease should be evaluated routinely in all patients seeking surgical treatment. In most instances, routine medical history and physical examination are sufficient to raise the possibility of a primary endocrine etiology, thus resulting in further evaluation as necessary. Laboratory indices for thyroid disease, such as serum TSH levels, are routinely obtained in all patients with obesity and should identify them at an early stage of the diagnostic work-up.

Patients with obesity presenting with Cushingoid features on physical examination should be questioned about their history of use of corticosteroid medications. Decisions about the eligibility of these patients for bariatric surgery may depend upon the etiology of Cushing's syndrome. For example, patients with a long history of steroid-dependent asthma may be considered appropriate candidates for gastric-bypass surgery because withdrawal of steroid medications is unlikely to reverse their obesity. On the other hand, patients with hypersecreting adrenal tumors often improve significantly with treatment of the primary disease. Presence of Cushingoid facial features with classical findings on physical examination, such as abnormal body-fat distribution and signs of skin fragility as well as masculinization in females, should trigger further screening with morning serum cortisol levels and 24-hour urinary excretion of free cortisol. These tests are usually sufficient to exclude adrenal hypersecretion (tumors and adrenal hyperplasia) in the majority

Table 4-2
Genetic Syndromes That Can Cause Morbid Obesity

Syndrome	Stature	Features
Prader-Willi	Short	Hypogonadism; short extremities
Angleman's	Normal	Movement disorder; happy affect
Albright's hereditary osteodystrophy	Normal/short	Bradydactyly; subcutaneous ossification
Bardet-Biedl	Normal/short	Cone dystrophy; polydactyly; renal structural defects
Alstrom	Normal/short	Deafness; cardiomyopathy; cone dystrophy
Carpenter's	Short	Acrocephaly; polydactyly; hypogonadism
Cohen	Normal/short	Facial features; retinal dystrophy: granulocytopenia
Down	Short	Facial features; cardiac malformations; hypotonia

of patients with morbid obesity. If inconclusive, the patient should be further tested and referred to an endocrinologist before he or she proceeds to bariatric surgery.

Genetic Syndromes

Patients with genetic obesity syndromes may pose more challenge in the appropriate selection of patients for bariatric surgery. In general, these patients present with obesity at an early age and are likely to present with other features, such as mental retardation and abnormal physical stature. Currently, sufficient information is not available to predict the outcome of bariatric surgery in patients with obesity and an identifiable genetic syndrome. Once committed to bariatric surgery, these patients need to be closely followed by a multidisciplinary team. In general, symptoms that point to the possibility of a genetic obesity syndrome include short stature, hypotonia, hypogonadism, movement disorders, and structural abnormalities such as bradydactyly (short fingers), structural cardiac defects, and peculiar facial features. A summary of autosomal and x-linked obesity syndromes is presented in Table 4-2.

It is important to note that a diagnosis of any of these syndromes does not necessarily preclude bariatric surgery if there is sufficient evidence that weight loss is medically necessary for the individual. However, because of the paucity of clinical experience in the surgical treatment of genetic-syndrome–related obesity, as well as the higher incidence of mental retardation and psychosocial and emotional issues in these patients, they must receive more intense scrutiny and observation before and after bariatric surgery. The PCP and the bariatric surgery team must be familiar with obesity-causing genetic syndromes and should order screening blood tests for karyotype identification as well as make appropriate referrals for further genetic assessment and counseling.

Health Benefits of Weight Loss and Obesity Surgery

Health improvement and prevention of chronic and debilitating comorbid conditions are the main indications for bariatric surgery. Therefore, making an accurate assessment of the health benefits of weight loss is a major determinant of the patient's eligibility for bariatric surgery. The patient's weight and height at presentation, expressed as body mass index (BMI), is the most important single criterion in making such an assessment. The 1991 National Institutes of Health (NIH) Consensus Development Conference Panel determined a BMI of 40 kg/m^2 as the degree of obesity that begins to justify surgical intervention.[3] While this number was chosen arbitrarily, substantial evidence documents the high prevalence rate of serious cardiovascular, metabolic, and skeletal comorbidities associated with a BMI ≥40.[4] However, assessment of the health hazards of obesity in a particular patient is also affected by other factors that need to be considered. In addition to the patient's BMI at presentation, the clinical assessment of obesity must consider the history of the condition's development, the number of years of uncontrollable body weight, the presence or absence of a weight-cycling phenomenon, as well as the physical pattern of body-fat distribution and existence of specific comorbid diagnoses. The physician must consider all of these factors before suggesting bariatric surgery as treatment for a particular patient with obesity.

Obesity and Dietary History

Although BMI is widely used to assess the degree of a patient's obesity and to make decisions about bariatric surgery, other parameters are also important in defining this disease in the patient. The patient's account of his or her sequence of body-weight changes can help clarify that patient's potential for success in further body-weight control. A patient's history of morbid obesity (BMI ≥40, also referred to as Class III obesity—see Chapter 1) that persists implies lack of previous attempts at medical and behavioral treatments, failure of these attempts, or a history of cycling between weight loss and regain. The latter is especially important as it may impact future behavioral patterns likely to affect the patient.

While the presence of weight-cycling behavior may be indicative of an eating disorder, it may also herald significant metabolic risk that may actually tilt the balance in favor of surgical treatment. Because weight cycling often involves periods of strong positive energy balance and rapid weight gain, it may impact the patient's health, although it is often ignored. Evidence of the harmful effects of rapid weight gain is mounting.

Evidence shows that weight gain is an important contributor to cardiovascular and metabolic pathophysiology in individuals with obesity.[5-7] At the same time, research shows that body-fat reduction by liposuction does not reduce the metabolic disorder of obesity, suggesting that it is negative energy balance, and not weight loss by any means, that is an important factor of metabolic and cardiovascular improvement associated with weight loss.[8-10] Additional research in this theory is needed; however, by raising circulating insulin and possibly leptin levels, positive energy balance may aggravate the basic pathophysiology that characterizes the disease of obesity. In as much as obesity surgery can lead to long-term body weight stabilization, patient's history of strong weight-cycling behavior may indeed be one of the determining factors that favor the surgical option.

Currently, there is no universal definition of what constitutes a medically significant weight cycle. Some physicians consider a weight loss and gain of 10% of the patient's stable weight to be significant enough in assessment of weight-cycling behavior. History of weight cycles of this magnitude, occurring less than twice within 10 years, is considered medically insignificant; however, weight cycling 5 or more times in 10 years should be considered significant and should be further investigated. Furthermore, no reliable data exist that addresses a patient's rate of weight gain in relationship to cardiovascular

Table 4-3
Metabolic Assessment of Obesity

Parameter	Measurement	Critical Value
Obesity	BMI	≥40 or ≥35 with comorbidities
Body-fat distribution	Waist circumference	Males: >40 in.; females: >35 in.
Fasting lipid profile	High-density lipid, triglycerides	High-density lipid (males: <40; females: <50), triglycerides: >150
Insulin resistance	Fasting blood glucose (mg/dL), fasting insulin (μU/mL)	HOMA-IR* ≥5
Hypertension	Blood pressure	Systolic >130, diastolic >85

*Homeostatic model assessment-insulin resistance (HOMA-IR) is calculated by this equation:

$$\frac{\text{fasting insulin } (\mu\text{U/mL}) \times \text{fasting glucose (mg/dL)}}{22.5}$$

and metabolic risk in obesity. Thus, assessment of the potential negative effects of weight cycling in a particular patient must be individualized. For example, weight cycling in a patient with congestive heart failure (CHF) could be detrimental in view of possible fluid retention during positive energy balance and weight gain. Similar arguments can also be made in the patient with fatty liver because positive energy balance can cause further lipid deposition in the liver, which can lead to irreversible liver pathology and cirrhosis.

Body-Fat Distribution and Metabolic Assessment

A large amount of literature relates the pattern of body-fat distribution to the cardiovascular and metabolic risks of obesity. This is best exemplified in the diagnosis of the "dysmetabolic syndrome" or "syndrome x," which can be a precursor of type 2 diabetes and a significant indicator of cardiovascular risk.[11] Central body fat, as measured by waist size and waist/hip ratio, is associated with insulin resistance, hypertension (HTN), and diabetes. Criteria for the diagnosis of the dysmetabolic syndrome, including body-fat distribution, are summarized in Table 4-3. These measurements are easy to perform and should be included in the preoperative assessment of all patients with obesity seeking obesity surgery.

In addition to waist circumference and waist/hip ratio, routine metabolic assessment of the patient with obesity should include assessment of the patient's cardiac risk, as relayed in the fasting lipid profile (Table 4-3) and measurement of fasting insulin and blood glucose levels. The latter also can be used to determine the degree of the patient's insulin resistance according to the homeostatic model assessment-insulin resistance (HOMA-IR).[12] (The equation for HOMA-IR is included in Table 4-3 footnotes.) Values of HOMA-IR

≥5 are indicative of significant insulin resistance. Therefore, the PCP can objectively assess the patient's metabolic status with readily available blood tests. In addition to HOMA-IR and blood lipid profiles, measurement of homocystine and C-reactive protein levels may also further expose effects of the patient's obesity on his or her health, thus assisting the PCP in assessing the potential benefit of bariatric surgery for an individual.

Comorbidities

Presence of significant comorbid conditions is an important factor in determining potential health benefits of bariatric surgery for an individual with obesity. As these conditions become resistant to medical treatment, the decision to proceed with gastric-bypass surgery may become more apparent to both physician and patient. Diabetes, HTN, sleep apnea, and coronary atherosclerotic heart disease are common comorbid conditions that often influence the PCP's recommendation for bariatric surgery, particularly because weight loss can dramatically improve these comorbidities. Occasionally, modest weight reductions (5% to 10% of initial body weight) produce significant improvements in glycemic and blood-pressure control among diabetic and hypertensive patients with obesity, respectively.[13-16] The use of preoperative weight loss of this magnitude to improve glycemic and blood pressure comorbidities may be beneficial in certain patients with morbid obesity. (See Preoperative Body Weight Changes.)

In addition to determining the presence of comorbid conditions, the preoperative assessment can help the PCP and the patient define the actual benefits expected from weight reduction. In situations in which the expected benefit is limited to improved metabolic status—such as better glycemic control in diabetic patients—a 5% to 10% weight reduction may be sufficient. However, the presence of multiple comorbidities may require more substantial weight reduction to achieve improvements in the patient's health. Such comorbid conditions are exemplified by degenerative joint disease in weight-bearing joints and obesity hypoventilation syndrome. Existence of these medical conditions in the patient with morbid obesity (Class III) should alert the PCP of the immediate need for the patient to lose 20% or more of his or her current weight, a loss that is typically only possible with bariatric surgery. A list of common comorbid conditions and evaluations for these comorbidities is presented in Table 4-4.

Other Options for Patients with Obesity

NIH criteria for selection of patients for bariatric surgery require that a patient has previously attempted to lose weight by diet and exercise. This addresses the question of whether bariatric surgery is the only treatment that might result in significant medical improvement because the patient's previous nonsurgical attempts of weight reduction and control were not successful. (The medical management of obesity is discussed in Chapter 2.)

While there are no concrete guidelines for this assessment, the patient's account of the number of attempts and the different diet and exercise programs attempted are generally sufficient. Patients are often able to provide detailed information about their dieting history and body-weight changes. However, patients driven by the hype to have surgery may have an exaggerated story of the medical therapy of their obesity. Thus, the clinician obtaining this information must critically assess the objective nature of the patient's report. The physician should examine available medical records that show the patient's sequential body-weight changes or, in the absence of documented participation in medi-

Table 4-4
Preoperative Assessment of Comorbidities

System	Condition	Minimal Evaluations	Additional Evaluations
Cardiovascular	Coronary artery disease, CHF	Physical examination, echocardiogram, chest x-ray (CXR)	Cardiac echogram, stress testing, cardiology consult
Metabolic	Diabetes, hypercholesterolemia	Fasting glucose and insulin, lipid profile, hemoglobin A1C	HOMA-IR calculation (Table 4-3)
Pulmonary	Obesity hypoventilation, sleep apnea, asthma, COPD*	Physical examination, CXR, pulmonary function test	Sleep study
Gastrointestinal	Fatty liver, gallstone, GERD†	Physical examination, abdominal ultrasound	Endoscopy
Musculoskeletal	Degenerative joint disease	Physical examination	Radiology, magnetic resonance imaging, orthopedic consultation

* chronic obstructive pulmonary disease (COPD)

† gastroesophageal reflux disease (GERD)

cally supervised weight-reduction programs, determine if the patient understands the basic principles of healthy eating and physical activity. If the assessing clinician feels that previous weight-reduction efforts reported by the patient seeking gastric-bypass surgery do not meet acceptable medical guidelines, then further assessment and dietary counseling by a registered dietitian are necessary before a final decision about the proposed surgical treatment can be made.

Risks of Bariatric Surgery

Final selection of patients for bariatric surgery depends on the balance of risks and benefits. Obesity surgery continues to have significant risks, often for the same medical reasons that justify the surgery in the first place. This situation, where risk and benefit are dictated by the same set of pathophysiologic conditions, is unique to bariatric surgery. Therefore, evaluation of the risk/benefit ratio associated with bariatric surgery should be undertaken only within the context of the surgeon's experience and availability of a multidisciplinary obesity-treatment team.

Despite the potential for large variations in surgical-risk assessment between different surgical institutions, there are general considerations that apply universally. A summary of risk factors in obesity surgery is presented in the following sections, and postoperative complications are discussed at length in Chapter 7.

Cardiovascular Disease

Morbid obesity is associated with high risk for coronary heart disease (CHD).[17,18] Postoperative cardiac complications are frequently associated with abnormal preoperative electrocardiograms.[19] Suspicion of cardiovascular pathophysiology warrants further evaluation and risk stratification for the identification of reversible factors. However, assessment of CHD may be difficult because of weight limitations imposed by diagnostic equipment used in noninvasive testing and cardiac catheterization. The value of preoperative myocardial perfusion imaging and dobutamine stress echocardiography in the cardiovascular risk stratification of patients undergoing noncardiac surgery has been studied extensively. The positive predictive value for myocardial perfusion imaging is 4% to 20% and for dobutamine stress echocardiography is 7% to 25%; negative predictive values for both studies range from 95% to 100%.[20] Current evidence suggests deferring coronary arteriography prior to noncardiac surgery unless the patient's clinical status otherwise warrants—eg, unstable angina, recent myocardial infarction, or strongly positive noninvasive stress testing.[21]

A recent review of 11 randomized controlled trials concluded that perioperative beta-blocker therapy reduced the risk of perioperative cardiac death or myocardial infarction by 75% and 80%, respectively.[22] While no currently available data addresses cardiovascular risk reduction in bariatric surgery, it would be reasonable to consider perioperative beta-blocker therapy in individuals with coronary artery disease and 2 or more risk factors—BMI ≥50, low forced expiratory volume, previous abdominal surgery, abnormal echocardiogram[17]—or with a history of prior myocardial infarction. The American College of Cardiology and the American Heart Association, in a combined position paper, prompts strong consideration of empiric therapy in reducing the risk of cardiac events in patients undergoing high-risk noncardiac surgery.[23]

Pulmonary Disease

Obesity is an independent risk factor for deep vein thrombosis (DVT) or pulmonary embolism (PE) in ambulatory persons[24,25] and in hospitalized medical and surgical patients.[26,27] Additional risk factors relevant to bariatric-surgery patients are prior history of venous thromboembolism (VTE),[28] abdominal-fat distribution,[29] smoking,[29] advanced age,[30] venous insufficiency,[24,28] venous stasis due to immobilization,[24] obesity hypoventilation syndrome or severe sleep apnea,[24] CHF,[24] use of oral contraceptives and hormone replacement containing estrogen,[25,30] and inborn or acquired hypercoagulable states.[26] In retrospective reviews of bariatric-surgery case series in which patients clinically suspected to have VTE after surgery were assessed, it was suggested that both DVT and PE occur in <1%, although in high-risk subgroups, such as those with severe venous stasis or other risk factors, incidence of DVT has been up to 8% and PE to 4%.[31-33] Larger and more recent surveys find generally lower rates. A recent systematic review of Roux-en-Y gastric bypass (RYGB) and laparoscopic adjustable gastric banding (LAGB) found average rates of PE of 0.21 and 0.16, respectively, and rates of DVT of 0.05 and 0.01, respectively.[34] Between 1990 and 1997, a nationwide survey demonstrated declining rates of PE, with the 1997 rates of 0.07%.[35] However, although the incidence of PE after obesity surgery is low, PE accounts for 25% to 66% of postoperative mortality.[36,37]

Several specific risk factors for VTE deserve mention. There are parallel general trends toward greater overall complication rates after surgery and greater general VTE risk in patients who are older, heavier, and male. However, the low incidence of VTE may preclude definitive associations in clinical series. Patients with severe venous stasis appear to be at increased risk for VTE.[28] The predominance of females of childbearing age undergoing surgery underscores the importance of identifying oral-contraceptive use to ensure cessation prior to surgery. The duration of time prior to surgery that oral contraceptives should be withheld remains controversial.

Obstructive Sleep Apnea

Obstructive sleep apnea (OSA) is considered to be a serious and potentially life-threatening pulmonary disorder that may be caused by repeated cessation of breathing, either from collapse of the upper airways during sleep or lack of respiratory effort. OSA pathophysiology associated with obesity involves anatomic and functional aspects of the pharyngeal airway, the central nervous system, central obesity, and possibly hormonal regulators such as leptin and ghrelin. OSA has been associated with the initiation and progression of cardiovascular diseases, and some data implicate OSA as contributing to the development of HTN, cardiac ischemia, CHF, arrhythmias, and possibly cerebrovascular accidents.[38]

It is well established that there is a high prevalence of OSA in patients with obesity (12% to 40%)[39] and a high prevalence of obesity in patients with OSA.[40] OSA is also among the most underdiagnosed weight-related comorbidities: it is estimated that up to 93% of middle-aged females and 82% of males of the same age are undiagnosed.[41] In studies in which patients were evaluated with polysomnography prior to weight-loss surgery, OSA was diagnosed in 35% to 71%.[42-44] BMI does not correlate with nor is it a predictor of OSA, as one study indicates[39]; in a study of 170 patients presenting for weight-loss surgery, sleep apnea was prevalent in 77% independent of BMI. The data from this study and others[41] support the use of routine screening polysomnography in patients with symptoms of OSA. Another study investigating the incidence of OSA during preoperative assessment conducted polysomnography in all patients, regardless of symptoms, and found that patients with obesity had 88% incidence of obstructive-related breathing disorder, and 71% of those had OSA.[45]

Based on physiologic rationale, presence of OSA is thought to be a predisposing factor for perioperative cardiovascular and pulmonary complications,[46,47] especially in patients with obesity and those who also have other comorbidities. However, data from multivariate statistical models do not consistently support OSA as an independent risk factor in perioperative morbidity.[48] Currently, there is no support for the routine use of continuous positive airway pressure in the immediate postoperative period following bariatric surgery. Rather, decisions about the use of positive pressure ventilation should be individualized.

Liver Disease

Obesity increases a patient's risk for nonalcoholic fatty-liver disease, which includes steatosis, nonalcoholic steatohepatitis, fibrosis, and cirrhosis. The disease is estimated to occur in 10% to 24% of the population worldwide and in 30% to 100% of adults with obesity.[49] Up to 25% of cases of patients with nonalcoholic steatohepatitis may progress to cirrhosis.[50] In patients undergoing bariatric surgery, intraoperative liver biopsies revealed hepatic steatosis in 65% to 89% of patients, nonalcoholic steatohepatitis in 10% to 56%, fibrosis in 1% to 51%, and cirrhosis in 0% to 6%.[51-54] Of note, cirrhosis is often detected unexpectedly at the time of surgery.

Nonalcoholic fatty-liver disease is most commonly associated with type 2 diabetes mellitus, insulin resistance or hyperinsulinemia, older age, male gender, and elevated BMI. It was associated somewhat less consistently with other components of the metabolic syndrome, ie, abdominal obesity as measured by anthropometry or imaging.[55,56] In patients undergoing bariatric surgery, histological severity of nonalcoholic fatty-liver disease has been best predicted by the presence of type 2 diabetes, level of glycemia, insulin resistance, HTN, and older age.[51-53] Hepatic transaminase concentrations are unreliable predictors of histological severity of nonalcoholic fatty-liver disease, and normal or elevated concentrations have been observed across the spectrum, although increased concentration of aspartate aminotransferase (AST) or a ratio of AST to alanine aminotransferase >1 have been associated with more advanced inflammation or fibrosis.[57] Hyperferritinemia has also been associated with more advanced nonalcoholic fatty-liver disease histology in some studies.[58] Reports of patients with cirrhosis who underwent surgery are rare, but early postoperative mortality was increased in one report and complications appear to be more frequent.[59,60]

Other Risk Factors

Smoking

Cigarette smoking has been implicated as a risk factor for postoperative pulmonary, wound, and other complications.[61,62] Evidence demonstrating a clear benefit of preoperative smoking cessation prior to any type of surgery, including obesity surgery, is inconclusive. However, despite this paucity of objective evidence, smoking cessation is universally recommended in all patients undergoing bariatric surgery.

Preoperative Body Weight Changes

Changes in body weight, reflecting positive and negative energy balance, may play a role in the perioperative risk associated with bariatric surgery. Many obesity-surgery–treatment programs require that patients lose weight by dieting before being selected. This practice encourages compliance with food restriction and tests the motivation of the patient to begin a long process of behavioral changes imposed by the surgery. Extensive evidence already shows that modest weight loss improves cardiopulmonary function[15,16,63] and leads to significant metabolic improvements.[13-15] However, the relative contributions of the actual reduction in body fat and of the negative energy associated with weight loss to the metabolic and cardiovascular improvements attributed to weight loss remain incompletely understood. Recent reports point to the possibility that negative energy balance plays the crucial role in determining the benefits of weight loss.[8] For the most part, the actual benefits of weight reduction before bariatric surgery have not been documented by controlled clinical trials. However, a recent study documented shortened operative times in patients with BMI >50 who had intragastric balloons placed to induce weight loss before gastric-bypass surgery.[64] It is also important to note that, while the current literature is replete with studies documenting the benefits of weight loss, much less is known about the physiologic effects and clinical hazards of weight gain. This is especially important in view of the possibility that body weight can be gained more rapidly than it is usually lost in the morbidly obese with high prevalence rates of binge-eating behavior. Thus, efforts to optimize weight loss, or at least to prevent preoperative weight gain, must be intensified, especially in patients with cardiovascular and pulmonary comorbidities.

Contraindications of Bariatric Surgery

Another important question for preoperative assessment of the patient with obesity is whether there are identifiable contraindications for bariatric surgery. The most common reason for declining obesity-surgery treatment is the patient's lack of understanding of the procedure and inability to comprehend the need for behavioral adaptation or demonstrate commitment to follow postoperative instructions. While the clinician conducting the general preoperative assessment needs to be aware of prospective patient's understanding of the surgery, it is important that behavioral contraindications be identified by formal psychological and behavioral assessments (Chapter 12).

Medical conditions that could exclude a patient from bariatric surgery should be considered on a patient-by-patient basis. In general, advanced and/or unstable cardiac disease, irreversible pulmonary conditions that are unlikely to improve with weight loss, and conditions that seriously complicate anesthesia and hemostasis or wound healing are considered contraindications. While gastrointestinal pathology is not necessarily an exclusion criterion for bariatric surgery, it is important that patients with inflammatory bowel disease and intestinal motility disorders undergo further evaluations before their final selection.

Readiness of the Patient Considering Bariatric Surgery

Although preoperative psychological factors are not proven to consistently predict outcomes, there are multiple reasons to conduct psychological assessment prior to surgery (Chapter 12). Diet and lifestyle changes that the patient must adopt are profound, and physical well-being and long-term weight-loss success depend on adherence to these changes. Patients who choose to have weight-loss surgery carry with them the psychological consequences of years of obesity, which may influence the success of the surgery itself.

Extreme obesity is associated with increased prevalence of depression and increased incidence of major depression,[65] diminished quality of life,[66] marked effects on self-esteem,[67] and impaired psychological and psychosocial functioning of the affected individual.[68] In patients presenting for weight-loss surgery, binge-eating behavior has been reported to occur in >50%, and diagnostic criteria for binge-eating disorder was found in 11% to 47%.[69,70] Binge-eating disorder is associated with increased risk for depression, lower self-esteem, symptoms of borderline personality disorder, and a higher incidence of all psychiatric disorders.[71]

Patients seeking surgery comprise a self-selected, psychologically "vulnerable" group, and, while the great majority of these subjects appear to have normal psychological functioning, in clinical settings, 10% to 20% are likely to suffer from clinically significant symptoms of depression, negative body image, or impaired quality of life. These problems are most frequently present in females with a high BMI and with binge-eating disorder.

Pre-existing Nutritional Deficiencies

Patients undergoing bariatric surgery are at a high risk of developing deficiencies in several nutrients. Therefore, the usual preoperative work-up of the patient being considered for obesity surgery should also include an assessment of the nutritional status, especially for the nutrients known to be affected by diet or surgery. This is particularly important if the patient has a history of disordered eating behaviors, unsupervised dieting, or previous bariatric surgery. Preoperative nutritional deficiencies will add significant comorbidities to the surgery, and the nutritional problem can be compounded if postoperative nutritional complications are added. A review of the nutritional problems that can arise following gastric-bypass surgery is presented in Chapter 8.

Briefly, there is sufficient evidence to show that the nutritional status of iron, vitamin B12, folic acid, and vitamin D may each become compromised within the first year following bariatric surgery. Therefore, at minimum, preoperative evaluation of patients selected for bariatric surgery should include an assessment of the nutritional stores of each of these nutrients. If not optimal, nutritional supplements should be instituted to replenish the body stores prior to the surgery.

Summary

Preoperative assessment of patients with obesity seeking surgical treatment is a necessity in correctly identifying those patients who are appropriate candidates for weight-loss surgery. Evaluation of these patients includes consideration of the cause of obesity, health benefits and risks of weight-loss surgery in each patient, and contraindications of the surgical procedure. As the number of individuals seeking bariatric treatment increases, PCPs must be prepared to evaluate these patients and assist in the selection of those qualified to undergo bariatric surgery.

References

1. Steinbrook R. Surgery for severe obesity. *N Engl J Med.* 2004;350(11):1075-1079.
2. Hedley AA, Ogden CL, Johnson CL, Carroll MD, Curtin LR, Flegal KM. Prevalence of overweight and obesity among US children, adolescents, and adults, 1999-2002. *JAMA.* 2004;291(23):2847-2850.
3. Gastrointestinal surgery for severe obesity: National Institutes of Health Consensus Development Conference statement. *Am J Clin Nutr.* 1992;55(2 suppl):615S-619S.
4. Kral JG. Selection of patients for anti-obesity surgery. *Int J Obes Relat Metab Disord.* 2001;25(suppl 1):S107-S112.
5. Wannamethee SG, Shaper AG, Walker M. Overweight and obesity and weight change in middle aged men: impact on cardiovascular disease and diabetes. *J Epidemiol Community Health.* 2005;59(2):134-139.
6. Field AE, Manson JE, Laird N, Williamson DF, Willett WC, Colditz GA. Weight cycling and the risk of developing type 2 diabetes among adult women in the United States. *Obes Res.* 2004;12(2):267-274.
7. Field AE, Coakley EH, Must A, et al. Impact of overweight on the risk of developing common chronic diseases during a 10-year period. *Arch Intern Med.* 2001;161(13):1581-1586.
8. Kelley DE. Thermodynamics, liposuction, and metabolism. *N Engl J Med.* 2004;350(25):2542-2544.
9. Kelley DE, Wing R, Buonocure C, Sturis J, Polonsky K, Fitzsimmons M. Relative effects of calorie restriction and weight loss in noninsulin-dependent diabetes mellitus. *J Clin Endocrinol Metab.* 1993;77(5):1287-1293.
10. Klein S, Fontana L, Young VL, et al. Absence of an effect of liposuction on insulin action and risk factors for coronary heart disease. *N Engl J Med.* 2004;350(25):2549-2557.
11. Klein S, Burke LE, Bray GA, et al. Clinical implications of obesity with specific focus on cardiovascular disease: a statement for professionals from the American Heart Association Council on Nutrition, Physical Activity, and Metabolism: endorsed by the American College of Cardiology Foundation. *Circulation.* 2004;110(18):2952-2967.

12. Abbasi F, Reaven GM. Evaluation of the quantitative insulin sensitivity check index as an estimate of insulin sensitivity in humans. *Metabolism.* 2002;51(2):235-237.
13. Bosello O, Armellini F, Zamboni M, Fitchet M. The benefits of modest weight loss in type II diabetes. *Int J Obes Relat Metab Disord.* 1997;21(suppl 1):S10-S13.
14. Wedick NM, Mayer-Davis EJ, Wingard DL, Addy CL, Barrett-Connor E. Insulin resistance precedes weight loss in adults without diabetes: the Rancho Barnardo Study. *Am J Epidemiol.* 2001;153(12):1199-1205.
15. Muscelli E, Camastra S, Catalano C, et al. Metabolic and cardiovascular assessment in moderate obesity: effect of weight loss. *J Clin Endocrinol Metab.* 1997;82(9):2937-2943.
16. Mavri A, Alessi MC, Bastelica D, et al. Subcutaneous abdominal, but not femoral fat expression of plasminogen activator inhibitor-1 (PAI-1) is related to plasma PAI-1 levels and insulin resistance and decreases after weight loss. *Diabetologia.* 2001;44(11):2025-2031.
17. Gonzalez R, Bowers SP, Venkatesh KR, Lin E, Smith CD. Preoperative factors predictive of complicated postoperative management after Roux-en-Y gastric bypass for morbid obesity. *Surg Endosc.* 2003;17(12):1900-1904.
18. Eckel RH, Krauss RM. American Heart Association call to action: obesity as a major risk factor for coronary heart disease. AHA Nutrition Committee. *Circulation.* 1998;97(21):2099-2100.
19. Wilson PW, D'Agostino RB, Sullivan L, Parise H, Kannel WB. Overweight and obesity as determinants of cardiovascular risk: the Framingham experience. *Arch Intern Med.* 2002;162(16):1867-1872.
20. Eagle KA, Berger PB, Calkins H, et al. ACC/AHA guideline update for perioperative cardiovascular evaluation for noncardiac surgery. Available at: http://www.acc.org/clinical/guidelines/perio/update/periupdate_index.htm. Accessed March 22, 2005.
21. Fleisher LA, Eagle KA. Clinical practice. Lowering cardiac risk in noncardiac surgery. *N Engl J Med.* 2001;345(23):1677-1682.
22. Stevens RD, Burri H, Tramer MR. Pharmacologic myocardial protection in patients undergoing noncardiac surgery: a quantitative systematic review. *Anesth Analg.* 2003;97(3):623-633.
23. Grayburn PA, Hillis LD. Cardiac events in patients undergoing noncardiac surgery: shifting the paradigm from noninvasive risk stratification to therapy. *Ann Int Med.* 2003;138(6):506-511.
24. Samama MM. An epidemiologic study of risk factors for deep vein thrombosis in medical outpatients: the Sirius study. *Arch Intern Med.* 2000;160(22):3415-3420.
25. Goldhaber SZ, Grodstein F, Stampfer MJ, et al. A prospective study of risk factors for pulmonary embolism in women. *JAMA.* 1997;277(8):642-645.
26. Blaszyk H, Bjornsson J. Factor V leiden and morbid obesity in fatal postoperative pulmonary embolism. *Arch Surg.* 2000 Dec;135(12):1410-1413.
27. Blaszyk H, Wollan PC, Witkiewicz AK, Bjornsson J. Death from pulmonary thromboembolism in severe obesity: lack of association with established genetic and clinical risk factors. *Virchows Arch.* 1999;434(6):529-532.
28. Sugerman HJ, Sugerman EL, Wolfe L, Kellum JM Jr, Schweitzer MA, DeMaria EJ. Risks and benefits of gastric bypass in morbidly obese patients with severe venous stasis disease. *Ann Surg.* 2001;234(1):41-46.
29. Hansson PO, Eriksson H, Welin L, Svardsudd K, Wilhelmsen L. Smoking and abdominal obesity: risk factors for venous thromboembolism among middle-aged men: "the study of men born in 1913". *Arch Intern Med.* 1999;159(16):1886-1890.
30. Lowe GD, Haverkate F, Thompson SG, et al. Prediction of deep vein thrombosis after elective hip replacement surgery by preoperative clinical and haemostatic variables: the ECAT DVT Study. European Concerted Action on Thrombosis. *Thromb Haemost.* 1999;81(6):879-886.
31. Westling A, Bergqvist D, Bostrom A, Karacagil S, Gustavsson S. Incidence of deep venous thrombosis in patients undergoing obesity surgery. *World J Surg.* 2002;26(4):470-473.
32. Eriksson S, Backman L, Ljungstrom KG. The incidence of clinical postoperative thrombosis after gastric surgery for obesity during 16 years. *Obes Surg.* 1997;7(4):332-335.
33. Printen KJ, Miller EV, Mason EE, Barnes RW. Venous thromboembolism in the morbidly obese. *Surg Gynecol Obstet.* 1978;147(1):63-64.

34. Chapman AE, Kiroff G, Game P, et al. Laparoscopic adjustable gastric banding in the treatment of obesity: a systematic literature review. *Surgery*. 2004;135(3):326-351.

35. Pope GD, Birkmeyer JD, Finlayson SR. National trends in utilization and in-hospital outcomes of bariatric surgery. *J Gastrointest Surg*. 2002;6(6):855-860.

36. Livingston EH, Huerta S, Arthur D, Lee S, De Shields S, Heber D. Male gender is a predictor of morbidity and age a predictor of mortality for patients undergoing gastric bypass surgery. *Ann Surg*. 2002;236(5):576-582.

37. Peltier G, Hermreck AS, Moffat RE, Hardin CA, Jewell WR. Complications following gastric bypass procedures for morbid obesity. *Surgery*. 1979;86(4):648-654.

38. Shamsuzzaman AS, Gersh BJ, Somers VK. Obstructive sleep apnea: implications for cardiac and vascular disease. *JAMA*. 2003;290(14):1906-1914.

39. O'Keeffe T, Patterson EJ. Evidence supporting routine polysomnography before bariatric surgery. *Obes Surg*. 2004;14(1):23-26.

40. Young T, Shahar E, Nieto FJ, et al. Predictors of sleep-disordered breathing in community-dwelling adults: the Sleep Heart Health Study. *Arch Intern Med*. 2002;162(8):893-900.

41. Young T, Evans L, Finn L, Palta M. Estimation of the clinically diagnosed proportion of sleep apnea syndrome in middle-aged men and women. *Sleep*. 1997;20(9):705-706.

42. Frey WC, Pilcher J. Obstructive sleep-related breathing disorders in patients evaluated for bariatric surgery. *Obes Surg*. 2003;13(5):676-683.

43. Serafini FM, MacDowell Anderson W, Rosemurgy AS, Strait T, Murr MM. Clinical predictors of sleep apnea in patients undergoing bariatric surgery. *Obes Surg*. 2001;11(1):28-31.

44. van Kralingen KW, de Kanter W, de Groot GH, et al. Assessment of sleep complaints and sleep-disordered breathing in a consecutive series of obese patients. *Respiration*. 1999;66(4):312-316.

45. Guardiano SA, Scott JA, Ware JC, Schechner SA. The long-term results of gastric bypass on indexes of sleep apnea. *Chest*. 2003;124(4):1615-1619.

46. Benumoff JL. Obstructive sleep apnea in adult obese patient: implications for airway management. *J Clin Anesth*. 2001;13(2):144-156.

47. Peiser J, Ovnat A, Uwyyed K, Lavie P, Charuzi I. Cardiac arrhythmias during sleep in morbidly obese sleep-apneic patients before and after gastric bypass surgery. *Clin Cardiol*. 1985;8(10):519-521.

48. Fernandez AZ Jr, Demaria EJ, Tichansky DS, et al. Multivariate analysis of risk factors for death following gastric bypass for treatment of morbid obesity. *Ann Surg*. 2004;239(5):698-702.

49. Angulo P, Lindor KD. Treatment of non-alcoholic steatohepatitis. *Best Pract Res Clin Gastroenterol*. 2002;16(5):797-810.

50. Scheen AJ, Luyckx FH. Obesity and liver disease. *Best Pract Res Clin Endocrin Metab*. 2002;16(4):703-716.

51. Luyckx FH, Desaive C, Thiry A, et al. Liver abnormalities in severely obese subjects: effect of drastic weight loss after gastroplasty. *Int J Obes Relat Metab Disord*. 1998;22(3):222-226.

52. Gholam PM, Kotler DP, Flancbaum LJ. Liver pathology in morbidly obese patients undergoing Roux-en-Y gastric bypass surgery. *Obes Surg*. 2002;12(1):49-51.

53. Beymer C, Kowdley KV, Larson A, Edmonson P, Dellinger EP, Flum DR. Prevalence and predictors of asymptomatic liver disease in patients undergoing gastric bypass surgery. *Arch Surg*. 2003;138(11):1240-1244.

54. Spaulding L, Trainer T, Janiec D. Prevalence of non-alcoholic steatohepatitis in morbidly obese subjects undergoing gastric bypass. *Obes Surg*. 2003;13(3):347-349.

55. Marchesini G, Bugianesi E, Forlani G, et al. Nonalcoholic fatty liver, steatohepatitis, and the metabolic syndrome. *Hepatology*. 2003;37(4):917-923.

56. Dixon JB, Bhathal PS, O'Brien PE. Nonalcoholic fatty liver disease: predictors of nonalcoholic steatohepatitis and liver fibrosis in the severely obese. *Gastroenterology*. 2001;121(1):91-100.

57. Angulo P, Keach JC, Batts KP, Lindor KD. Independent predictors of liver fibrosis in patients with nonalcoholic steatohepatitis. *Hepatology*. 1999;30(6):1356-1362.

58. Hsiao TJ, Chen JC, Wang JD. Insulin resistance and ferritin as major determinants of nonalcoholic fatty liver disease in apparently healthy obese patients. *Int J Obes Relat Metab Disord*. 2004;28(1):167-172.

59. Brolin RE, Bradley LJ, Taliwal RV. Unsuspected cirrhosis discovered during elective obesity operations. *Arch Surg.* 1998;133(1):84-88.

60. Dallal RM, Mattar SG, Lord JL, et al. Results of laparoscopic gastric bypass in patients with cirrhosis. *Obes Surg.* 2004;14(1):47-53.

61. Sorensen LT, Jorgensen T. Short-term pre-operative smoking cessation intervention does not affect postoperative complications in colorectal surgery: a randomized clinical trial. *Colorectal Dis.* 2003;5(4):347-352.

62. Moller AM, Villebro N, Pedersen T, Tonnesen H. Effect of preoperative smoking intervention on postoperative complications: a randomised clinical trial. *Lancet.* 2002;359(9301):114-117.

63. Gokce NG, Vita JA, McDonnell M, et al. Effect of medical and surgical weight loss on endothelial vasomotor function in obese patients. *Am J Cardiol.* 2005;95(2):266-268.

64. Busetto L, Segato G, De Luca M, et al. Preoperative weight loss by intragastric balloon in super-obese patients treated with laparoscopic gastric banding: a case-control study. *Obes Surg.* 2004;14(5):671-676.

65. Onyike CU, Crum RM, Lee HB, Lyketsos CG, Eaton WW. Is obesity associated with major depression? Results from the Third National Health and Nutrition Examination Survey. *Am J Epidemiol.* 2003;158(12):1139-1147.

66. Kolotkin RL, Crosby RD, Williams GR. Health-related quality of life varies among obese subgroups. *Obes Res.* 2002;10(8):748-756.

67. Wadden TA, Womble LG, Stunkard AJ, Anderson DA. Psychosocial consequences of obesity and weight loss. In: Wadden TA, Stunkard AJ, eds. *Handbook of Obesity Treatment.* New York, NY: The Guilford Press; 2002:144-169.

68. De Zwaan M, Mitchell JE, Howell LM, et al. Two measures of health-related quality of life in morbid obesity. *Obes Res.* 2002;10(11):1143-1151.

69. Adami GF, Gandolfo P, Bauer B, Scopinaro N. Binge eating in massively obese patients undergoing bariatric surgery. *Int J Eat Disord.* 1995;17(1):45-50.

70. Saunders R. Binge eating in gastric bypass patients before surgery. *Obes Surg.* 1999;9(1):72-76.

71. Williamson DA, Martin CK. Binge eating disorder: a review of the literature after publication of DSM-IV. *Eat Weight Disord.* 1999;4(3):103-114.

5

Anesthesia Issues in Patients Undergoing Gastric-Bypass Surgery

Keith P. Lewis, RPh, MD

Introduction

A thorough and complete preoperative assessment is critical in all patients considered for bariatric surgery. The laboratory information obtained must be carefully reviewed in conjunction with a thorough physical examination. Particular attention to the airway and comorbid conditions is key so the bariatric surgeon can develop a complete plan with the patient and family prior to the day of surgery. All organ systems must be thoroughly reviewed to avoid intraoperative and postoperative problems that should be anticipated in advance. Issues such as antibiotic dosing and timing, approach to intubation, central venous pressure versus pulmonary-artery–catheter (PAC) monitoring, need for postoperative ventilation, as well as the location and type of postoperative monitoring must be discussed and determined. Active dialogue between the surgeon and anesthesiologist is of the utmost importance in bariatric surgery.

Bariatric patients raise special issues in the detection of signs of cardiac or pulmonary failure. Even when clinically significant hepatomegaly, peripheral edema, and pulmonary rales are present, they may not be detectable because of the patient's body habitus. Other special issues include the weight capacity of the operating-room table, risk of nerve injury, pressure sores from prolonged surgery, and injury to the staff from lifting the patient in the operating room or postoperatively. Mask ventilation of the patient may be difficult with standard equipment and a second anesthesiologist may be necessary during securement of the airway. Dosing of muscle relaxants may pose special issues and highly lipophilic drugs may exhibit prolonged activity. All the information obtained from the preoperative assessment is compiled into a well-designed anesthetic plan.

Physiologic Changes in Obesity That Impact the Anesthesiologist

Cardiac Issues

Both blood volume and cardiac output increase with obesity. As a result, the stroke volume is elevated to perfuse the additional tissue. The higher cardiac output and larger blood volume in patients with obesity often result in hypertension (HTN) and cardiac hypertrophy.[1] Actual weight loss has been shown to successfully reduce blood pressure[2]; therefore, one of the major preoperative strategies to lower postoperative risk for bariatric patients is a weight-reduction program prior to the actual procedure.

Even without elevations in systemic pressure, the preload and afterload may be increased with an elevated mean pulmonary artery pressure and increased right and left ventricular stroke work. Careful assessment of ventricular function is key to determine the degree of left ventricular dysfunction prior to surgery. Left ventricular dysfunction can be present in young, asymptomatic patients with obesity. Both an echocardiogram and a multigated acquisition scan may offer valuable information. About 10% of patients with obesity develop signs and symptoms of congestive heart failure (CHF). Obesity is also a risk factor for coronary artery disease and sudden death.

Patients with obstructive sleep apnea (OSA) may have pulmonary HTN, signs of which include exertional dyspnea, fatigue, and syncopal episodes.[3] Valvular heart disease must be addressed in patients who received phentermine/fenfluramine (Phen-Fen) for weight loss. Phen-Fen was removed from clinical usage in 1997 (Chapter 2). The electrocardiogram, or ECG, must be closely examined for evidence of left ventricular hypertrophy, cardiac conduction abnormalities, arrhythmias, and previous myocardial infarction. Conduction abnormalities can occur because of fatty infiltration of the heart muscle itself. Utilizing all the cardiac information obtained will aid the anesthesiologist in determining the type of monitoring required. The blood-pressure cuff must be the correct size for the arm to avoid erroneous readings. If there is difficulty in obtaining reliable numbers with a standard blood-pressure cuff, it may necessitate the insertion of a radial artery catheter.

Respiratory Function

An increased body mass index (BMI) directly impacts respiratory mechanics.[4] The additional body mass puts additional weight on the rib cage, which lowers chest-wall compliance while the pressure from the increased abdominal girth pushes on the diaphragm and thus decreases total lung compliance. The result of the bariatric patient's additional weight is abnormal pulmonary function due to the elevated work required for breathing. Patients with obesity have a high metabolic demand coupled with an increase in oxygen consumption and carbon-dioxide production. Weight loss decreases the work required by the patient's lungs and thus may, to some degree, improve reversible pulmonary dysfunction.

Most important to the anesthesiologist is the change in pulmonary function associated with changes in posture. Assuming the supine position will reduce the patient's functional residual capacity (FRC) and thus increase his or her susceptibility to hypoxemia. The Trendelenburg position further reduces the expiratory reserve volume, lowering the FRC, which can lead to airway closure, especially in the dependent lung regions, and can

Table 5-1
Respiratory Changes in Patients With Morbid Obesity

- Decreased chest-wall compliance
- Increased work for breathing
- Impaired respiratory muscle function
- Airway closure during normal ventilation
- Decreased total lung capacity
- Decreased vital capacity
- Decreased functional residual capacity
- Decreased expiratory reserve volume

produce a ventilation/perfusion mismatch. Going from the sitting to the supine position is associated with an increase in cardiac output and pulmonary artery wedge pressure and a decrease in heart rate and peripheral vascular resistance.[5,6]

Careful examination of preoperative arterial blood gas (ABG) is important because it can significantly alter the intraoperative and postoperative management of the patient. The most common abnormality found on ABG examination is hypoxemia. In patients with morbid obesity, there may be premature airway closure secondary to a markedly reduced expiratory reserve volume coupled with an increase in cardiac output and circulating blood volume. This can produce hypoxemia from the low ventilation/perfusion ratio.[7] Typically, the ABG indicates mild degrees of hypoxemia (PaO_2 of 75 to 90 mmHg) and of hypocarbia ($PaCO_2$ 30 to 35 mmHg) secondary to alveolar hyperventilation.[8] Patients may maintain normocarbia during the day but develop hypercarbia at night secondary to OSA.

The impact of the high BMI on pulmonary function is summarized in Table 5-1.

Obstructive Sleep Apnea

There are three types of sleep apnea: OSA, central, and mixed. The definition of OSA includes episodes of complete apnea with cessation of air movement for greater than 10 seconds despite continued respiratory effects against a closed airway, with 5 or more apneic episodes per hour. Individuals with OSA can experience intermittent airway obstruction, hypoxemia, arrhythmias, and resultant sleep disturbances. Obstructive sleep hypopnea is present when there is a 50% decrease in airflow for more than 10 seconds, occurring 15 or more times per hour, which is usually associated with a drop in oxygen saturation of greater than 4% from baseline.[8] As a result of the snoring and apnea, daytime somnolence is not uncommon.

Most bariatric patients with sleep apnea have the obstructive type. It is estimated that as many as 70% of the patients with morbid obesity undergoing bariatric surgery have OSA. About 60% to 90% of those patients with OSA are obese and about 5% of patients with obesity develop OSA.[7] Of significance is the fact that there is no direct relationship between OSA and BMI.

OSA is a major concern in the anesthetic management of patients with obesity who are undergoing bariatric surgery. One reason OSA is of such concern to the anesthesiologist is that postoperatively, patients may experience episodes of apnea and even death.

Table 5-2
Problems Seen in Patients With Obstructive Sleep Apnea

- Obstructive snoring
- Restless sleep pattern
- Episodes of apnea/hypopnea at night
- Arterial O_2 desaturation
- Hypoxemia/hypercarbia
- Daytime somnolence
- Right-sided heart failure
- Pulmonary artery HTN
- Polycythemia

Performing a preoperative sleep study and an echocardiogram will help the anesthesiologist define the severity of the OSA and pulmonary HTN. Table 5-2 summarizes those problems seen in patients with OSA.

Two major factors make patients with morbid obesity particularly prone to develop OSA. The first factor is a decrease in pharyngeal area in patients with obesity secondary to the deposition of adipose tissue within the lateral pharyngeal walls. This fat deposition increases the likelihood for collapse of the oropharynx between the uvula and epiglottis, with resultant airway obstruction. If the upper airway muscles relax during sleep, there will be a resultant decrease in pharyngeal patency secondary to the increased fat deposited in the lateral pharyngeal walls. The second factor is that the extraluminal pressure in the pharynx is increased by the fat deposition resulting in external compression of the upper airway. The difference between the extraluminal and intraluminal pressures in the pharynx determines its patency (Figure 5-1). These 2 factors can increase the likelihood of collapse of the oropharynx. In addition to the fat deposition in the lateral pharyngeal walls, it is also deposited in the uvula, tonsils, tonsillar pillars, aryepiglottic folds, and the tongue. Neck circumference is frequently increased in patients with obesity and OSA. Comparison between patients with obesity who have and who do not have OSA shows a greater average neck circumference in the former group.[9]

The treatment for OSA is continuous positive airway pressure (CPAP).[10] In certain situations, an elective tracheostomy can be performed. Performing the tracheostomy prior to the surgery may relieve the airway obstruction, may improve the pulmonary HTN, and will reduce the risk of airway obstruction in the postoperative period following extubation. The tracheostomy can be removed when the patient is stable.

Two important syndromes that can be encountered in patients with morbid obesity include the Pickwickian syndrome and obesity-hypoventilation syndrome (OHS) (Table 5-3). Pickwickian syndrome was named after Joe, the obese somnolent boy described by Charles Dickens in the 1800s in his novel, *The Pickwick Papers*. The syndrome's primary symptom is sleep apnea. In contrast, OHS represents a long-term sequela of OSA.[11]

Two major concerns of the anesthesiologist and surgeon when operating on a patient with OSA include the patient's sensitivity to CNS depressants, which are commonly used for premedication and postoperative pain relief. Airway obstruction and respiratory

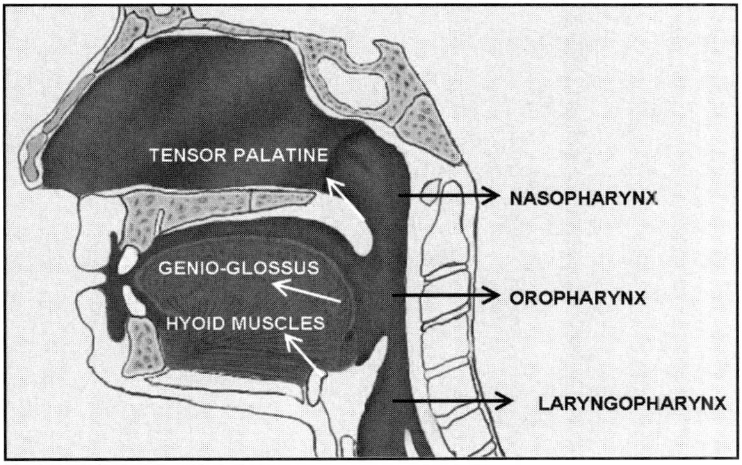

Figure 5-1. Upper airway dilator muscles. *For a full-color version, see page CA-III of the Color Atlas.*

arrest can occur with even small doses of sedative drugs.[12] In addition to the above concerns, OSA patients with obesity have a higher percentage of difficult intubations (up to 25%) than do nonobese patients. Dangerous episodes of apnea and arterial desaturation can occur throughout the entire postoperative period. Fortunately, successful bariatric surgery can be associated with significant improvement in OSA and the associated pulmonary and cardiovascular abnormalities.

Gastrointestinal Issues

The risk of pulmonary aspiration of gastric contents is increased in patients with obesity. The elevated intra-abdominal pressure, gastric volume, and acidity put them at additional risk over nonobese controls. Patients with morbid obesity also have a higher incidence of gastroesophageal reflux, hiatal hernia, and a prolonged gastric-emptying time. The volume of gastric juice in patients with obesity may exceed 25 ml, and the pH may be less than 2.5, making these patients particularly vulnerable to aspiration pneumonitis during the induction of anesthesia with the loss of consciousness and resultant airway reflexes.[13] This—coupled with a potentially difficult airway, a markedly decreased FRC, and an increased total body oxygen consumption—makes this part of the procedure particularly dangerous.

Although the potential risk may be high, the actual supporting evidence for a higher incidence of aspiration pneumonitis in patients with obesity is sparse. One study that compared patients with obesity to nonobese controls found lower gastric residual volumes in the patients with obesity.[14] This raises the question of the protective value of a rapid-sequence induction with its inherent risks in these patients. In contrast, diabetic patients with obesity and gastroparesis may be at risk for aspiration. Finally, fatty infiltration of the liver may result in abnormalities of liver-function tests with the potential for delayed drug metabolism with commonly used agents such as midazolam and vecuronium.

For patients at risk for aspiration, rapid-sequence induction is used for intubation. This process involves preoxygenation, followed by administration of the induction agent (ie, propofol) and succinylcholine, and application of cricoid pressure. The patient does not receive assisted ventilation until the endotracheal tube is placed.

Table 5-3
Pickwickian Syndrome and Obesity-Hypoventilation Syndrome

Pickwickian Syndrome	OHS
Massive obesity	Long-term consequence of OSA
Sleep deprivation	Central apneic episodes
Periodic respiration	Desensitization of respiratory center to nocturnal hypercarbia
Hypoxemia	Treated with progestational agents
Daytime somnolence	
Alveolar hypoventilation	
Secondary polycythemia	
Right-heart failure/hypertrophy	

Metabolic Issues

Total body metabolic rate in patients with obesity is often normal. These patients can have an absolute increase in total oxygen consumption and carbon-dioxide production because of the elevated total body mass.

Diabetes mellitus is not as prevalent as one would expect in patients with obesity. Obesity is typically characterized by insulin resistance secondary to tissue insensitivity associated with a high level of insulin secretion.

Premedication

Patients with morbid obesity, and especially those with Pickwickian syndrome, are exquisitely sensitive to the effects of sedative drugs. This may result in somnolence and respiratory depression and can necessitate the need for urgent control of a potentially difficult airway. A thorough preoperative visit can often allay or minimize any patient anxiety and fears, which can reduce the need for preoperative sedation. If sedation is given, it should be in small, titrated doses with the application of supplemental oxygen and with close direct observation.

Midazolam 0.5 to 1.0 mg is usually well tolerated. If a fiber-optic intubation is planned while the patient is awake, he or she should be given glycopyrrolate 0.2 mg intravenously 30 minutes prior to airway manipulation. To reduce the risk of aspiration pneumonitis, an H_2 antagonist can be given, such as cimetidine 300 mg orally the night prior to surgery and 300 mg intravenously 1 hour before the patient enters the operating room. Alternatively, ranitidine can be administered, which has less impact on the metabolism of other drugs.[15] In addition, metoclopramide and 30 ml of a nonparticulate antacid can be considered.

A preoperative antibiotic must be given to the patient intravenously in an appropriate dosage and time prior to the incision to ensure adequate tissue concentrations, and administration must be repeated at the appropriate intervals. Patients undergoing bariatric surgery have significant risk of infection; therefore, it is important to administer the antibiotic and wait until it is adequately concentrated in the tissue involved in the surgical procedure. In addition, deep vein thrombosis prophylaxis should be administered.

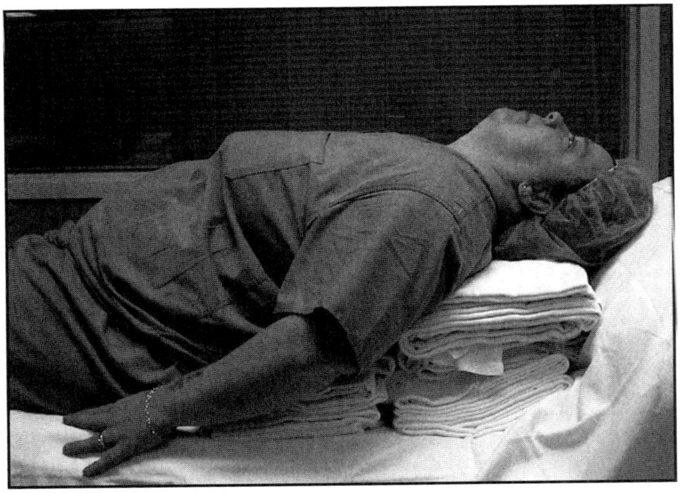

Figure 5-2. Positioning for intubation. The head, neck, and shoulders should be properly elevated with the external auditory canal—at the same level as the top of the sternum—to facilitate intubation. *For a full-color version, see page CA-III of the Color Atlas.*

Airway Issues

Careful and thorough examination of the airway is essential in the care of patients with morbid obesity. It is crucial that the anesthesiologist, before inducing anesthesia, has all the necessary airway equipment present in the operating room: endotracheal tubes of many different sizes, different laryngoscopes, a variety of oral and nasopharyngeal airways, intubating stylets, intubating and nonintubating laryngeal mask airways, a fiber-optic bronchoscope, and equipment for urgent intervention including transtracheal ventilation and cricothyrotomy capability. Patients with obesity desaturate quickly; therefore, if the physician experiences difficulty in securing the airway during the induction of anesthesia, all equipment and necessary personnel must be immediately available.

A patient with obesity usually has large cheeks and excessive facial tissue, a prominent tongue, a short thick neck, and smaller mouth opening due to submental fat with poor extension of the neck and atlantoaxial joint. These patients also have excess tissue of the palate and pharyngeal walls and large amounts of suprasternal fat with prominent breasts, all of which may be in the way during intubation and securing a neck line. These factors can increase the anesthesiologist's difficulty in securing the airway if not anticipated in advance.

It is estimated that as many as 13% of patients with obesity present with difficult laryngoscopic intubation.[16] Perhaps the most helpful predictors of a difficult intubation in this group include a high Mallampati score and a large neck circumference.[17,18] Of note is the fact that increasing BMI is not a risk factor for difficult laryngoscopy.[19] Still, patients with obesity often have high Mallampati scores (III and IV), with higher and more anterior laryngeal position. Key to successful intubation of such patients is proper positioning of the patient with elevation of the head, neck, and shoulders; this is accomplished with stacked blankets or towels to bring the chin to the level of the sternum (Figure 5-2).

For patients expected to be difficult to intubate, the best method is the awake fiber-optic approach. The airway should be prepared with topical local anesthetic and a drying agent such as glycopyrrolate. Either cetacaine or 4% lidocaine is effective as a topical local anesthetic. Certain anesthesiologists prefer to take an "awake" look and determine if they feel comfortable putting the patient to sleep first as opposed to proceeding to the awake fiber-optic intubation.

Another available option is an inhalation induction that maintains spontaneous ventilation with use of the fiber-optic bronchoscope for securing the sleeping patient's airway, as opposed to direct laryngoscopy where the view may be impaired by excessive pharyngeal tissue.

If a rapid-sequence technique is selected, adequate preoxygenation for several minutes is necessary prior to the induction of anesthesia.[20] Patients with obesity will desaturate quickly because of their high metabolic rate and the markedly reduced FRC and oxygen reserves. Mask ventilation can be extremely difficult for a single anesthesiologist; therefore, it is beneficial to have assistance readily available.

Monitoring

American Society of Anesthesiologists standards should be used to monitor all patients undergoing bariatric surgery. Urine output is monitored with a Foley catheter and the degree of muscle paralysis is checked with a peripheral nerve stimulator. Blood pressure should be monitored at the patient's upper arm if he or she has minimal comorbidities and an uncomplicated operation is anticipated. The appropriate size of cuff must be utilized to avoid erroneous readings; for larger patients, a 42-cm long bladder is the largest available. If the patient's arm is too large for a blood-pressure cuff, the patient's blood pressure can be monitored at the forearm. The surgical approach (open versus laparoscopic versus robotic) may impact the use of a standard blood-pressure cuff as opposed to a radial arterial catheter. In more complicated surgical procedures, blood pressure can be monitored through arterial lines. Securement of an arterial line allows frequent blood gas analysis if necessary.

When securing vascular access, even the peripheral intravenous access can be difficult.[21] For patients with difficult intravenous access, a central line may be indicated. There are no available prospective randomized trials establishing the need or efficacy of invasive monitoring in patients with obesity.[22] In reference to PAC monitoring, it is usually restricted to those patients with left ventricular dysfunction and/or pulmonary HTN. The risk/benefit ratio of a PAC must be considered because placement of a central line can be extremely difficult with the potential for significant morbidity. Routine landmarks are often not evident to help with the placement of a central line; ultrasound can help the surgeon or anesthesiologist locate the vessel to avoid excessive probing. It is often necessary to place the central line after the patient is intubated, as he or she may not be able to tolerate being placed in Trendelenburg position for a long time.

Induction of Anesthesia

There are many different successful techniques available to induce anesthesia for bariatric surgery. Techniques used include a standard intravenous induction, rapid-sequence induction, a spontaneous breathing-mask induction, or a pure-awake fiber-optic technique. The skill set of the anesthesiologist and any unique patient characteristics all impact the plan. Many institutions have a dedicated team of anesthesiologists performing all of their cases to maintain their skill set and assure consistency and safety for the procedure.

Key to any technique is ideal positioning of the patient prior to intubation (Figure 5-2). Placing the head in the optimal position for laryngoscopy can be achieved with the

Table 5-4

Factors Affecting Drug Dosing in Patients With Obesity

- Increased adipose tissue
- Increased blood volume
- Elevated cardiac output
- Decreased total body water
- Altered protein binding
- Increased renal blood flow and glomerular filtration rate

"stacking" technique described previously or with a special foam elevation pillow.[23] Making sure the head is in the ideal position will markedly increase the likelihood of a successful intubation.[24] Certain patients with obesity do not tolerate the supine position from a respiratory and hemodynamic standpoint, and it can be fatal if their cardiac reserve is limited.[25] Inferior vena cava compression can occur when the patient is in the supine position, in which case tilting the table to the left may be necessary to avoid systemic hypotension. Taking advantage of the reverse Trendelenburg position (head up-feet down) will minimize the risk of aspiration of gastric contents. Electric tables facilitate rapid position changes that may be necessary.

In reference to preoxygenation, patients with morbid obesity are particularly prone to desaturation with the induction of anesthesia because of their low FRC and high oxygen consumption. Comparing a 3-minute preoxygenation technique with a 4-maximum-breath procedure, the former was found to be more effective in lengthening the time until a saturation of 90% was obtained (3½ versus 6½ minutes, respectively).[26] One author describes the use of CPAP at 10 cm H_2O for 5 minutes during the administration of oxygen, followed by ventilation via face mask with positive and expiratory pressure (PEEP) at 10 cm H_2O for 5 minutes to minimize the risk of atelectasis formation following the induction of general anesthesia.[27]

Drug Dosing

In the nonobese patient population, drug dosing is based on a particular dose per body weight. The same relationship does not hold for patients with obesity. Nonlipophilic drugs are administered on a lean body weight basis.[28] Some of the factors that impact drug dosing in patients with obesity[8] are summarized in Table 5-4. In reference to lipophilic drugs, the patients with obesity requires larger doses due to their elevated volume of distribution compared to nonobese patients, although their elimination half-lifes are prolonged.[29]

The impact of the above-cited changes can be significant, and drugs like the benzodiazepines, barbiturates, and propofol will need to be administered in larger doses. A dose of 7.5 mg/kg of thiopental may be necessary for the induction of anesthesia in a bariatric patient, compared to 5 mg/kg for a nonobese patient.[30]

Maintenance of Anesthesia

Significant concern exists about fluoride toxicity in patients with obesity who have been given inhalation agents. Increased serum fluoride levels secondary to elevated biotransformation have occurred with methoxyflurane, halothane, and enflurane anesthesia.[31,32] Hepatic dysfunction due to fatty infiltration of the liver may potentiate the hepatotoxicity, especially with agents like halothane, which has been associated with postoperative jaundice.[33] The best choice for an inhalation agent is most frequently considered to be isoflurane or desflurane. Since nitrous oxide has low lipid solubility, it is an attractive option; however, its usage may be limited by the need for higher inspired oxygen concentrations in patients with obesity, as well as the concern about bowel distention and interference with the surgical view.

In reference to narcotics, the pharmacokinetic profile of fentanyl is unchanged in patients with obesity. In contrast, drugs like remifentanil have prolonged elimination half-lifes.[34] Despite the concerns cited above, the use of an inhalation agent (such as isoflurane) combined with a muscle relaxant allows titration of the inhalation agent to affect the patient and thus avoid use of large doses of narcotic and nitrous oxide that may be required for a typical balanced anesthetic technique.

Maintenance of adequate oxygenation may be a major issue with patients undergoing bariatric surgery. The patient's total dead space will increase during anesthesia, and air will be trapped distal to the closed alveoli, which produces venous admixture and the risk of hypoxemia.[35] In patients with obesity, there is an overall decrease in lung compliance coupled with a lower FRC beyond the closing volume.[36] FRC is negatively affected by the patient being in the supine position, as is general anesthesia. Other factors that may negatively impact FRC include abdominal insufflation, abdominal packs, retractors, and the lithotomy and Trendelenburg positions. PEEP may be helpful in maintaining or improving oxygenation during anesthesia and surgery. Because of the ventilation/perfusion mismatch, the dependant lung zones may be closed, and the majority of the gas will be distributed to the upper lung zones. The application of PEEP may recruit these collapsed lung areas and improve oxygenation.[37]

To ventilate the patient, the anesthesiologist should administer a tidal volume of 12 to 15 ml/kg based on the patient's ideal body weight. To assure adequate oxygenation, high-peak inspiratory pressures may be necessary. The addition of higher tidal volumes may have a minimal impact on improving oxygenation but may result in significant hypocapnia.[38] Addition of PEEP (10 to 15 cm H_2O) may improve oxygenation but can decrease cardiac output with high tidal volumes.

The physiologic impact of pneumoperitoneum must be carefully assessed because it can produce hypercarbia and a resultant respiratory acidosis. It is critical that the anesthesiologist reverify the position of the endotracheal tube if hypoxemia develops intraoperatively; shifting the patient's body or neck in conjunction with the pneumoperitoneum and resultant diaphragmatic elevation could advance the endotracheal tube from the correct position in the trachea into a mainstem bronchus.[39] Another strategy shown to improve oxygenation includes the reverse Trendelenburg position.[40] In certain situations, the only strategy that improves oxygenation is increasing the inspired oxygen concentration.

Muscle Relaxants

A key part of successful bariatric surgery is adequate muscle relaxation for both open and closed procedures. In laparoscopic procedures, inadequate paralysis may result in loss of gas from the peritoneum or in difficulty in exposure due to "tightness." Ease of maneuverability of laparoscopic instruments is essential for the surgeon; inadequate relaxation of the patient may severely limit the physician's surgical access and success.

If a rapid-sequence induction is planned, a depolarizing agent such as succinylcholine must be given in an adequate dose (1.5 mg/kg) to assure complete paralysis prior to direct laryngoscopy. Patients with obesity often have increased pseudocholinesterase activity.[41] They require larger doses of pancuronium than do patients of normal weight, but if the dose is related to body surface area it is similar to doses for nonobese patients.[42] In patients with obesity, drugs like vecuronium require a longer recovery time (hepatic clearance may be altered) than they require in nonobese patients. Atracurium has significant advantages because it is not dependent on hepatic metabolism and has a constant recovery time in obese and nonobese patients alike. Careful assessment of neuromuscular function with a nerve stimulator is mandatory. Using incremental dosing is an effective strategy to avoid excessive paralysis and difficulty reversing the paralytic agent upon completion of the surgery.

Regional Anesthesia

With the widespread use of laparoscopic techniques, as opposed to open procedures, patients experience significantly less postoperative pain and pulmonary dysfunction. The use of rapid emergence agents such as propofol, remifentanil, and desflurane also allows for quick emergence and extubation in many patients. With laparoscopic procedures, the use of thoracic epidurals for intraoperative management and postoperative analgesia is usually not necessary. When a thoracic epidural is utilized, the anesthesiologist can titrate the local anesthetic intraoperatively to improve the abdominal-wall relaxation and to minimize the requirement for inhalation agents.[43] One author successfully used a technique of continuous spinal/general anesthesia with continuation of the spinal analgesia into the postoperative period for patients undergoing gastroplasty.[44] The use of an epidural, besides producing profound muscle relaxation, can keep the bowel contracted and undistended, which improves surgical exposure. When performing regional blocks in patients with morbid obesity, the actual procedure can be extremely difficult and in some cases dangerous because of the absence of traditional landmarks. Longer needles are commercially available, and adding the nerve stimulator with insulated needles to locate the nerve fibers will aid in improving block efficacy and safety.

When performing a thoracic epidural for postoperative analgesia, placing the patient in the sitting position may help the anesthesiologist to identify the midline, which may be difficult to assess in the lateral position.[16] The use of an ultrasound guidance device may help the physician identify the epidural space in a patient with obesity.[45] In reference to the dose of local anesthetic, it must be reduced for both spinal and epidural blocks. The dose of local anesthetic should be reduced by 20% to 25%.[46] The actual volume of the epidural space is reduced in bariatric patients because of the elevated intra-abdominal pressure, which shifts blood from the inferior vena cava into the epidural veins. The size of the epidural space can be further reduced by fatty infiltration. With spinal anesthesia, the onset time may be delayed, the level achieved may be higher, and the block may drift upward, which produces the possibility of respiratory compromise.[47] Inadequate spontaneous ventilation may be an issue in a patient with obesity who is supine with paralyzed abdominal muscles during spinal anesthesia. Many of these patients also get anxious with the higher level of anesthesia and may have difficulty tolerating the procedure for an extended time. The combination of light general and epidural anesthesia offers true advantages, such as control of ventilation accompanied with blunting of the cardiovascular stress response and stable hemodynamics.[48] When spinal anesthesia is indicated for a procedure, like hip surgery, having the patient on his or her side as opposed to supine may be better tolerated.

With the usage of short-acting drugs and careful titration of muscle relaxants, the anesthesiologist can achieve excellent anesthesia with a rapid wake-up, avoiding the potential risks and difficulties with regional anesthesia in patients with morbid obesity. For gastric-bypass surgery, securing the airway with an endotracheal tube is routine, and performing the procedure with epidural or spinal anesthesia while the patient is awake would present significant challenges to the surgeon, anesthesiologist, and patient.

Fluid Requirements

In determining fluid requirements, the physician must consider if the patient received a preoperative bowel preparation, which causes some degree of dehydration and increases the total amount of fluid required. Surgery may be prolonged, with extensive tissue manipulation, which results in significant third-space losses. Third-space losses are also frequently greater than is the patient's actual blood loss during the procedure. Because a patient with morbid obesity has an elevated glomerular filtration rate (GFR) and renal blood flow (RBF), maintaining the typically desired intraoperative urine output of 0.5 ml/kg/hr may not be adequate.[49] During surgery, the creation of a pneumoperitoneum will decrease the GFR and RBF, a circumstance which usually resolves when the abdomen is deflated at the end of the procedure.

Calculating fluid requirements is often difficult because these patients often have an increased total circulating volume, although their total body water may be reduced from 65% to 40%. (Fat itself has relatively little water [6% to 10%].[6]) Certain patients with obesity have some degree of cardiac dysfunction, and a rapid infusion of fluid may result in hypoxemia and CHF.

Giving an adequate amount of fluid is crucial to avoid postoperative acute tubular necrosis. One author usually administers 4 to 5 L of crystalloid for an average 2-hour operation.[50] Using the 4-2-l formula, the fluid replacement is twice the calculated maintenance-fluid requirement plus the calculated deficit on a 12-hour fasting period for a 70-kg patient for the first hour. The author uses twice the calculated maintenance requirement that is based on lean body mass and gives 200 ml/hour overnight. Utilizing central venous pressure or pulmonary artery catheter may help the anesthesiologist and surgeon to determine fluid needs and thus avoid postoperative complications such as acute tubular necrosis or CHF with the need for prolonged intubation.

For additional information on fluid replacement, see Chapter 7.

Positioning and Nerve Injury

Putting the patient in the proper position for successful intubation is of extreme importance, as discussed previously with difficult intubation and the airway. The patient's head and shoulders are elevated significantly above the chest with blankets and/or pillows. To maximize the incidence of successful intubation, Brodsky and colleagues imagine a horizontal line from the patient's sternal notch to the external auditory canal.[24,51] In their study, Brodsky et al successfully intubated 99% of patients with obesity using direct laryngoscopy.[24] No patient required a bougie, and 75% of the patients had a Cormack Grade I view. A second study by Keller and colleagues reports a 97% success rate of intubation with a 8-cm elevation of the patient's head; 15% of their patients required a bougie, and 33% of their patients had a Grade I Cormack view.[52] It appears from the data available that significant elevation of the head above the chest—as described using the external auditory meatus as a marker with the sternum—results in a high success rate of intubation by laryngoscopy alone.

A major issue for anesthesiologists caring for bariatric patients is the availability of appropriately-sized equipment during the entire perioperative experience. Even the weight capacity of the operating-room table must be determined. Operating-room tables often have a weight limit of 205 kg, but tables capable of holding up to 455 kg are commercially available. Although 2 regular operating-room tables can be joined together, having an electric table allows for easy maneuverability of the patient into different positions that may be necessary during the operation. Patients with obesity are prone to sliding off operating-room tables, so carefully strapping the patient to the table or using bean bags may be necessary to avoid slippage.[50] The concerns about the weight capacity of equipment does not end in the operating room. Chairs, beds, and even toilets need to be assessed so that breakage will not occur with potential significant injury to the patient and/or staff. A complete evaluation of all phases of the patient's hospital visit is essential—from the preadmission clinic to the final discharge from the hospital.

Of major concern is compression and stretch nerve injury to the patient. The neural structures at particular risk are the brachial plexus, ulnar, and sciatic nerves.[53] In addition, unusual injuries have been described such as bilateral occipital nerve injury in thyroid surgery secondary to positioning of a patient with obesity.[54] Patients at additional risk would include diabetics and those with a BMI >55 kg/m^2. Injury to the brachial plexus is most likely to occur from turning the head excessively to the side or abduction of the arm during the procedure. This may occur if the surgeon pushes the arm while trying to get closer to the patient or excessively moves the arm boards cephalad to move the patient's arms out of the way. In one series, ulnar neuropathy was more common in patients with a BMI >38 than in control subjects (29% versus 1%).[55]

Damage to the sciatic nerve can occur from prolonged pressure on the nerve itself during a lengthy procedure. Rhabdomyolysis has been reported in patients who have undergone bariatric surgery (Chapter 7) and may result from prolonged direct compression of the dorsal and gluteal muscles against the operating-room table. One series had an incidence of 1.4%.[56] Even with the best padding and protection of the patient, nerve injuries occur, and most will improve over time.

Careful documentation of the extent and nature of the injury is crucial, and consultation with neurology is helpful to make a precise diagnosis utilizing electromyography and nerve conduction studies. In addition, the physician should provide adequate follow-up when the patient is discharged from the hospital.

When positioning the bariatric patient for surgery, the operating-room staff should give special attention to pressure points. Pressure sores can occur and are often difficult to heal.

Special Intraoperative Issues

Pneumoperitoneum can produce significant changes in the hemodynamic and respiratory status of the bariatric patient. The increase in intra-abdominal pressure produced by pneumoperitoneum can decrease venous return to the heart and can lower cardiac output.[57] The decreased venous return results most likely from compression of the inferior vena cava. Of note is the fact that at lower insufflation pressures (<10 mmHg) there may be an actual increase in venous return and cardiac output, while at higher insufflation pressures (>20 mmHg) there is typically a lowering of venous return and cardiac output. In addition, the higher insufflation pressures lower the GFR and RBF.[58]

Hypercarbia can occur because of the pneumoperitoneum, which results in a respiratory acidosis. Oxygenation can worsen from the cephalad movement of the diaphragm secondary to the insufflation of the abdomen with carbon dioxide. Ventilation/perfusion mismatch can occur from uneven distribution of ventilation to the lung. Other risks of insufflation of the abdomen with carbon dioxide include pneumothorax, gas embolism, and mediastinal emphysema,[50] as well as deep vein thrombosis secondary to lowered femoral blood flow resulting from the pneumoperitoneum and the Trendelenburg position.[59]

If the patient undergoing bariatric surgery requires cardiac defibrillation, the maximum 400 J of energy that can be delivered by the device should be adequate.[60] In some patients who are classified as "super obese," the transthoracic impedance from chest-wall fat may make defibrillation difficult.

Patients with obesity are at risk of retained foreign bodies in the abdomen, such as instruments and surgical packs. In one recent review, obesity was found to be an independent risk factor, and the recommendation was for an intraoperative radiograph to rule out retained foreign bodies in patients with obesity. In addition, the conversion from a closed to an open procedure, change of nursing staff during the case, and emergency surgery were identified as risk factors.[61] This issue is discussed in detail in Chapter 7.

One unique function for the anesthesiologist during bariatric surgery is the placement of an intragastric balloon and nasogastric (NG) tube for sizing of the gastric pouch. A special leak test is performed intraoperatively to assess the integrity of the surgical anastomosis (Chapter 7). When utilizing methylene blue for the leak test to assess the integrity of the anastomosis, the endotracheal tube cuff must be adequately inflated to prevent the dye from leaking into the lungs, which would cause chemical pneumonitis. All the devices inserted by the anesthesiologist should be withdrawn from the stomach during the stapling to avoid incorporation into the staple line. At the completion of the gastric pouch, a NG tube is reinserted; this should not be placed blindly because doing so could result in damage to the new surgical anastomosis.[50] The surgeon should aid the anesthesiologist in the final placement of the NG tube, which should be secured to the nose in a manner that guarantees it will not migrate postoperatively.

Postoperative Anesthetic Concerns

The transition from the operating room to the postoperative-care setting is a critical part of the care for the bariatric patient. Some of the major challenges include timing of extubation, pain control, and location of the patient for postoperative monitoring—on the floor versus in the intensive care unit (ICU). Communication between the surgeon, anesthesiologist, and postoperative-care providers is essential so that all critical information is transferred effectively. At some institutions, the anesthesiologist labels the endotracheal tube with a bright sticker that says "Difficult Intubation." This ensures that any health care provider directly interacting with the patient is informed of the difficult intubation and thus knows that accidental extubation could be life threatening. Noting this in the patient's chart or anesthesia record does not assure that all providers caring for that patient are aware of the difficult-intubation status, especially if the patient remains intubated for a prolonged time. Transfer of information during transfer of care is crucial.

Timing of Extubation

Whenever possible, extubation in the operating room is preferable. There, it is completed in a controlled environment with all the necessary airway equipment and experienced staff immediately available if a problem occurs. Certain patients who were difficult to intubate and those with OSA and Pickwickian syndrome may be left intubated overnight to be extubated in the ICU at a later point. Many postoperative bariatric patients have residual effects from the inhalation agents, increased sensitivity to the opioids, and the potential for lingering paralysis from the muscle relaxants. The anesthesiologist must carefully assess each individual to determine if the patient is ready for extubation. To be successfully extubated, the patient must: (1) be awake, alert, and responding appropriately to verbal commands; (2) have adequate oxygenation; (3) be fully reversed from the muscle relaxants; (4) be hemodynamically stable; and (5) have adequate respiratory mechanics. In reference to respiratory mechanics, a maximum inspiratory force of 25 to 30 cm H_2O, a vital capacity ≥10 ml/kg, and a tidal volume >5 ml/kg must be present.[62] Since the timing of extubation is so critical, certain groups have elevated the standard they set for extubation in patients with super obesity (BMI ≥50). For extubation in the operating room, they have 2 anesthesiologists present, use a nonrebreathing mask with high concentrations of oxygen after extubation, and assure direct observation of the patient for at least 5 minutes following extubation. If the anesthesiologist is unable to meet any of the above criteria, the patient is transported intubated to the postanesthesia care unit or ICU, where the endotracheal tube will be removed by normal extubation criteria. Part of this strategy is to avoid placing the patient immediately in the supine position, which can result in hypoxemia and hypoventilation. In the recovery room, the patient is placed in the semirecumbent position for extubation.[63] Just changing from the supine to semirecumbent position can increase the FRC by as much as 30%.[64] In those patients requiring a laparotomy, the procedure itself can decrease the FRC postoperatively by 25%. It is recommended that, after extubation, a bariatric patient be positioned with the head and upper body elevated 30 to 45 degrees and that the supine position be avoided.

Prevention of Atelectasis

With upper abdominal surgery, as many as 45% of patients may experience postoperative atelectasis.[65] Bilevel CPAP has been found to be helpful in reducing pulmonary problems after upper abdominal surgery in bariatric patients, utilizing 12 cm H_2O of inspiratory positive airway pressure with 4 cm H_2O of expiratory pressure. Using the above approach can significantly reduce postoperative pulmonary dysfunction.[66]

Concern exists about the negative impact of pressurized air from CPAP on the new surgical anastomosis, as this could result in leakage and possible sepsis. One investigator studied the impact of postoperative CPAP in patients who had a gastrojejunostomy as part of a Roux-en-Y gastric bypass (commonly called the RYGB) and found no negative impact of CPAP on anastomotic leakage.[67] Fortunately, laparoscopic procedures are associated with fewer postoperative complications such as pulmonary dysfunction and postoperative pain.[68]

Despite widespread support for incentive spirometry, there is relatively little data to support its usage.[69] In addition, the actual restoration of pulmonary dysfunction may take several days.[70] One study found that patients with morbid obesity develop more atelectasis during general anesthesia than do nonobese patients. Atelectasis in patients with obesity persisted at 24 hours after completion of surgery, whereas there was complete

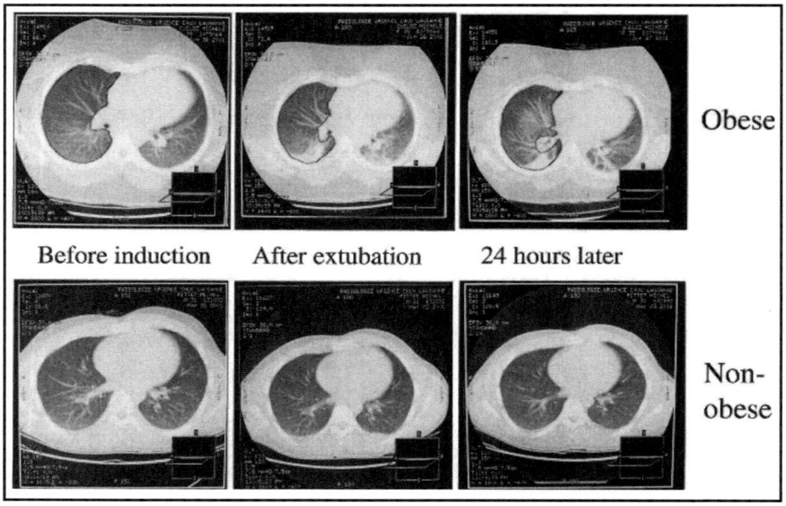

Figure 5-3. Atelectasis following surgery in obese and nonobese patients. Computerized tomography scans in one nonobese patient and in one morbidly obese patient before anesthesia induction, after extubation, and 24 hours postsurgery. The slices are at the level of the interventricular septum. (Reproduced, with permission of Dr. L. Magnusson and Lippincott Williams & Wilkins, from Eichenberger A, Proietti S, Wicky S, et al.[71]) *For a more detailed version, see page CA-IV of the Color Atlas.*

reversal of atelectasis in nonobese patients (Figure 5-3).[71] Bariatric patients may be slower to ambulate, which would delay the resolution of the postoperative atelectasis. The surgical procedure in itself may be lengthier in patients with obesity, but no correlation was found between duration of surgery and degree of atelectasis.

Because hypoxemia and atelectasis are so common in bariatric patients after abdominal surgery, supplemental oxygen by mask or nasal cannula is critical.[72] Even with supplemental-oxygen therapy, wound and tissue hypoxemia are common in these patients, which makes them more susceptible to postoperative infections.[73] In addition, postoperative pain medications will help avoid splinting and hypoventilation, which can worsen atelectasis and hypoxemia. Strategies utilized to minimize postoperative atelectasis include preoperative CPAP, intraoperative PEEP, and postoperative CPAP or bilevel positive airway pressure.

Postoperative Obstructive Apnea

Patients with OSA can be safely extubated in the operating room but can experience problems (eg, acute airway obstruction) in the postoperative period. Postoperatively, the patient may experience lingering effects from sedative and analgesic agents as well as the inhalation agents that were administered during the procedure. One study found that, with benzodiazepine-induced general anesthesia, there could be a reduction in tonic pharyngeal muscle support, which results in postoperative airway obstruction.[74] Narcotics administered may precipitate apnea that could result in respiratory arrest. Use of postoperative pulse oximetry coupled with monitoring in an intermediate care or ICU setting will assure close observation and immediate support of the airway if necessary.

Thromboembolic Complications

Thromboembolism is a major concern in patients undergoing bariatric surgery. It is estimated that as many as 5% to 12% of patients undergoing laparotomy may develop pulmonary emboli.[75,76] Factors that increase the risk of thromboembolism in patients with morbid obesity include their greater blood volume and relative polycythemia, elevated levels of fatty acids and cholesterol, and accelerated fibrin formation and fibrinogen-platelet interaction.[8] The procoagulant effects of surgery itself may be potentiated with slower resumption of ambulation seen in bariatric patients. Anticoagulation or other prophylactic measures should be initiated to minimize the risk of thromboembolism. There are no differences in the pharmacokinetics of antithrombotic agents in patients with obesity.

Miscellaneous Postoperative Issues

Other problems seen postoperatively in bariatric patients include infection, pressure sores, protein malnutrition, and rhabdomyolysis. Certain patients may remain intubated for prolonged periods because of sepsis or cardiovascular complications (eg, myocardial infarction, CHF, pulmonary embolism). Failure to wean from the ventilator may result from protein loss and subsequent muscle wasting. Lipid stores may remain unaffected, despite significant protein loss in the postoperative period. Bariatric patients are quite susceptible to pressure ulceration because they can remain in the same position for long periods with excessive weight placed on edematous tissue that has lower-than-normal perfusion. Ulcers in patients with obesity are often extremely difficult to heal. Infections can occur and may be difficult to localize because of limitations in radiographic equipment and the diagnostic studies available with regard to the patient's weight; many scanning devices only tolerate patients ≤180 kg. Abdominal ultrasound may also be extremely difficult.[77] Cases of neuroleptic malignant syndrome have been described in patients with morbid obesity who received neuroleptic agents (eg, haloperidol).

Postoperative complications in patients with obesity are discussed at length in Chapter 7.

Postoperative Pain Control

With the majority of cases being performed laparoscopically, the severity of the bariatric patient's postoperative pain has decreased dramatically compared to that after open procedures. For those patients requiring a laparotomy (planned or conversion from closed), the degree of postoperative pain can be severe, necessitating use of a thoracic epidural to avoid pulmonary deterioration from splinting. When using intravenous narcotics, the anesthesiologist must use caution to provide excellent postoperative analgesia rather than cause oversedation and potential respiratory depression. Holding back on narcotic dosing in fear of respiratory depression may markedly compromise the patient's ability to breath spontaneously and ambulate aggressively. Sedative agents are sometimes added postoperatively to ease the patient's anxiety or agitation, but they may potentiate the chance of respiratory depression seen with the narcotics. In certain situations, an agent like ketorolac may add significant analgesia without associated respiratory compromise.

When patient-controlled analgesia (PCA) with an opioid is combined with infiltration of the wound with local anesthetic, the patient can experience excellent pain relief. It should be noted that serious respiratory depression could occur with just PCA alone.[78] It is generally not recommended to use a continuous opioid background infusion PCA mode for patients with morbid obesity because of their risk of respiratory compromise. One can also add a nonsteroidal anti-inflammatory drug.[79]

Thoracic epidural anesthesia can provide excellent pain relief and beneficial cardiovascular effects including decreased left-ventricular stroke work.[43] Thoracic epidural anesthesia will improve gastrointestinal motility and respiratory function and allow for earlier ambulation and shortened hospital stay.[80] Other techniques used include continuous postoperative spinal analgesia and patient-controlled thoracic epidural analgesia.

Because of concerns about delayed respiratory depression with epidural narcotics, these patients must recover in a monitored setting. Patients with sleep-apnea syndrome may have sudden postoperative respiratory arrest when receiving epidural opioids.[81] The risk of respiratory depression with neuraxial opioids can occur after prolonged periods of time when the patient appears to be completely stable. To minimize the risk of postoperative respiratory depression, providers should limit preoperative sedation, maintain a heightened level of awareness about the possibility of acute airway obstruction postoperatively, and assure close monitoring in the postoperative setting.

Other Important Factors

With the change from open to laparoscopic procedures for patients undergoing bariatric surgery, patient satisfaction and postoperative course have significantly improved. When reviewing outcomes in laparoscopic gastric bypass, the factors associated with major complications were age (>50 years) and operative experience of the surgeon. Also, male gender was associated with more postoperative complications compared to women (19% versus 9%). Laparoscopic surgery is technically more difficult in males because of their android body habitus with a larger intra-abdominal concentration of adipose tissue than in women. Patients who had laparoscopic gastric bypass during their surgeons' initial 75 laparoscopic procedures also had a greater risk of major complication than did those whose had surgery after their surgeons' first 75 cases.[82]

Robotics

As we move forward, robotic bariatric surgery is an option that still utilizes small incisions to perform certain technical procedures that previously could only be performed in an open approach. The hand movements made by the robot are natural and intuitive and are transmitted directly through the robot's arms to the patient. The robot's arms offer several degrees of freedom that are more than those achieved by the surgeon's hands using conventional techniques. In addition, the 3D virtual operating field allows for precise maneuverability and surgical suturing. With bariatric procedures, the robot performs a primary anastomosis as opposed to using a stapling device.

The use of the robot in bariatric surgery will add certain potential challenges to the anesthesiologist. When the robot is in place, the anesthesiologist's access to the patient will be limited; therefore, all monitors and IVs must be secured safely prior to the procedure. In addition, the patient will have to be meticulously positioned to avoid accidental injury.[83] With robotic surgery, the length of the procedure may be prolonged, so one author recommends bispectral index monitoring to avoid awareness during surgery and to minimize the excessive use of drugs.[84] Not enough data is available at this time to access the full impact of the robot on outcomes and recovery profile.

The Future

As weight-loss surgery moves forward, research will aid in the development of drugs and devices to improve the safety and outcomes of patients undergoing bariatric procedures. Development of new analgesics without respiratory depression will offer real advantages over the current regimens. The development of evidence-based evaluation systems for both preoperative assessment and risk stratification will be crucial. Developing safe and effective approaches for the care and evaluation of patients with OSA will be critical. In reference to technology, the development of devices that are created for specific usage in patients with morbid obesity—such as blood pressure monitors, intubating pillows, and padding devices—will assure safe positioning to avoid the devastating consequences of pressure ulcers and nerve injury. There is much work to be done to improve the safety and outcome for patients undergoing bariatric procedures. Anesthetic implications in the patient undergoing bariatric surgery are vital to the overall surgical plan to assure a successful and uneventful outcome for all patients.

References

1. Alpert MA, Hashimi MW. Obesity and the heart. *Am J Med Sci.* 1993;306(2):117-123.
2. Kochar MS. Hypertension in obese patients. *Postgrad Med.* 1993;93(4):193-195.
3. Schiller NB. Pulmonary artery pressure estimation by Doppler and two-dimensional echocardiography. *Cardiol Clin.* 1990;8(2):277-287.
4. Pelosi P, Croci M, Ravagnan I, et al. The effects of body mass on lung volumes, respiratory mechanics, and gas exchange during general anesthesia. *Anesth Analg.* 1998;87(3):654-660.
5. Paul DR, Hoyt JL, Boutros AR. Cardiovascular and respiratory changes in response to change of posture in the very obese. *Anesthesiology.* 1976;45(1):73-78.
6. Oberg B, Poulsen TD. Obesity: an anaesthetic challenge. *Acta Anaesthesiol Scand.* 1996;40(2):191-200.
7. Yao F-S F. *Yao and Artusio's Anesthesiology: Problem-Oriented Patient Management.* 5th ed. Philadelphia, Pa: Lippincott Williams & Wilkins; 2005.
8. Brodsky, JB. Anesthesia for bariatric surgery, *ASA Refresher Courses.* 2004:506.
9. Benumof, JL. Obesity, sleep apnea, the airway and anesthesia. *ASA Refresher Courses* 2003:234.
10. O'Keeffe T, Patterson EJ. Evidence supporting routine polysomnography before bariatric surgery. *Obes Surg.* 2004;14(1):23-26.
11. Bickelmann AG, Burwell CS, Robin, ED, Whaley RD. Extreme obesity associated with alveolar hypoventilation: a Pickwickian syndrome. *Am J Med.* 1956;21(5):811-818.
12. Strollo PJ Jr, Rogers RM. Obstructive sleep apnea. *N Engl J Med.* 1996;334(2):99-104.
13. Vaughan RW, Bauer S, Wise L. Volume and pH of gastric juice in obese patients. *Anesthesiology.* 1975:43(6):686-689.
14. Harter RL, Kelly WB, Kramer MG, Perez CE, Dzwonczyk RR. A comparison of the volume and pH of gastric contents of obese and lean surgical patients. *Anesth Analg.* 1998:86(1):147-152.
15. Manchikanti L, Roush JR, Colliver JA. Effect of preanesthetic ranitidine and metoclopramide on gastric contents in morbidly obese patients. *Anesth Analg.* 1986;65(2):195-199.

16. Buckley FP, Robinson NB, Simonowitz DA, Dellinger EP. Anaesthesia in morbidly obese. A comparison of anaesthetic and analgesic regimens for upper abdominal surgery. *Anaesthesia*. 1983;38(9):840-851.

17. Juvin P, Lavaut E, Dupont H, et al. Difficult tracheal intubation is more common in obese than in lean patients. *Anesth Analg*. 2003;97(2):595-600.

18. Brodsky JB, Lemmens HJ, Brock-Utne JG, Vierra M, Saidman LJ. Morbid obesity and tracheal intubation. *Anesth Analg*. 2002;94(3):732-736.

19. Erzi T, Medalion B, Weisenberg M, Szmuk P, Warters RD, Charuzi I. Increased body mass index per se is not a predictor of difficult laryngoscopy. *Can J Anaesth*. 2003;50(2):179-183.

20. Goldberg ME, Norris MC, Larijani GE, Marr AT, Seltzer JL. Preoxygenation in the morbidly obese: a comparison of two techniques. *Anesth Analg*. 1989;68(4):520-522.

21. Juvin P, Blarel A, Bruno F, Desmonts JM. Is peripheral line placement more difficult in obese patients than in lean patients? *Anesth Analg*. 2003;96(4):1218.

22. Ledgerwood AM, Harrigan C, Saxe JM, Lucas CE. The influence of an anesthetic regimen on patient care, outcome, and hospital charges. *Am Surg*. 1992;58(9):527-533.

23. Rich JM. Use of an elevation pillow to produce the head-elevated laryngoscopy position for airway management in morbidly obese patients and large-framed patients. *Anesth Analg*. 2004;98(1):264-265.

24. Brodsky JB, Lemmens HJ, Brock-Utne JG, Saidman LJ, Levitan R. Anesthetic considerations for bariatric surgery: proper positioning is important for laryngoscopy. *Anesth Analg*. 2003;96(6):1841-1842.

25. Tseuda K, Debrand M, Zeok SS, Wright BD, Griffin WO. Obesity supine death syndrome: reports of two morbidly obese patients. *Anesth Analg*. 1979;58(4):345-347.

26. Gambee AM, Hertzka RE, Fisher DM. Preoxygenation techniques: comparison of three minutes and four breaths. *Anesth Analg*. 1987;66(5):468-470.

27. Coussa M, Proietti S, Schnyder P, et al. Prevention of atelectasis formation during the induction of general anesthesia in morbidly obese patients. *Anesth Analg*. 2004;98(5):1491-1495.

28. Ogunnaike BO, Jones SB, Jones DV, Provost D, Whitten CW. Anesthetic considerations for bariatric surgery. *Anesth Analg*. 2002;95(6):1793-1805.

29. Servin F, Farinotti R, Haberer JP, Desmonts JM. Propofol infusion for maintenance of anesthesia in morbidly obese patients receiving nitrous oxide. A clinical and pharmacokinetic study. *Anesthesiology*. 1993;78(4):657-665.

30. Buckley, FP. Anesthetizing the morbidly obese patient. *ASA Refresher Courses*. 1989; 243:1-6.

31. Bentley JB, Vaughan RW, Gandolfi AJ, Cork RC. Halothane biotransformation in obese and nonobese patients. *Anesthesiology*. 1982;57(2):94-97.

32. Bentley JB, Vaughan RW, Miller MS, Calkins JM, Gandolfi AJ. Serum inorganic fluoride levels in obese patients during and after enflurane anesthesia. *Anesth Analg*. 1979;58(5):409-412.

33. Walton B, Simpson BR, Strunin L, Doniach D, Perrin J, Appleyard AJ. Unexplained hepatitis following halothane. *Br Med J*. 1976;1(6019):1171-1176.

34. Bentley JB, Borel JD, Gillespie MS, Baughan RW, Gandolfi AJ. Fentanyl pharmacokinetics in obese and non obese patients. *Anesthesiology*. 1981;55:A177.

35. Vaughan RW, Wise L. Intraoperative arterial oxygenation in obese patients. *Ann Surg*. 1976;184(1): 35-42.

36. Agarwal N, Shibutani K, SanFilippo JA, Del Guercio LR. Hemodynamic and respiratory changes in surgery of the morbidly obese. *Surgery*. 1982;92(2):226-234.

37. Santesson J. Oxygen transport and venous admixture in the extremely obese. Influence of anaesthesia and artificial ventilation with and without positive end-expiratory pressure. *Acta Anaesthesiol Scand*. 1976;20(4):387-394.

38. Bardoczky GI, Yernault JC, Houben JJ, d'Hollander AA. Large tidal volume ventilation does not improve oxygenation in morbidly obese patients during anesthesia. *Anesth Analg*. 1995;81(2):385-388.

39. Ezri T, Hazin V, Warters D, Szmuk P, Weinbroum AA. The endotracheal tube moves more often in obese patients undergoing laparoscopy compared with open abdominal surgery. *Anesth Analg*. 2003;96(1):278-282.

40. Perilli V, Sollazzi L, Bozza P, et al. The effects of the reverse Trendelenburg position on respiratory mechanics and blood gases in morbidly obese patients during bariatric surgery. *Anesth Analg*. 2000;91(6):1520-1525.

41. Bentley JB, Borel JD, Vaughan RW, Gandolfi AJ. Weight, pseudocholinesterase activity, and succinylcholine requirement. *Anesthesiology*. 1982;57(1):48-49.
42. Tsueda K, Warren JE, McCafferty LA, Nagle JP. Pancuronium bromide requirement during anesthesia for the morbidly obese. *Anesthesiology*. 1978;48(6):438-439.
43. Gelman S, Laws HL, Potzick J, Strong S, Smith L, Erdemir H. Thoracic epidural vs balanced anesthesia in morbid obesity: an intraoperative and postoperative hemodynamic study. *Anesth Analg*. 1980;59(12):902-908.
44. Michaloudis D, Fraidakis O, Petrou A, et al. Continuous spinal anesthesia/analgesia for perioperative management of morbidly obese patients undergoing laparotomy for gastroplastic surgery. *Obes Surg*. 2000;10(3):220-229.
45. Wallace DH, Currie JM, Gilstrap LC, Santos R. Indirect sonographic guidance for epidural anesthesia in obese pregnant patients. *Reg Anesth*. 1992;17(4):233-236.
46. Hodgkinson R, Husain FJ. Obesity and the cephalad spread of analgesia following epidural administration of bupivicaine for Cesarean section. *Anesth Analg*. 1980;59(2):89-92.
47. Pitkanen MT. Body mass and spread of spinal anesthesia with bupivacaine. *Anesth Analg*. 1987;66(2):127-131.
48. Hamm CW, Koehler LS. The implications of morbid obesity for anesthesia: report of a series. *Anesth Rev*. 1979;6:29-35.
49. Ribstein J, du Cailar G, Mimran A. Combined renal effects of overweight and hypertension. *Hypertension*. 1995;26(4):610-615.
50. Ogunnaike BO, Jones SB, Jones DB, Provost D, Whitten CW. Anesthetic considerations for bariatric surgery. *Anesth Analg*. 2002;95(6):1793-1805.
51. Brodsky JB, Lemmens HJ, Brock-Utne JG, Saidman LJ, Levitan R. Anesthetic considerations for bariatric surgery: proper positioning is important for laryngoscopy. *Anesth Analg*. 2003;96(6):1841-1842
52. Keller C, Brimacombe J, Kleinsasser A, Brimacombe L. The Laryngeal Mask Airway ProSeal ™ as a temporary ventilatory device in grossly and morbidly obese patients before laryngoscope-guided tracheal intubation. *Anesth Analg*. 2002;94(3):737-740.
53. Sawyer RJ, Richmond MN, Hickey JD, Jarratt JA. Peripheral nerve injuries associated with anaesthesia. *Anaesthesia*. 2000;55(10):980-991.
54. Schulz-Stubner S. Bilateral occipital neuropathy as a rare complication of positioning for thyroid surgery in a morbidly obese patient. Acta *Anaesthesiol Scand*. 2004;48(1):126-127.
55. Warner MA, Warner ME, Martin JT. Ulnar neuropathy. Incidence, outcome, and risk factors in sedated or anesthetized patients. *Anesthesiology*. 1994;81(6):1332-1340.
56. Khurana RN, Baudendistel TE, Morgan EF, Rabkin RA, Elkin RB, Aalami OO. Postoperative rhabdomyolyis following laparoscopic gastric bypass in the morbidly obese. *Arch Surg*. 2004;139(1):73-76.
57. Chui PT, Gin T, Oh TE. Anaesthesia for laparoscopic general surgery. *Anaesth Intensive Care*. 1993;21(2):163-171.
58. Harman PK, Kron IL, McLachlan HD, Freedlender AE, Nolan SP. Elevated intra-abdominal pressure and renal function. *Ann Surg*. 1982;196(5):594-597.
59. Rosen DM, Chou DC, North L, et al. Femoral venous flow during laparoscopic gynecologic surgery. *Surg Laparosc Endosc Percutan Tech*. 2000;10(3):158-162.
60. DeSilva RA, Lown B. Energy requirement for defibrillation of a markedly overweight patient. *Circulation*. 1978;57(4):827-830.
61. Gawande AA, Studdert DM, Orav EJ, Brennan TA, Zinner MJ. Risk factors for retained instruments and sponges after surgery. *N Engl J Med*. 2003;348(3):229-235.
62. Barash PG, Cullen BF, Stoelting RK, eds. *Clinical Anesthesia*. 4th ed. Philadelphia, Pa: Lippincott Williams & Wilkins; 2001,1035-1041.
63. Rosenblatt MA, Reich DL, Roth R. Bariatric surgery and the prevention of postoperative respiratory complications. *Anesth Analg*. 2004;98(6):1810.
64. Vaughan RW, Bauer S, Wise L. Effect of position (semirecumbent versus supine) on postoperative oxygenation in markedly obese patients. *Anesth Analg*. 1976;55(1):37-41.
65. Soderberg M, Thomson D, White T. Respiration, circulation and anaesthetic management in obesity. Investigation before and after jejunoileal bypass. *Acta Anaesthesiol Scand*. 1977;21(1):55-61.

66. Joris J, Sottiaux TM, Chiche JD, Desaive CJ, Lamy ML. Effect of bi-level positive airway pressure (BiPAP) nasal ventilation on the postoperative pulmonary restrictive syndrome in obese patients undergoing gastroplasty. *Chest.* 1997;111(3):665-670.

67. Huerta S, DeShields S, Shpiner R, et al. Safety and efficacy of postoperative continuous positive airway pressure to prevent pulmonary complications after Roux-en Y gastric bypass. *J Gastrointest Surg.* 2002;6(3):354-358.

68. Nguyen NT, Lee SL, Goldman C, et al. Comparison of pulmonary function and postoperative pain after laparoscopic versus open gastric bypass: a randomized trial. *J Am Coll Surg.* 2001;192(4):469-476.

69. Celli BR, Rodriguez KS, Snider GL. A controlled trial of intermittent positive pressure breathing, incentive spirometry, and deep breathing exercises in preventing pulmonary complications after abdominal surgery. *Am Rev Respir Dis.* 1984;130(1):12-15.

70. Eriksen J, Andersen J, Rasmussen JP. Postoperative pulmonary function in obese patients after upper abdominal surgery. *Acta Anaesthesiol Scand.* 1977; 21:336-341.

71. Eichenberger A, Proietti S, Wicky S, et al. Morbid obesity and postoperative atelectasis: an underestimated problem. *Anesth Analg.* 2002;95(6):1788-1792.

72. Vaughan RW, Engelhardt RC, Wise L. Postoperative hypoxemia in obese patients. *Ann Surg.* 1974;180(6): 877-882.

73. Kabon B, Nagele A, Reddy D. Obesity decreases perioperative tissue oxygenation. *Anesthesiology.* 2004;100(2):274-280.

74. Dhonneur G, Combes X, Leroux B, Duvaldestin P. Postoperative obstructive apnea. *Anesth Analg.* 1999;89(3):762-777.

75. Fox GS. Anaesthesia for intestinal short circuiting in the morbidly obese with reference to the pathophysiology of gross obesity. *Can Anaesth Soc J.* 1975;22(3):307-315.

76. Fox GS Whalley DG, Bevan DR. Anaesthesia for the morbidly obese. Experience with 110 patients. *Br J Anaesth.* 1981;53(8):811-816.

77. Neligan PJ. Bariatric medicine: clinical implications of morbid obesity. *ASA Refresher Courses.* 2004:121.

78. VanDercar DH, Martinez AP, De Lisser EA. Sleep apnea syndromes: a potential contraindication for patient-controlled analgesia. *Anesthesiology.* 1991;74(3):623-624.

79. Schummann R, Shikora S, Weiss JM, Wurm H, Strassels S, Carr DB. A comparison of multimodal perioperative analgesia to epidural pain management after gastric bypass surgery. *Anesth Analg.* 2003;96(2):469-474.

80. Rawal N, Sjostrand U, Christoffersson E, Dahlstrom B, Arvill A, Rydman H. Comparison of intramuscular and epidural morphine for postoperative analgesia in the grossly obese: influence on postoperative ambulation and pulmonary function. *Anesth Analg.* 1984;63(6):583-592.

81. Ostermeier AM, Roizen MF, Hautkappe M, Klock PA, Klafta JM. Three sudden postoperative respiratory arrests associated with epidural opioids in patients with sleep apnea. *Anesth Analg.* 1997;85(2):452-460.

82. Nguyen NT, Rivers R, Wolfe BM. Factors associated with operative outcomes in laparoscopic gastric bypass. *J Am Coll Surg.* 2003;197(4):548-555.

83. Parr KG, Talamini MA. Anesthetic implications of the addition of an operative robot for endoscopic surgery: a case report. *J Clin Anesth.* 2002;14(3):228-233.

84. Myles P, Leslie K, McNeil J, Forbes A, Chan MT. Bispectral index monitoring to prevent awareness during anaesthesia: the B-Aware randomized controlled trial. *Lancet.* 2004;363(9423):1757-1763.

6

Gastric Bypass Surgery in the Pediatric and Elderly Patient

Caroline M. Apovian, MD

Pediatric/Adolescent Weight-Loss Surgery

Introduction and Rationale

In children and adolescents, classification by body mass index (BMI) is assessed with consideration of pediatric growth curves. Individuals younger than 18 years of age are considered "overweight" if their BMIs are at or above the 95th percentile for their ages. Charts showing BMI percentiles for US children by age and sex are published by and available from the Centers for Disease Control and Prevention.[1] According to these definitions, an estimated 16.1% of adolescents 12 to 19 years of age in the United States are overweight.[2] Fifty percent to 77% of these adolescents will go on to become adults with obesity, while 80% of those with 1 parent with obesity will do so.[3-6]

The prevalence of overweight in pediatric and adolescent age groups has nearly tripled in the last 30 years, paralleling the increase in adult obesity. Because of this, the comorbidities of obesity—such as type 2 diabetes mellitus, lipid disorders, hypertension (HTN), and sleep apnea—are being seen in patients at younger ages.[7-9]

For adults with extreme obesity who have failed medical therapy, weight-loss surgery is a relatively safe and extremely effective option for the treatment of obesity and its comorbidities. In children and adolescents, data on the safety and efficacy of weight-loss surgery are scant, and decisions to proceed with surgery are justifiably made difficult by concerns of proper nutrition and attainment of maximal growth potential. Even so, there are cases of severe obesity in adolescence for which bariatric surgery should be considered to resolve obesity-related comorbidities and to reduce the early mortality that is certain to occur. The most serious conditions prompting surgical intervention for obesity in adolescents are type 2 diabetes, HTN, sleep apnea, hyperlipidemia, and pseudotumor cerebri. Other serious conditions include steatohepatitis, slipped capital femoral epiphysis, polycystic ovary syndrome, Blount's disease, cholelithiasis, and early severe degenerative joint disease.

Definitions

BMI (weight in kilograms divided by height in meters squared), when adjusted for age and sex and expressed as a percentile within the reference population, is the standard method to assess adiposity in the office setting for pediatrics and adolescents.[10] Data used to construct the 2000 BMI reference charts were collected through the National Health and Nutrition Examination Surveys (NHANES) and pre-date the rapid increase in obesity in the US population (Chapter 1). The 85th and 95th percentiles of BMI for age from these references have been used to define the lower limit of "at risk of overweight" and "overweight" in children and adolescents.[11] These charts and percentiles, while helpful for deciding on interventions in most children, are not useful for those with extreme overweight who might warrant weight-loss surgery. Children and adolescents with BMI >40 kg/m^2 were poorly represented in NHANES, and thus there are no reliable population-based data by which percentile boundaries can be calculated.[12] Therefore, a conservative cut-off point—BMI ≥40—was determined by experts in the field as the threshold with which to consider surgical options.[13] This measure has been incorporated into guidelines for adolescent bariatric surgery.[14] This is consistent with the adult threshold for surgical intervention but without the consideration of lesser BMI with comorbidities.

Case Studies of Weight-Loss Surgery in Adolescents and Selection of Procedure

Table 6-1 summarizes the case series reports of adolescent bariatric surgery published since 1980: 9 papers in all.[13,15-22] These papers have reported on short- and long-term morbidity, mortality, and success with adolescents undergoing vertical banded gastroplasty (VBG); jejunoileal bypass (JIB); laparoscopic adjustable gastric banding (LAGB); and Roux-en-Y gastric bypass (RYGB), including open and laparoscopic approaches and short-limb, long-limb, and distal variants. To date, no data on the use of biliopancreatic diversion (BPD) in adolescents are available. The number of subjects operated on in all case series total 139, with an average sample size of 17 subjects per report. The average length of follow-up across the case reports is 5.5 years, with approximately 100 patients followed beyond 5 years. Based on these 10 reports and data from adult bariatric-surgery studies, pediatric/adolescent guidelines recommend consideration of RYGB or LAGB in those adolescents who are candidates for surgery, because of the relative safety of both procedures and the reversibility of LAGB.[14] The significant malabsorptive effects of the BPD make this procedure undesirable for adolescent populations, and the VBG has largely been abandoned and is no longer a recommended weight-loss procedure in adults. The JIB has been abandoned for many years because of its severe malabsorptive side effects.

The available literature that reports results of RYGB in adolescents documents weight losses of 62% to 77% with few complications.[17-24] Laparoscopic RYGB subjects also did well in 1 series by Stanford et al, losing 87% of excess body weight with follow-up of up to 22 months.[18] There are 2 studies in the literature documenting results of the LAGB in adolescents.[20,22] One reported on 17 adolescents, 12 to 19 years of age, who underwent the LAGB procedure with an average of 2 years follow-up. Excess weight loss in this series was 59.3%, and there was a significant improvement in obesity-related comorbidities.[22] Longer follow-up is necessary to determine the acceptability of LAGB versus RYGB in terms of safety and efficacy in the adolescent population.

None of the published case series report procedure-related mortality in adolescents undergoing RYGB or LAGB. Early complications of RYGB in adolescents have included

Table 6-1

Case Series Reports of Adolescent Bariatric Surgery Reported Since 1980 (Category C Data)

Reference	Subject Age, Gender	Initial mean BMI	Type of Surgery	Postop Results	Complications	Follow-up
13	13-18 y Total: 10	51-54	8 lap RYGB; 2 open RYGB	53% excess weight loss	7/10: partial obstruct Roux limb, leak, DVT, dumping syndrome, dehydration, thiamine deficiency	Up to 2 y
15	11-22 y 8F/3M	None listed (154 kg)	JIB	Avg wt: 107 kg	3 deaths; hepatic failure, renal failure, sepsis	10 y
16	11-19 y 27F/7M	47	30 RYGB, 4 VBG	Avg BMI: 32; 66% wt loss	1 staple-line failure; 3 inadequate wt loss (revision); hypoglycemia; anemia; gallbladder disease	6 y
17	15-17 y 7F/3M	52.4	RYGB	62% wt loss	3 pregnancies; 1 protein-calorie malnutrition; 2 cholelithiasis	1 y
18	17-19 y 3F/1M	55.1	Lap RYGB	87% wt loss	1 persistent sleep apnea	4-22 mo
19	13-17 y Total: 19	49	VBG, RYGB	BMI mean: 28	2 gastrogastric fistulas; 2 cholelithiasis; 1 ulcer; 3 anemia	10 y
20	11-17 y 8F/3M	46.6	LAGB	BMI mean: 33.1	4 iron-deficient anemia	23 mo
21	12-18 y 19F/14M	52	1 HG*; 2 VBG; 17 RYGB; 10 LLGB†; 3 DGB‡	77% weight loss	1 PE; 1 wound infection; 3 stomal stenoses; 4 marginal ulcers; 2 deaths; 1 SBO; 6 incisional hernia	14 y
22	12-19 y Total: 17	42.2	LAGB	BMI: 30	None	2 mo

* HG: horizontal gastroplasty

† LLGB: long-limb gastric bypass

‡ DGB: distal gastric bypass

pulmonary embolism, wound infection, stomal stenoses, and marginal ulcers. Late complications have included small-bowel obstruction, incisional hernias, cholelithiasis, gastrogastric fistulas, and protein-calorie malnutrition, as well as vitamin and mineral deficiencies.[13,15-23] These complications are similar to those seen in the adult population undergoing these procedures.

Criteria for Patient Selection and Considerations in the Adolescent Population

Adolescent candidates for bariatric surgery should be referred to centers with multidisciplinary weight-management teams experienced with treatment of adolescent obesity. Ideally, the team should include pediatricians, dietitians, surgeons, psychologists, psychiatrists, and an exercise specialist, if possible. Additional expertise that is readily available at the center should include endocrinology, pulmonology, gastroenterology, cardiology, orthopedics, and ethics. The team should meet regularly to review candidates and make recommendations for whether or not surgery is indicated and appropriate and on optimal time for surgical intervention.

There are not adequate data to determine if bariatric surgery adversely affects pubertal development and growth before full maturity has been reached. Adolescent candidates who have not reached physiological maturity before bariatric surgery may experience delay of or failure to attain full potential growth and sexual development because of post-surgical nutrient deficiencies.

For adolescents, psychological maturity is required to comprehend the consequences of bariatric surgery, to give an informed consent for the procedure, and to ensure optimal compliance with lifestyle changes necessary before and after surgery.

A special consideration for adolescent female candidates for bariatric surgery is the effect of the procedure on future pregnancy. Weight-loss surgery may potentially affect fertility, the pregnancy itself, and the health of the offspring. Adolescent recipients of bariatric surgery should be counseled on birth control and monitored closely for nutritional deficiencies during pregnancy and the peripartum period. There have been case reports of successful pregnancies after bariatric surgery in adolescence.[17]

Because of the above concerns, the following guidelines have been developed recently as criteria for eligibility for weight-loss surgery in adolescents.[14,24]

Body Mass Index Criteria

Bariatric surgery can be considered in adolescents with BMI ≥40 in the presence of at least 1 serious comorbidity (such as type 2 diabetes, obstructive sleep apnea, HTN, or pseudotumor cerebri) and for adolescents with BMI ≥50 who have less serious comorbidities. Those adolescents with lower BMI and with life-threatening comorbidities and quality-of-life issues should also be considered on a case-by-case basis. These BMI criteria in adolescents are more stringent than are those for adults (NIH guidelines[24,25]) so adolescents can spend ample time in medical-treatment programs to try to achieve lifestyle changes before resorting to bariatric surgery. Surgery should be considered only after failed attempts at medical management.

Physiological Maturity

Physiological maturity should be attained before bariatric surgery is performed in an adolescent. Height and pubertal maturity have been deemed reasonable markers of metabolic and physiologic maturity. Those adolescents who have not attained Tanner stage IV and 95% of predicted adult height based on estimates from bone age should be excluded from weight-loss surgery. Cases in which it is difficult to assess the patient for maturity should be referred to a specialist in pediatric endocrinology, and bone age should be determined via x-ray analysis by pediatric radiology.

Organic Causes of Obesity

Syndromic obesity should be excluded or diagnosed prior to establishing an individual's eligibility for bariatric surgery. If syndromic obesity is diagnosed, there should be a reasonable expectation that the syndrome will not adversely affect the outcome of bariatric surgery.

Psychological Maturity

An extensive evaluation by the multidisciplinary team before bariatric surgery should include elements of psychological maturity. The goal of the evaluation is to assess the adolescent's understanding of: (1) the procedure—including the risks, benefits, and complications; (2) the commitment to treatment adherence before and after the procedure; and (3) the support available to the adolescent during the procedure and follow-up. Table 6-2 lists questionnaires and tools to facilitate the psychological evaluation of an adolescent. After the psychological evaluation and a preparatory education process, the patient and at least 1 family member should undergo a written examination to evaluate their understanding of the commitment to undergo bariatric surgery. The examination should test the patient's and family member's knowledge of the following:

1. The change in anatomy expected from the procedure
2. The basic risks and benefits of the procedure
3. Potential problem areas for the individual that were identified during psychological evaluation (eg, binge eating, depression, conflict with parents, impulsivity) and the recommended treatment for these problems
4. Potential short- and long-term complications and the preventive measures
5. Rationale for and contracting for compliance with long-term follow-up and treatment (monthly for the first 6 to 12 months or until weight is stable; quarterly for the 2nd and 3rd years; and twice yearly indefinitely)
6. The importance of utilizing support services such as individual and family or group therapy
7. Rationale for and contracting for nutritional compliance, which includes taking vitamin and mineral supplementation to avoid deficiencies that may lead to metabolic bone disease, iron-deficiency anemias, and folate and B12 deficiencies

Table 6-2

Psychological Evaluation in Adolescent Candidates for Bariatric Surgery

1. Evaluate ability to consent to the procedure; assess family agreement, support, or coercion *(use interview, mental status exam, visual analogue scales).*
2. Evaluate motivation, compliance, knowledge about the procedure and postop requirements, and expectations *(use repeated interviews, homework between appointments, and "test" of knowledge/understanding).*
3. Evaluate psychological factors that could interfere with treatment or negatively impact surgical outcome or adjustment *(talk with counselor or therapist if available)*:
    - Eating disorder symptoms *(use interview and self-report instrument such as the EDE-Q or EDI subscales or QEW-P for adolescents*[26-28]*)*
    - Mood *(use interview and self-report instrument such as the CDI)*
    - Smoking and substance abuse *(use interview and self-report questions)*
    - Psychosis and borderline personality disorder *(use interview, treatment and symptom history, and talk with current/past clinicians if possible)*
    - Abuse, post-traumatic stress disorder *(use interview)*
4. Assess family environment, school environment, social support, and barriers to adherence *(use interviews with patient, parents, other family members living in home, and teachers or coaches if an appropriate reference is available).*

Adapted from Apovian CM, Baker C, Ludwig DS, et al.[14]

8. Rationale for and contracting for compliance to avoid pregnancy for at least 2 years postoperatively, which includes evaluation of the need for aggressive contraceptive methods for sexually active adolescent females undergoing bariatric surgery

Surgery should not be recommended until the adolescent and at least one member of her immediate family pass the written examination.

Postoperative Complications—Considerations in the Adolescent Patient

The postoperative complications of bariatric surgery in adults (Chapter 7) can be extrapolated to occur in the same manner in adolescents. However, nutritional deficiencies and vitamin and micronutrient deficiencies (Chapter 8) would be more harmful in this population than in adults because of adolescents' growth potential in general and because of pregnancy in females. The most common vitamin deficiencies seen in adults after bariatric surgery are of vitamin B12, calcium, and iron. Vitamin-B12 absorption is impaired because of the lack of acidity in the gastric pouch, which is needed to release vitamin B12 bound to food. This can be ameliorated with oral B12 replacement, but at times, intranasal and parenteral B12 is required. Calcium and iron absorption occurs in the duodenum, which is bypassed after RYGB. In adolescents, resulting calcium and iron deficiencies can negatively impact bone development and erythropoesis. In fact, recent studies have shown a correlation between obesity in children and anemia,[29] so adolescents undergoing RYGB may already be at risk for anemia because of their obesity. Bone density increases because of progressive bone mineralization up to the middle of the third decade of life. Bone mineralization is dependent on adequate intake of vitamin D and calcium, and these requirements are higher in adolescent years than in any other stage of development. In addition, obesity in adults is correlated with low vitamin-D levels,[30] which may also be the case in adolescents. Therefore, the concern of negatively impacting bone mineralization and erythropoesis after RYGB in adolescents is high. The necessity for compliance with supplementation and intensive follow-up postsurgery is crucial in adolescents.

Female adolescents postsurgery will soon be in their childbearing years, and thus, for these young women, B12, iron, and calcium supplementation is crucial. In addition, folate will be important for prevention of fetal malformations, notably neural tube defects. This vitamin may also become deficient postsurgery, and thus micronutrient supplementation must be stressed during future pregnancies, especially the first trimesters.

The common deficiencies seen in adults after RYGB are vitamins A, B12, C, D, and E; folic acid; and iron.[31-33] In addition, there have been reports of beriberi (thiamine-B1 deficiency) in adults and recently 3 cases of dry beriberi in adolescents after RYGB.[34] Thiamine plays a role in the metabolism of simple sugars and keto acids. It is possible that beriberi can therefore occur in adolescents who have been used to eating sweets and then undergo gastric-bypass surgery and are subjected to a prolonged ketotic state after surgery.

Postoperative Patient Management

Special considerations of the postoperative care of the adolescent bariatric patient include risk of nutritional deficiencies, pregnancy issues, and compliance with care and follow-up.

It is recommended by expert guidelines that pregnancy should be avoided for at least 2 years postoperatively in adolescent female patients, and thus, both pre- and postoperatively, there should be an evaluation of the need for aggressive contraceptive methods for sexually active adolescent females.[14]

Follow-up after bariatric surgery in adolescence is intensive, and patients should be apprised of this prior to surgery: patients are seen weekly for the first month, monthly for 6 to 12 months or until weight stabilizes, quarterly for the 2nd and 3rd years, and then twice yearly for an indefinite time. Patients must comply with a low-calorie, low-carbohydrate dietary plan that focuses on adequate intake of protein (0.5 to 1 0 g/kg/day, calculated by actual weight) to spare lean mass during the rapid weight-loss period. The diet begins as a protein-supplemented liquid diet and progresses slowly after the first month toward a goal of eating a variety of foods in small portions, averaging about 1 cup per meal. Patients should be instructed to eat 3 to 4 small meals per day and to consume 64 to 96 oz of fluids per day, continually sipping water throughout the day except 30 minutes before and after each meal.

Consistently prescribed medications are ursodiol and ranitidine because of an increased risk of gallstone formation from rapid weight loss and peptic-ulcer development after RYGB. Nonsteroidal anti-inflammatory agents, such as ibuprofen and indocin, should be avoided for life to reduce the risk of intestinal ulceration. Chewable vitamins, a calcium supplement, and an iron supplement for females are prescribed, as is a B-complex vitamin to avoid the possibility of B6 and thiamine deficiencies and to increase thiamine intake above the usually recommended daily intake of 1.5 mg/day.[34] It is also advisable to begin daily multivitamins several months prior to surgery in adolescents.

Biochemical parameters to follow postoperatively include a complete blood count; prothrombin time for vitamin-K adequacy; iron studies; B1, B12, and folate levels; and calcium, thiamine, 25-hydroxy vitamin D, and PTH levels. Periodic bone-density measurements via dual energy x-ray absorptiometry (DEXA) should be performed if possible (not an option for patients over 300 lb) after 3 and 6 months (during the rapid weight-loss period) and then again at 12 months after weight stabilization. DEXA can also assess body composition, which provides information regarding rate and relative amounts of fat and lean body mass loss. This information is useful when adjusting the dietary program to preserve lean body mass during the rapid weight-loss period.[13,14]

Data Collection

Prospective collection of data on outcomes of adolescents undergoing weight-loss surgery is imperative to advance the field and improve the ability to predict outcomes and manage adolescents after weight-loss surgery in the future. Programs offering pediatric bariatric surgery should be engaged in data collection. The minimum requirements for data collection are listed in Table 6-3.

Summary—Adolescent Bariatric Surgery

Adolescent bariatric surgery is being offered at a growing rate to select adolescent patients in the United States because of the epidemic of obesity and failure of medical management in the adolescent population. The selection process and preoperative education for bariatric surgery in this population is rigorous to ensure the safety of these patients. Guidelines consider BMI, comorbidities, and physiological and psychological maturity, in addition to family support and ability for compliance with postoperative follow-up. All programs offering bariatric surgery to adolescents should be involved in data collection to further progress in this growing area.

Bariatric Surgery in the Older Patient

The 1991 NIH consensus conference on bariatric surgery did not specify age limits for consideration of eligibility for bariatric surgery, although most of the trials supporting bariatric surgery involve adults less than 55 years old.[35] In addition, the obesity epidemic has spared neither the young nor the old, with 30.5% of men and 34.7% of women over 60 years of age meeting the criteria for obesity (BMI ≥30). The prevalence of extreme obesity (BMI ≥40) in individuals over 60 years of age is 1.7% in men and 5.6% in women; these persons would meet the BMI criteria for bariatric surgery.[36]

Concerns for offering bariatric surgery to older (>60 years) persons include higher operative morbidity and mortality and possible inadequacy of weight loss due to the relative immobility of older persons with obesity and with osteoarthritis of the weight-bearing joints. A third concern is economic: is performing bariatric surgery on an older patient cost-effective? At what postoperative time point is the cost of bariatric surgery overtaken by the decrease in health care dollars experienced because of weight loss? For younger patients, several papers have demonstrated the cost-effectiveness of bariatric surgery.[37,38] Christou et al estimate that the total direct health care cost for managing a patient with

Table 6-3

Minimum Requirements for Data Collection in Adolescent Weight-Loss Surgery

1. Preoperative assessments
   - Anthropometrics, including past measurements to determine age of onset of overweight if available
   - Medical comorbidities and laboratory screening to include TSH, BUN/Cr, LFTs, total cholesterol, triglycerides, HDL-C, LDL-C, fasting glucose or 2-hour OGTT, insulin, PTH, 25 (OH) vitamin D, pregnancy test
   - Psychological measures (standardized written measures and expert assessment)
   - Family history of obesity and the major obesity-related comorbidities in first- and second-degree relatives
2. Perioperative data
   - Surgical procedure(s)
   - Intraoperative findings and complications
   - Postoperative recovery time and setting
3. Short-term outcomes (0 to 1 year postoperative)
   - Weight change, height velocity pre- and postsurgery, symptoms (vomiting, pain, other complaints), menstrual patterns
   - Surgical complications
   - Cosmetic complications: assessment of pannus formation
   - Medical complications: laboratory assessment of micronutrient deficiencies [iron studies, vitamin B12, 25(OH) vitamin D, prothrombin (PT), calcium, PTH, thiamine] and periodic bone-density measurements
   - Status of medical comorbidities (repeated measures)
   - Compliance with prescribed supplements, follow-up visits, eating and exercise requirements, and contraception
   - Social adjustment (return to school, repeat written measures of depression, eating attitudes and eating disorders, self-esteem, and body image, assessment of substance abuse)
4. Long-term outcomes—all of the above plus:
   - Pregnancies
     - Timing, laboratory assessment during, complications
     - Long-term follow-up of offspring, whenever possible: anthropometrics, medical problems, school performance
   - Male reproductive function, erectile function
   - Social outcomes
     - Further education
     - Stable relationships
     - Employment

Adapted from Apovian CM, Baker C, Ludwig DS, et al.[14]

morbid obesity may be reduced by 45% within 5 years after surgery.[37] For older patients, the answer to the cost-effectiveness question will require the collection of long-term data in older postsurgical patients.

Several published case reports address the efficacy and safety of bariatric surgery in older patients, and one of these (Sugerman et al, 2004)[39] compared results in older patients versus younger patients. All case series in older patients reported that bariatric surgery is safe and effective for weight loss, in addition to facilitating improvement in obesity comorbidities.[39-42] In Sugerman et al, the weight loss (60% excess body weight) and improvements in comorbidities were less in the older compared with those in younger patients, but all weight losses were clinically significant.[39]

Which procedure should be recommended for the older population? As in the adolescent population, class II evidence regarding the use of RYGB compared to the LAGB for the older patient will require long-term randomized prospective trials.

Regarding the laparoscopic versus open approach to RYGB, a recent review of 52 patients older than 50 years who underwent RYGB compared the 2 approaches and found that the laparoscopic technique resulted in fewer intensive-care admissions and shorter length of stay than did the open approach for RYGB in the cohort.[43] Currently, among surgeons whose expertise is bariatric surgery, the laparoscopic RYGB is the procedure of choice in older patients.[39]

In summary, the available data show that bariatric surgery in persons over 60 years of age results in less weight loss and less improvement in comorbidities than does surgery performed in younger groups. Nevertheless, in the case series published to date, bariatric surgery was effective for older patients with low morbidity and mortality. It may be considered in selected patients over 55 to 60 years of age on a case-by-case basis.

References

1. 2000 CDC Growth Charts: United States. DHHS Centers for Disease Control and Prevention Web site. Available at: http://www.cdc.gov/growthcharts. Accessed January 29, 2005.
2. Hedley AA, Ogden CL, Johnson CL, Carroll MD, Curtin LR, Flegal KM. Prevalence of overweight and obesity among US children, adolescents, and adults, 1999-2002. *JAMA*. 2004;291(23):2847-2850.
3. Freedman DS, Khan LK, Dietz WH, Srinivasan SR, Berenson GS. Relationship of childhood obesity to coronary heart disease risk factors in adulthood: the Bogalusa Heart Study. *Pediatrics*. 2001;108(3):712-718.
4. Whitaker RC, Wright JA, Pepe MS, Seidel KD, Dietz WH. Predicting obesity in young adulthood from childhood and parental obesity. *N Engl J Med*. 1997;337(13):869-873.
5. Guo SS, Huang C, Maynard LM, et al. Body mass index during childhood, adolescence and young adulthood in relation to adult overweight and adiposity: the Fels Longitudinal Study. *Int J Obes Relat Metab Disord*. 2000;24(12):1628-1635.
6. Serdula MK, Ivery D, Coates RJ, Freedman DS, Williamson DF, Byers T. Do obese children become obese adults? A review of the literature. *Prev Med*. 1993;22(2):167-177.
7. Must A, Jacques PF, Dallal GE, Bajema CJ, Dietz WH. Long-term morbidity and mortality of overweight adolescents. A follow-up of the Harvard Growth Study of 1922 to 1935. *N Eng J Med*. 1992;327(19):1350-1355.
8. Fontaine KR, Redden DT, Wang C, Westfall AO, Allison DB. Years of life lost due to obesity. *JAMA*. 2003;289(2):187-193.
9. Pinhas-Hamiel O, Dolan LM, Daniels SR, Standiford D, Khoury PR, Zeitler P. Increased incidence of non-insulin-dependent diabetes mellitus among adolescents. *J Pediatr*. 1996;128(5 Pt 1):608-615.
10. Himes JH, Dietz WH. Guidelines for overweight in adolescent preventive services: recommendations from an expert committee. The Expert Committee on Clinical Guidelines for Overweight in Adolescent Preventive Services. *Am J Clin Nutr*. 1994;59(2):307-316.

11. Cole TJ, Bellizzi MC, Flegal KM, Dietz WH. Establishing a standard definition for child overweight and obesity worldwide: international survey. *BMJ.* 2000;320(7244):1240-1243.

12. Kuczmarski RJ, Ogden CL, Guo SS, et al. 2000 CDC growth charts for the United States: methods and development. *Vital Health Stat 11.* 2002;246:1-190.

13. Inge TH, Garcia V, Daniels S, et al. A multidisciplinary approach to the adolescent bariatric surgical patient. *J Pediatr Surg.* 2004;39(3):442-447.

14. Apovian CM, Baker C, Ludwig DS et al. Best practice guidelines in pediatric/adolescent weight loss surgery. *Obes Res.* 2005;13(2):274-282.

15. Silber T, Randolph J, Robbins S. Long-term morbidity and mortality in morbidly obese adolescents after jejunoilial bypass. *J Pediatr.* 1986;108(2):318-322.

16. Rand CS, Macgregor AM. Adolescents having obesity surgery: a 6-year follow-up. *South Med J.* 1994;87(12):1208-1213.

17. Strauss RS, Bradley LJ, Brolin RE. Gastric bypass surgery in adolescents with morbid obesity. *J Pediatr.* 2001;138(4):499-504.

18. Stanford A, Glascock JM, Eid GM, et al. Laparoscopic Roux-en-Y gastric bypass in morbidly obese adolescents. *J Pediatr Surg.* 2003;38(3):430-433.

19. Capella JF, Capella RF. Bariatric surgery in adolescence. Is this the best age to operate? *Obes Surg.* 2003;13(6):826-832.

20. Abu-Abeid S, Gavert N, Klausner JM, Szold A. Bariatric surgery in adolescence. *J Pediatr Surg.* 2003;38(9):1379-1382.

21. Sugerman HJ, Sugerman EL, DeMaria EJ, et al. Bariatric surgery for severely obese adolescents. *J Gastrointestinal Surg.* 2003;7(1):102-108.

22. Dolan K, Fielding G. A comparison of laparoscopic adjustable gastric banding in adolescents and adults. *Surg Endosc.* 2004;18(1):45-47.

23. Soper RT, Mason EE, Printen KJ, Zellweger H. Gastric bypass for morbid obesity in children and adolescents. *J Pediatr Surg.* 1975;10(1):51-58.

24. Inge T, Krebs NF, Garcia VF, et al. Bariatric surgery for severely overweight adolescents: concerns and recommendations. *Pediatrics.* 2004;114(1):217-223.

25. Gastrointestinal surgery for severe obesity: National Institutes of Health Consensus Development Conference Statement. *Am J Clin Nutr.* 1992;55(Suppl 2):615S-619S.26.

26. Decaluwe V, Braet C. Assessment of eating disorder psychopathology in obese children and adolescents: interview versus self-report questionnaire. *Behav Res Ther.* 2004;42(7):799-811.

27. Kalarchian MA, Marcus MD, Wilson GT, Labouvie EW, Brolin RE, LaMarca LB. Binge eating among gastric bypass patients at long-term follow-up. *Obes Surg.* 2002;12(2):270-275.

28. Engelsen BK, Laberg JC. A comparison of three questionnaires (EAT-12, EDI, and EDE-Q) for assessment of eating problems in healthy female adolescents. *Nord J Psychiatry.* 2001;55(2):129-135.

29. Nead KG, Halterman JS, Kaczorowski JM, Auinger P, Weitzman M. Overweight children and adolescents: a risk group for iron deficiency. *Pediatrics.* 2004;114(1):104-108.

30. Wortsman J, Matsuoka LY, Chen TC, Lu Z, Holick MF. Decreased bioavailability of vitamin D in obesity. *Am J Clin Nutr.* 2000;72(3):690-693.

31. Halverson JD. Vitamin and mineral deficiencies following obesity surgery. *Gastroenterol Clin North Am.* 1987;16(2):307-315.

32. Halverson JD. Micronutrient deficiencies after gastric bypass for morbid obesity. *Am Surg.* 1986;52(11):594-598.

33. MacLean LD, Rhode BM, Shizgal HM. Nutrition following gastric operations for morbid obesity. *Ann Surg.* 1983;198(3):347-355.

34. Towbin A, Inge TH, Garcia VF, et al. Beriberi after gastric bypass surgery in adolescence. *J Pediatr.* 2004;145(2):263-267.

35. NIH conference. Gastrointestinal surgery for severe obesity. Consensus Development Conference Panel. *Ann Intern Med.* 1991;115(12):956-961.

36. Hedley AA, Ogden CL, Johnson CL, Carroll MD, Curtin LR, Flegal KM. Prevalence of overweight and obesity among US children, adolescents, and adults, 1999-2002. *JAMA.* 2004;291(23):2847-2850.

37. Christou NV, Sampalis JS, Liberman M, et al. Surgery decreases long-term mortality, morbidity, and health care use in morbidly obese patients. *Ann Surg.* 2004;240(3):416-424.

38. Flum DR, Dellinger EP. Impact of gastric bypass operation on survival: a population-based analysis. *J Am Coll Surg.* 2004;199(4):543-551.

39. Sugerman HJ, DeMaria EJ, Kellum JM, Sugerman EL, Meador JG, Wolfe LG. Effects of bariatric surgery in older patients. *Ann Surg.* 2004;240(2):243-247.

40. Macgregor AM, Rand CS. Gastric surgery in morbid obesity. Outcome in patients aged 55 years and older. *Arch Surg.* 1993;128(10):1153-1157.

41. Murr MM, Siadati MR, Sarr MG. Results of bariatric surgery for morbid obesity in patients older than 50 years. *Obes Surg.* 1995;5(4):399-402.

42. Printen KJ, Mason EE. Gastric bypass for morbid obesity in patients more than fifty years of age. *Surg Gynecol Obstet.* 1977;144(2):192-194.

43. Gonzalez R, Lin E, Mattar SG, Venkatesh KR, Smith CD. Gastric bypass for morbid obesity in patients 50 years or older: is laparoscopic technique safer? *Am Surg.* 2003;69(7):547-554.

7

Immediate Postoperative Complications

Donald T. Hess, Jr, MD and R. Armour Forse, MD, PhD

Introduction

Surgery for obesity has risen dramatically in the last decade, with over 140,000 operations performed in the United States in 2004. The majority of these were Roux-en-Y gastric-bypass (RYGB) surgeries, followed by gastric banding and the biliopancreatic diversion (BPD). The average body mass index (BMI) of patients who underwent bariatric surgery was 48 kg/m^2, which equals approximately 150 pounds overweight. Performing bariatric surgery on the obese is considered a high-risk procedure in a high-risk patient population. Associated with obesity are restrictive lung disease and cardiomyopathy characterized by diastolic dysfunction. Patients with obesity also present with numerous associated clinical comorbidities, such as type 2 diabetes mellitus, hypertension (HTN), sleep apnea, and hypercholesterolemia.

Despite surgeons' increasing experience with bariatric surgery and improvements in related anesthetic care (Chapter 5), many known risks continue to be associated with these procedures. When caring for bariatric patients, the health care provider must be familiar with the common clinical scenarios associated with these complications. These not only include those complications associated with correctable morbidities but also surgery-specific complications such as bleeding, leak, and obstruction, which are associated with mortality. All of these are addressed in this chapter.

Common Postoperative Complications

Hypovolemia in the Bariatric Patient

Hypovolemia is a very common and under-recognized problem in patients who have undergone bariatric procedures. The symptoms of hypovolemia are low urine output, tachycardia, and (as it progresses) hypotension, but these are late manifestations and represent a deficit of >8% of total body water. Early symptoms, such as thirst and signs of decreased skin turgor and dry mucous membranes, should be sought, and the provider must remember that even these represent liters of water deficit in these patients. Although hypovolemia and its symptoms may be warning signs of a postoperative complication, such as bleeding (a direct cause of hypovolemia) or a leak (an indirect cause of hypovolemia), the most common cause is inadequate fluid replacement. The first step in treating hypovolemia is fluid replacement, and the bariatric patient's volume deficit is usually very large; therefore, a bolus of an isotonic solution, such as lactated Ringer's solution, should be ordered immediately, even as the bariatric patient's fluid needs are calculated.

When calculating the fluid needs of a postoperative patient, the provider must address the 3 areas: preoperative deficits, operative losses, and postoperative needs. Fluids need to be calculated according to the patient's weight. For an individual with morbid obesity (Chapter 1), the provider should calculate with an adjusted body weight (ABW): the ideal body weight (IBW) plus 40% of the excess body weight (EBW). The fluid deficits of a larger patient who has undergone a gastric-bypass procedure, and therefore who has not consumed anything by mouth since the day prior to surgery, will be over 4 L (Sidebar 7-1). This replacement should be readily found on the anesthesia record.

After a gastric-bypass procedure, urine output can be used to help determine a patient's fluid requirements. The caveat is that the standard of 30-cc/hour urine output is insufficient as a guide in the bariatric patient. This is based on the formula of 0.5 to 1.0 cc/kg per hour of urine output as a minimum for the kidney to secrete nitrogenous waste in maximum concentration. For bariatric patients, one must use the ABW, which often places adequate urine output in the range of 50 to 100 cc/hour.

Using urine output as a way to monitor fluid requirements is not useful during a laparoscopic procedure because of increased intra-abdominal pressure (IAP) of the pneumoperitoneum after surgery. With increasing pressure comes compression of the renal arteries and renal veins, which results in obstruction to flow as well as direct compression to the renal parenchyma. At pressures above 10 mmHg, renal function decreases. This is compounded by elevated levels of rennin, angiotensin II, aldosterone, and catecholamines. The added effect of decreased cardiac output from the inhaled anesthetics and increased abdominal and thoracic pressures from the pneumoperitoneum result in a further decrease of urine output. Research supports this: in a group of 104 patients with morbid obesity who were randomly assigned to either open or laparoscopic gastric bypass, the laparoscopic group had 64% lower urine output at 1 hour compared to those undergoing open procedures. Additionally, urine output continued to be 31% to 50% lower in the laparoscopic patients during their operations.[1] After release of the pneumoperitoneum, urine output will increase, as measured by blood urea nitrogen and creatinine, with no kidney dysfunction.[2]

Pulmonary Complications

Postoperative pulmonary complications can be seen in the morbidly obese. Most large series specifically track pneumonia to represent pulmonary complications, and the incidence of postoperative pneumonia can be estimated at 2.6%.[3] However, when considering other pulmonary complications—including effusion, atelectasis, respiratory insufficiency, and pneumonia—the incidence rises to 5.8%[4] or more as atelectasis is underdiagnosed and underreported.

The etiology of pulmonary complications can best be understood in terms of changes in pulmonary-function tests. Most patients with obesity have a higher oxygen consump-

Sidebar 7-1

How to Calculate the Fluid Needs of a Bariatric Patient

1. ***Determine the patient's ABW.*** The patient's actual weight overestimates fluid needs because of the proportionately lower percentage of cardiac output going to the fat stores, but the IBW alone underestimates the patient's fluid requirements.
   - EBW = actual weight – IBW
   - ABW = IBW + 0.40(EBW)
2. ***Determine the patient's fluid deficits before, during, and after surgery.***
   - Deficits coming into the operating room are calculated at 70% of the maintenance fluid for each hour NPO.
   - Add 1200 cc for a bowel prep.
   - Insensible fluid loss during the operation is 8cc/kg/h for an open case and 2 cc/kg/h for a laparoscopic case.
   - The crystalloid replacement for blood loss should be calculated using a 3:1 ratio.
3. ***Maintenance fluid should be calculated using the 4/2/1 rule:*** 4 cc/kg for the first 10 kg ABW, 2 cc/kg for the next 10 kg, and 1 cc/kg for the remainder.

❖ ***For example:*** Calculate the fluid requirement for a 34-year-old, 5′6″, 350-lb woman undergoing a 3-hour laparoscopic gastric bypass with 150 cc of blood loss who has been NPO for 12 hours prior to surgery. (Her IBW is 140 lb.)

EBW = 350 lb – 140 lb = 210 lb

ABW = 140 lb + 0.40(210 lb) = 224 lb

Pounds to kilograms: 224 lb x (1 kg/2.2 lb) = 102 kg

Maintenance fluid (4/2/1 rule): 140 cc/h

Deficit: Bowel prep—1200 cc

NPO prior to surgery: 140 cc/h x 0.7 x 12 h = 1176 cc

OR losses:

140 cc/h x 4 h (3 h OR + 1 h pre- and postsurgery) = 560 cc

Insensible losses: laparoscopic—2 cc/kg/h x 3 x 102 kg = 612 cc

Blood loss: 150 cc x 3 = 450 cc

Total replacement: 1200 cc + 1176 cc + 560 cc + 612 cc + 450 cc = 3998 cc (approximately 4 L)

tion and carbon-dioxide production from the work of moving the obese body. Most patients classified as obese are eucapneic preoperatively and they, therefore, have higher minute ventilation.

Routine spirometry conducted in patients with obesity consistently demonstrates a decrease in the functional residual capacity (FRC), or the volume of air left in the lung after a normal breath. This occurs because there is a thick, noncompliant chest wall with elevation of the diaphragm due to increased IAP from increased visceral fat.

FRC is comprised of 2 components: the expiratory reserve volume plus the residual volume in the lungs. The residual volume cannot change significantly; therefore, most changes to the FRC are due to the changes in expiratory reserve volume. Expiratory

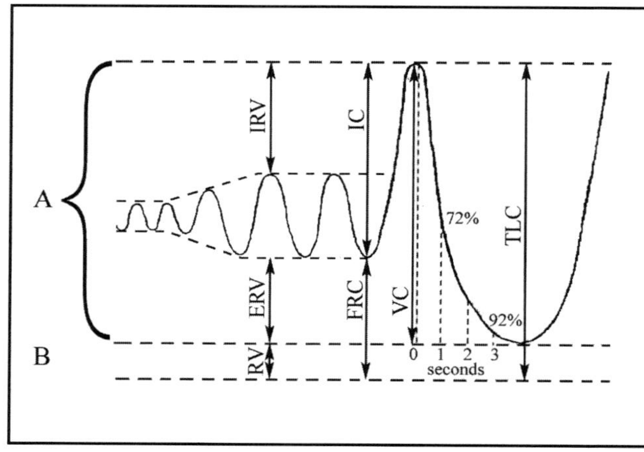

Figure 7-1 (A and B). Normal spirogram. IRV=inspiratory reserve volume; ERV=expiratory reserve volume; RV=residual volume; IC=inspiratory capacity; VC=vital capacity; FRC=functional residual capacity; TLD=total lung capacity. (A) Measured during spirometry. (B) Measured by washout or equilibrium techniques. (Adapted from Vaughn RW.[6])

reserve volume is decreased to 35% of that predicted for a body weight/height ratio greater that 0.7 kg/cm and 60% for a body weight/height ratio greater than 1 kg/cm.[5] The clinical significance of a decreasing expiratory reserve volume with increasing weight gain is evident when one compares it to the closing volume of the lung.

Closing volume is the volume at which dependent lung zones are no longer ventilated because of closure of small airways. Airways that are less than 1.0 mm in diameter do not have cartilaginous support, and they are held open with the resting negative pressure in the lung. (Pleural pressures are typically less than atmospheric pressure.) In patients with a decreased functional residual capacity, negative pressures do not exist in these dependent areas of the lung, resulting in small airways closure. These airways are most dependent in the lung with the greatest amount of blood supply. Perfusion continues in these dependent areas, resulting in a severe ventilation/perfusion mismatch and results in hypoxemia. This has particular importance when one considers body position, especially for the positions a patient might be in on an operating room table (Figures 7-1 and 7-2). When an individual with obesity is in the supine or the Trendelenburg position, the patient's tidal volume will be below the closing capacity, causing small airway closure. The consequence is further ventilation-perfusion mismatch and hypoxemia.

Another important problem is that, after an extended time with the dependent airways closed, this section of the patient's lung collapses, producing atelectasis. Keeping the patient with morbid obesity flat or in the reverse Trendelenburg position for much of the surgery will minimize atelectasis. These concepts are also important in the patient's postoperative care: specialized beds with footboards can allow heavy patients to assume a sitting position to optimize their pulmonary mechanics. Indeed, one of the first lines of treatment for a bariatric patient in respiratory distress is to assume a head-up position. The most important method of prevention is early ambulation.

When the abnormalities of spirometry become more pronounced, a patient with obesity suffers from the obesity hypoventilation syndrome (OHS). OHS is characterized by hypoxia and hypercapnea while the patient breathes room air. One half of these patients will have polycythemia from the hypoxia as well as pulmonary HTN. The presence of OHS increases a patient's risk of anesthesia-related, as well as postoperative respiratory, complications.

General anesthesia in the bariatric surgical patient worsens the dysfunction of an already compromised pulmonary system. Anesthetic agents such as sedatives or narcotics can decrease the drive to breathe. The induction of general anesthesia with intubation

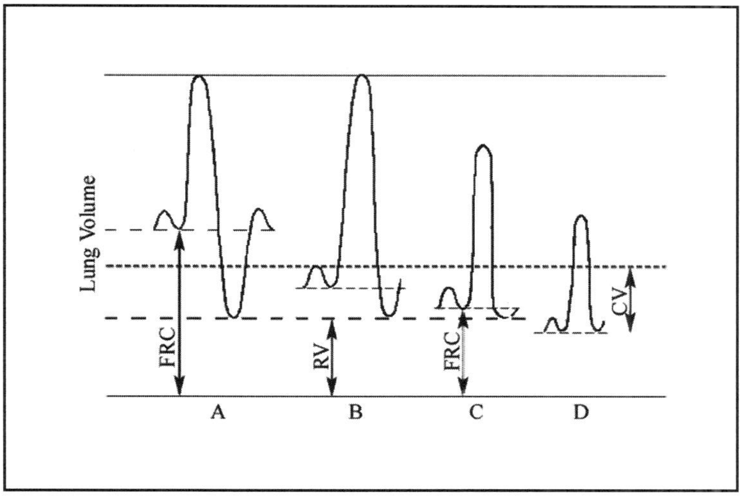

Figure 7-2 (A, B, C, and D). Spirograms with changing weights and body positions. FRC=functional residual capacity; RV=residual volume; CV=closing volume. (A) Lung volume in nonobese patient. (B) Lung volume in patient with obesity in upright position. (C) Lung volume in patient with obesity in supine position. (D) Lung volume of patient with obesity in Trendelenburg position. (Adapted from Vaughn RW.[6])

and paralysis will further reduce the FRC. The monotonous tidal ventilation provided with mechanical ventilation results in a gradual collapse of the alveoli and atelectasis. (See Chapter 5 for details.)

Other risk factors that the provider should consider when evaluating a bariatric patient's risk of pulmonary problems are incision type, surgical technique, and length of operation. Studies show that an upper-midline abdominal incision is a risk factor for increased postoperative pulmonary complications most likely due to the associated splinting.[7] There have been no significant differences in pneumonia rate when comparing series of patients undergoing laparoscopic and open gastric bypasses; however, rates of other pulmonary complications are lower in laparoscopic groups.[8] Length of operation is associated with increased pulmonary complications, with a "longer" operation (increased risk) defined as one that lasts longer than 3 to 4 hours.[7]

Atelectasis is the first and most frequent pulmonary problem to be encountered postoperatively. The effects of anesthesia, the absence of sigh breaths to reinflate the lungs, and the use of narcotics to depress respirations continue to reduce the FRC after surgery. An upper abdominal incision will reduce tidal volumes by 20%, resulting in an increased respiratory rate to maintain minute ventilation. Atelectasis is suggested by arterial hypoxemia on a blood gas or low oxygen saturation with routine monitoring. Clinically significant atelectasis can be seen on a chest x-ray. Treatment is incentive spirometry, early ambulation, optimal pain management, and elevation of the patient's head and chest in bed. Early intervention is critical, as prolonged atelectasis can lead to pneumonia.

The same factors that put a patient at risk for atelectasis also put him or her at risk for pneumonia. Additional factors specific for pneumonia are the decreased ability to cough after surgery because of the incision and colonization of the respiratory tract with Gram-negative bacilli. Colonization can occur because of prolonged intubation, presence of a nasogastric (NG) tube, acidosis, and hypoxemia.[9]

Clinical presentation of pneumonia in a bariatric patient is fever, tachypnea, and low oxygen saturation. The diagnosis can be made by a 2-view chest x-ray or a chest computed tomography (CT) scan. Either will show consolidation and effusions. The treatment incorporates the same therapy as for atelectasis as sputum culture and broad-spectrum antibiotics. The postoperative pneumonias in the bariatric patient can be polymicrobial because of microaspiration. Other important treatment adjuncts are to support the patient with oxygen and to maintain the patient in a head-up position. Vigorous chest physiotherapy will help clear secretions, a problem that is more pronounced in the bariatric patient.

The key to reducing postoperative pulmonary complications in the obese is prevention. Patients should undergo pulmonary-function tests preoperatively, with arterial blood gases in patients with BMI >50 who have history of pulmonary dysfunction, OHS, or sleep apnea to help assess risk. More aggressive prevention should be prescribed in those with the greatest pulmonary dysfunction. As pulmonary risk is weight related, patients should be encouraged to lose weight before surgery. Smoking should be stopped at least 1 month prior to surgery. During the bariatric procedure, the patient should be kept in reverse Trendelenburg as much as possible to help prevent small-airway closure. (This requires proper placement of a footrest and support on the operating room table to prevent the patient from slipping.) The length of time the patient lies on the operating room table—including the pre- and post incision times—should be kept to a minimum. Long-acting local anesthetic, such as bupivicaine, should be used in the wounds.[10] Pain medication should be administered using patient-controlled analgesia to help optimize the amount of narcotic used. The patient should also use lung-expansion techniques including incentive spirometry and early ambulation.

Postoperatively, and particularly on the first night after surgery, patients with OHS or sleep apnea are at a high risk for respiratory distress because of their baseline hypercarbia. These patients will have redistribution of the lipid-soluble sedative medications, which can occur many hours after surgery. Fentanyl, a commonly used opioid, has a rapid distribution from plasma to skeletal muscle and fat. In bariatric patients, the fat serves as a reservoir, slowly releasing the drug back into the plasma. Plasma concentrations can be maintained for long periods, producing elimination half-life times of 3.1 to 7.9 hours.[11] This corresponds to when the patient leaves the recovery room. These patients should be transferred to an area of the hospital where continuous oxygen saturation and their pulses can be closely monitored.

For the patient who does develop respiratory distress, the initial treatment is supportive. Oxygen and bronchodilator should be administered immediately while data are gathered. Arterial blood gas and a chest x-ray will help determine if the problem is primarily pulmonary (atelectasis, pneumonia, etc) or is due to oversedation. It is very important that the physician remember that tachypnea, shortness of breath, and low oxygen saturation can also result from increasing lactic acidosis associated with an abdominal catastrophe, such as a leak.

Prolonged Mechanical Ventilation

As patients with morbid obesity have multiple comorbidities associated with their obesity—with pulmonary comorbidity documented in 49%—prolonged postoperative ventilatory support (for more than 24 hours) should be anticipated for some patients. Patients who are male and older than 50 years with a BMI >60 are more likely to require this.[12]

Revisional surgery and reoperation also increase the risk of prolonged ventilatory support. Revisional surgeries are often more complex that the initial operation, and additional adhesions formed since the initial operation can make these operations very long. The additional dissection will cause more tissue edema and fluid sequestration in the abdomen, which results in increased abdominal pressure; resulting increased IAP impinges on the lungs and negatively affects pulmonary mechanics. Because the full effects of tissue edema in the abdomen are not evident until hours after surgery, the physician should seriously consider leaving the patient intubated overnight in the intensive care unit until pulmonary mechanics can be optimized.

Leak

The most serious immediate postoperative complication is an intestinal leak. Leakage is the second most frequent cause of death in bariatric patients, after pulmonary embolism.[13] Numerous series have reported on this complication, with rates from less than 1% to as high as 6% and with a higher leak rate in a laparoscopic series, especially early in a surgeon's experience. Additionally, a higher rate of leaks is found in male bariatric patients. A leak can cause peritonitis, sepsis syndrome, multiorgan system failure, and death. The most important principle in addressing a leak is making an early diagnosis, which will lead to early treatment and reduce both the associated morbidities such as an abscess or fistula and death.

The most common site for a leak after a gastric bypass is the gastrojejunal anastomosis. All staple lines used in creating the pouch have the potential to leak including those on the remnant stomach side, on the side of the new pouch, or of the small-bowel anastomosis. These are rarely the source of a leak. When the gastrojejunal anastomosis leaks, it is often related to surgical technique, including excessive tension on the anastomosis, improper stapling, and narrowing or occluding the distal bowel.

Tension on the anastomosis occurs when the small bowel is placed in the upper abdomen to anastomose it to the gastric pouch. Patients with obesity—and especially those with central obesity—have thicker, more rigid small-bowel mesentery that makes placing the intestine in the upper abdomen more difficult. Whether a surgeon's approach is to bring the jejunum in front or behind the colon (ante- or retro-colic), the small bowel may be stretched; there are a number of surgical techniques that can be used to reduce this tension. If a stapled anastomosis is performed, a staple height that is too short for the thickness of the tissue will not allow the staples to fully close and, over time, will not hold the tissue together. A sutured anastomosis may cause ischemia of the tissue. If the bowel distal to the gastrojejunal anastomosis is narrowed or occluded, back pressure can cause a leak at the proximal (gastrojejunal) anastomosis. Common sites for narrowing or occlusion are as the bowel passes behind the transverse colon or at the jejunojejunostomy. These points emphasize the difficulties associated with this anastomosis and the reasons for its higher leak rate. Other, less technical issues associated with leaks are male gender, age, and BMI.[14]

Because the gastrojejunal anastomosis is the most common site of a leak, once it has been completed, its integrity is tested intraoperatively, either with methylene blue or oxygen. For the methylene-blue test, the patient is placed in reverse Trendelenburg with an NG tube in the new gastric pouch while the jejunum is occluded, usually with an instrument. Methylene blue is allowed to run into the pouch. Extravasation of methylene blue is monitored while the infusion is continued until the pouch is stretched with the dye. If no blue is seen, the test is considered negative. In the second test commonly employed—the oxygen test—oxygen is allowed to flow into the pouch. The anastomosis is held under a pool of irrigant to make sure there is no bubbling. If either test is positive, the site of the leak is identified and the anastomosis is reinforced with sutures until the test is negative.

Most surgeons leave a closed suction drain behind the anastomosis if the procedure is conducted laparoscopically. This has 2 purposes: first, to help early identification of a leak, and second, to drain the leak, which increases the chances of nonoperative management.[15]

To diagnose a leak, one must be vigilant for the clinical symptoms and signs. The morbidly obese are more difficult to examine and may not display the usual signs and symptoms of abdominal sepsis, especially in the postoperative period. Clinical symptoms

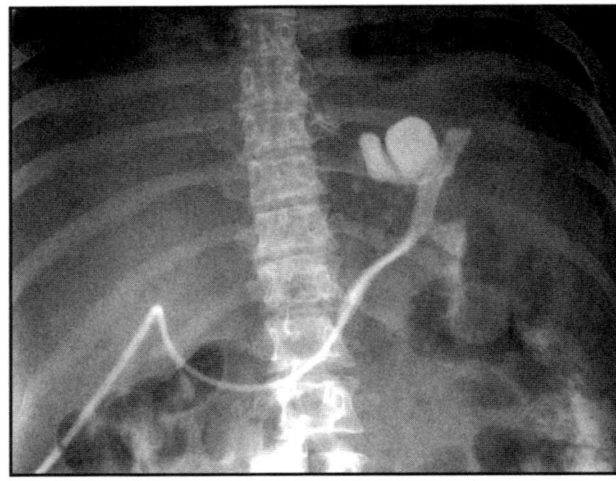

Figure 7-3. Nonoperative management of a leak at the gastrojejunal anastomisis. Contrast can be seen in the gastric pouch, distal small bowel and in the surgical drain. There is no undrained collection. This patient was fed via a G-tube (Foley balloon visible in remnant stomach), until the leak healed.

of a leak are abdominal pain, nausea, left shoulder pain, and shortness of breath. Signs of a leak include fever, tachycardia, tachypnea, pleural effusion, hyperglycemia, oliguria, or leukocytosis. The 2 most sensitive signs in predicting a leak are tachycardia (>120 beats per minute) and acute respiratory distress.[16]

When a leak is suspected, prompt diagnosis is mandatory. The 3 most common methods of diagnosis are an upper gastrointestinal (UGI) series, and an abdominal CT scan (Chapter 11), or to return to the operating room to either open the abdomen or investigate with a laparoscope. The UGI study is often used in diagnosing a leak at the gastrojejunal anastomosis; however, when routinely used, it may only detect 22% of leaks.[16] A CT scan can also detect leaks, better evaluate the other parts of the gastrointestinal (GI) tract, and give information about undrained fluid collections in the peritoneal cavity.[17] Another advantage of the CT scan is that any fluid collection can be percutaneously drained. If either test is equivocal, early laparoscopy or laparotomy can confirm the diagnosis and be the first step in treatment. A patient with unexplained tachycardia and respiratory distress should return to the operating room if a leak cannot be ruled out by CT or UGI.

The primary treatment of a leak is adequate drainage. Because surgeons (especially those who perform the surgery laparoscopically) routinely place closed suction drains near the anastomosis, some leaks require no further surgical therapy. This approach can be taken when there are no signs and symptoms of sepsis, and contrast can be seen evacuated by the drain on either CT or UGI (Figure 7-3).

When the leak is not controlled by the closed suction drain or a percutaneously placed catheter, or if the patient is clinically deteriorating, exploration is mandatory. The primary goal of the surgical procedure is adequate surgical drainage, usually accomplished by placement of more closed-suction drains. The secondary goal is repair of the leak. At reoperation, tissue is usually too friable or inflammation too intense for the surgeon to see the leak or to perform an adequate repair. The surgeon should place a gastrostomy tube (G-tube) in the remnant stomach for decompression and subsequent feeding. A patient with a leak will not be able to take food by mouth until the leak has sealed, which may be a prolonged period. Nutrition will either be parenteral (TPN) or, if a G-tube is placed, enteral. With the G-tube, a stable patient can feed himself or herself enterally at home while waiting for an adequately controlled leak to seal.

Obese patients have higher intra-abdominal resting pressure,[18] and the intraperitoneal effects of a leak are tissue edema and bowel distension. Consequently, the surgeon may consider leaving the patient's abdomen open after re-exploration. Closing the abdomen can result in intra-abdominal HTN and abdominal compartment syndrome, which can then lead to the cascade of tissue hypoperfusion, multisystem organ failure, and death. Once the sepsis has resolved and the edema has subsided, the abdomen can be closed. This often leaves the patient with a large ventral incisional hernia, which can be repaired successfully with the best results achieved after the bariatric surgical weight loss.

After a leak has been treated, supportive medical therapy should be initiated. Ventilatory support is often needed. Fluids must be adequately replaced according to the inflammatory response of the patient. Nutrition should be initiated, either intravenously through a central line or enterally if the patient has a G-tube or jejunostomy tube. Antibiotics and antifungal agents should be started, and deep venous thrombosis (DVT) prophylaxis should be continued. Often, these leaks can take a long time to seal; however, a majority of cases do seal with adequate drainage, optimal nutrition, and time. Successful closure should be confirmed by an UGI study. Once the leak has sealed, oral intake can be started, and the drains can be removed if oral intake is tolerated.

With a high index of suspicion, early diagnosis, and prompt therapy, morbidity and mortality can be greatly reduced.

Deep Venous Thrombosis/Pulmonary Embolism

Pulmonary embolism is the most common cause of death following gastric-bypass surgery.[13] Obesity and surgery are 2 of the cumulative risk factors for venous thromboembolism (VTE), as are increasing age, immobility, and heart or respiratory failure.[19] The incidence of VTE in series of open gastric-bypass surgeries is 0.36% to 3% and in laparoscopic series, 0.2% to 1.3%.[13] The risk increases with a history of venous stasis disease.[19]

The differences in incidences of pulmonary embolism between open and laparoscopic gastric bypass were not significant, despite the perceived risks of laparoscopy (eg, decreased flow in femoral veins due to the pneumoperitoneum, longer time positioned in reverse Trendelenburg, and potentially longer operative times). The theoretical benefits of laparoscopy—including decreased activation of the coagulation system and stimulation of fibrinolysis—have been demonstrated with differences in D-dimer, anti-thrombin III, and protein C.[20] Likely, the most important difference in favor of laparoscopy is the patient's ability to ambulate more easily after the operation.

Diagnosis of VTE in the obese is difficult. DVT may not be clinically evident in these patients; however, if suspected, it can be confirmed by duplex ultrasonography. To diagnose a pulmonary embolism, a contrast-enhanced spiral CT has been recommended as the test of choice.[21] In bariatric patients who exceed the table's weight limit, clinical suspicion alone warrants anticoagulation. A pulmonary angiogram can confirm the diagnosis if the patient does not exceed the weight limit of the fluoroscopy table.

The treatment of a pulmonary embolism is similar to that in other surgical patients—immediate initiation of intravenous unfractionated heparin with close monitoring of the partial thromboplastin time. Low-molecular-weight heparin should not be used in the obese because of the variable effects of standard weight-based dosing.[22] To properly dose low molecular weight heparin in the obese, continual monitoring of anti-factor Xa levels is necessary to titrate the effects. For patients who cannot be anticoagulated or who continue to have VTE while anticoagulated, vena cava filter is indicated.

There is no uniform consensus for thromboprophylaxis prior to bariatric surgery. Most bariatric surgeons use 1 or more of the 3 common forms of prophylaxis: sequential compression devices, unfractionated heparin, or low-molecular-weight heparin.[23] The first, sequential compression devices, has a theoretical advantage in a laparoscopic patient, as they partially reverse the reduced femoral return caused by the pneumoperitoneum.

Unfractionated heparin, the second prophylaxis, is given 3 times a day, in the usual dose of 5000 IU, and is given preoperatively for the patient to have full benefit. The third form is low-molecular-weight heparin, which comes in many forms and can be dosed once or twice a day. There is still controversy as to when the first dose should be initiated: either preoperatively or immediately after surgery. Studies comparing the dose of low-molecular-weight heparin tend to favor higher doses without increases in bleeding.[19,24] Regardless of the preoperative strategy used, all patients should be ordered to ambulate the first night after surgery. This requires nursing staff that know the importance of this order, as the patient may refuse. A nurse might be tempted to accept the refusal given the size of the patient, level of sedation, the number of tubes and lines, etc. Ambulating a patient with morbid obesity after surgery is not an easy task, is considered risky, and thus often requires more than one person. Good planning by the surgical team is required with limitations in personnel.

For particular high-risk patients, preoperative vena cava filter has been recommended. In 1 study, male patients who had BMI >60, obstructive sleep apnea, and venous stasis disease were at significantly increased risk to warrant consideration of a filter.[25] Other patients needing vena cava filters are those whose pulmonary comorbidities are great enough that even a small pulmonary embolism would not be survivable. In these patients, retrievable vena cava filters may be useful.

Postoperative Hemorrhage

The incidence of postoperative hemorrhage after RYGB ranges from 0.5% for the open procedure to 4.4% for the laparoscopic approach.[26] The difference in incidence is due to differences in technique between the 2 approaches. A stapled gastrojejunal anastomosis is more commonly used in the laparoscopic approach as opposed to a hand-sewn anastomosis with the open technique. Differences in tissue thickness and staple height can contribute to increased bleeding in a stapled anastomosis. Oversewing staple lines can decrease bleeding but can also increase tissue ischemia.

Postoperative hemorrhage will occur either inside the intestine (intraluminal), presenting as a GI bleed, or in the peritoneal cavity (intraperitoneal), presenting as bloody drainage output or more often as occult hypovolemia and/or shock. Intraluminal sites of bleeding are from any of the staple lines: the gastrojejunal anastomosis, the jejunojejunostomy, the gastric pouch, or the excluded stomach. When a staple line bleeds, it is either from the transected edge of tissue or at the point where a staple transects a vessel. Intraluminal bleeding may occur while the surgeon is still operating, but because the bleeding is taking place inside the stomach or small intestine, it is often not seen. Intraperitoneal causes of bleeding can be from the cut tissue edges of the gastric pouch or gastric remnant, the cut edges of mesentery, spleen or short gastric bleeding, or from the trocar sites (especially those near the epigastric vessels). Bleeding from these sites occurs after the surgeon has left the abdomen, and, in the case of laparoscopy, the bleeding may start when the pressure effect of the pneumoperitoneum has been removed.

The symptoms of postoperative hemorrhage are tachycardia, hypotension, and oliguria. These may be accompanied by hematemesis, melena, or bloody drainage output. More subtle bleeding can present as a decreasing hematocrit. There is no good diagnostic test for postoperative bleeding. Upper endoscopy can be used when the source is believed to be at the gastrojejunal anastomosis; however, this test poses the risk of perforation of the newly formed, small gastric pouch, especially if a therapeutic intervention is performed. Bleeding scans and angiograms have little place in the algorithm.

The treatment of bleeding relies on the principle that most occurrences of postoperative hemorrhage are self-limited and will respond to conservative measures. Initial treatment is volume resuscitation and discontinuation of heparin. Serial hematocrits should be used to guide the threshold for transfusion. Coagulopathy should be ruled out by routine laboratory tests. For the unstable patient or for ongoing bleeding, abdominal exploration is indicated, with either laparoscopy or a laparotomy. The time of presentation of the bleed after surgery often can predict the need for exploration. Those that present early (<24 hours postoperatively) are more likely to need exploration.[27]

Intra-abdominal bleeding sources are corrected by abdominal exploration. Often the source is not seen, but the decompression of the abdomen and the removal of the peritoneal clots stop the bleeding. Sources that are seen are easily corrected; these include mesenteric bleeding vessels that are oversewn and bleeding vessels from trocar sites that are ligated. A significant diagnostic dilemma occurs when the bleeding source is inside the bowel. An intraoperative upper endoscopy can help make a diagnosis and treat the problem if it is within reach of the scope. Clots that can potentially obstruct the gastrojejunal anastomosis can be cleared. If the bleeding cannot be seen endoscopically, the surgeon can oversew the staple lines in an effort to oversew the bleeding vessel. Most authors advocate that it is unnecessary to identify the source of the bleed, and treatment should be to oversew all staple lines at the time of reoperation.[28] If the remnant stomach is sufficiently dilated, a gastrostomy is made to evacuate clots. Most often, staple-line bleeding stops spontaneously.

Wound Infection

The incidence of wound-infection rates after gastric bypass varies from 3% for the laparoscopic approach to 6.6% in the open approach, with some laparoscopic series reporting rates as low as 0.1%[29] and some open series reporting rates as high as 20%.[30]

Patient's undergoing gastric-bypass surgery have a higher incidence of type 2 diabetes mellitus, which has shown to be an independent risk factor for surgical-site infections, as well as lower tissue-oxygen tension, because of the increase in fat-tissue mass without concomitant increase in blood flow per cell.[31] Gastric-bypass surgery is considered a clean contaminated operation because the surgeon opens the GI tract and thus puts patients at risk for infections from both skin and GI-tract flora. Wound-infection cultures are predominantly skin flora (*Staphylococcus aureus*) but can also contain Gram-negative rods. In laparoscopic cases, there is often a single trocar site that becomes infected more frequently than do others, this site often being the port through which intestinal trimmings and instruments used in the GI tract are extracted. Thus, there can be direct contamination of the subcutaneous tissue with GI-tract flora.

Treatment of a wound infection is the opening of the wound. When an infection is in a laparoscopic port, it involves the opening of the skin to allow adequate drainage down to the level of the fascia. This also applies to a midline incision, which, because of the wound's size, often requires skilled nurses to do the dressing changes with a longer healing time. Erythema of the wound or purulent drainage requires antibiotic coverage. This should be initially broad-spectrum coverage, using the Gram-stain and wound-culture results to narrow the antibiotic coverage. It should be noted that a wound infection after a laparoscopic procedure is not associated with an increased hernia rate, whereas there *is* an increased hernia rate with infection of the midline wound in an open case.

Prevention of a wound infection relies on proper use of preoperative antibiotics. Adequate antibiotic prophylaxis involves 3 components: antibiotic choice, dose, and dosing interval. For UGI surgery, the recommended antibiotic is kefzol, which primarily addresses skin flora. The UGI tract, where the surgeon is working, typically has a low rate of bacterial colonization. This can be altered by use of histamine-receptor blockers or proton pump inhibitors, which decrease stomach acid and promote bacterial overgrowth. Although it has not been studied prospectively, many groups also dose flagyl preoperatively to help decrease infection rate with Gram negatives. Tissue levels of kefzol have been studied in the obese, and the standard 1-g dose has been shown to be inadequate because of tissue levels below the minimum inhibitory concentration. It is suggested that antibiotic dose be based on BMI, using the following formula: dose of kefzol = 0.0422 x BMI.[32] For example, the dose of kefzol for a patient with a BMI of 50 (super obese) would be 0.0422 x 50 or 2.11 g, and for a BMI of 65 would be 2.7 g, usually rounded to 3 g.

The dosing interval of any prophylactic antibiotic should be 2 times the half-life of the antibiotic. The half-life of Kefzol is 1.8 hours; therefore, this antibiotic should be redosed after 3.5 to 4 hours of the original dose if the procedure is ongoing. Because the first dose of antibiotic should be given 30 minutes to 2 hours before an incision is made, redosing is often necessary. In most cases, antibiotics do not need to be continued beyond the operation.

Surgical technique also impacts wound-infection rate. Attempts at minimal spillage should be made during the operation. Instruments that have entered the bowel and surgical trimmings of stomach or small-intestinal tissue should be removed through trocars whenever possible. Protecting the wounds from direct contact with enteric contents is paramount. Copious irrigation of the wound before closure should be done. A separate closing table for open procedures should be entertained.

Recently, the comorbidity of diabetes has been associated with increased surgical complications—particularly infections. In patients with morbid obesity, it is important to control the blood glucose level. Difficulty controlling blood sugars may predispose the patient to complications; frequently, however, uncontrollable glucose levels indicate the presence of another complication, such as infection.

Renal Failure

Oliguria after obesity surgery may result because of many different causes. Hypovolemia should be the first cause considered, with immediate attention to adequate replacement of lost fluids (see above). Oliguria can also be a sign of sepsis from a leak, of acute tubular necrosis from intraoperative hypotension, or of rhabdomyolysis, which has become more frequently reported with obesity operations.

Rhabdomyolysis is a syndrome caused by injury to skeletal muscle that results in the release of intracellular muscle contents into the circulation. Prolonged positioning on an operating-room table has been implicated as a cause in other surgical patients with obesity as a risk factor.[33] Rhabdomyolysis represents a spectrum of disease ranging from no clinical symptoms to muscle pain, oliguria, renal failure, and possible death. It is also associated with major pressure or decubitus skin complications. There have been numerous recent articles in bariatric literature discussing this as a potential complication of surgery,[34-36] with an estimated incidence of up to 22.7% if defined by a rise in serum creatinine phosphokinase (CPK) greater than 1050 IU/L, but only 1.4% if defined by clinical symptoms such as muscle pain. It is more common in males, and, obviously, the incidence increases with longer operative times and elevated BMI.

Care providers should suspect this syndrome in patients with reddish-brown pigmented urine that tests heme negative on a urine dipstick that indicates myoglobinuria. It should also be in the differential diagnosis of oliguria in the bariatric patient. Diagnosis is easily made by measuring serum CPK levels. Prompt diagnosis is critical to avoid the more serious complication of renal failure.

Treatment for rhabdomyolysis is plasma volume expansion with intravenous isotonic saline, which should be done as soon as the diagnosis is made. This increases renal perfusion and the urine-flow rate, thus eliminating any obstructing casts. Patients will require large volumes of fluid because of third spacing in the injured muscle. Although controversial, traditional treatment has been a forced alkaline-mannitol diuresis.[37] The addition of sodium bicarbonate to the resuscitative fluid increases the solubility of the myoglobin, whereas the mannitol increases the diuresis and acts as a free radical scavenger. During the treatment phase, the patient's health care provider should monitor serum potassium, calcium, phosphate, and creatinine. If a patient develops acute renal failure, dialysis should be initiated.

To prevent this complication, operative time should be minimized whenever possible, particularly for the super obese. In patients with longer operative times and high BMI, a postoperative CPK should be checked.

Retained Foreign Body

In any abdominal surgery, a retained foreign body, such as a surgical instrument or a sponge, is more likely when a patient is obese (increasing incidence with increasing BMI), when the surgical plan changes, or when the surgery is emergent.[38] The conversion of a laparoscopic procedure to an open operation meets 2 of the 3 listed criteria and thus increases the chances of a retained instrument. When the conversion is done because of bleeding, a third criterion is added and thus the risk is significantly increased. In these situations, it is recommended that the surgeon obtain a routine abdominal x-ray at the end of the case to ensure that no foreign body is retained, even if the procedure counts are correct. With a laparoscopic case, instruments are never completely placed in the abdominal cavity and sponges are usually always outside the abdomen. However, other objects, such as a Penrose drain or ruler, may be routinely placed in the abdomen during a laparoscopic procedure; they should be part of the procedure count because of the possibility for retention.[39]

Small-Bowel Obstruction

Small-bowel obstruction in the immediate postoperative period is an unusual occurrence in an open gastric bypass but is more common with the laparoscopic approach, with incidences in the range of 1% to 2%.[13] The etiology of the obstruction is either a narrowing of the small-bowel anastomosis, a narrowing at the level of the transverse mesocolon, or a twisted limb of bowel.[40] Diagnosis is usually first made on clinical grounds with nausea, vomiting, and the inability to tolerate fluids often demonstrated very early in the postoperative period. An abdominal or UGI series or a CT scan can confirm the clinical suspicions; these tests may require that contrast pass through the 100 cm of the small-bowel limb to see the point of obstruction at the jejunojejunostomy (Chapter 11).

Once identified, an immediate postoperative obstruction requires immediate treatment, and the surgeon must take the patient back to the operating room. Narrowing of the bowel as it passes through the mesentery of the colon can be fixed by widening the opening, and if the jejunojejunostomy is narrowed or the small-bowel limb twisted, its anastomosis will need to be revised. Either procedure can be done laparoscopically.

Sepsis

The most common cause of sepsis in the bariatric patient is a postoperative leak, which can trigger severe systemic inflammation and cause organ dysfunction. The treatment of a bariatric patient who shows signs of sepsis are to search for and correct, if necessary, any leak, while critical, nonsurgical supportive measures are taken to prevent progression of the syndrome and potential death.

An early sign of the sepsis is acute respiratory deterioration often requiring immediate resuscitation including intubation, a procedure that can be very difficult in an unstable patient with morbid obesity. Ventilating the septic bariatric patient will be very challenging. The patient's pulmonary compliance is decreased because of a heavy chest wall, which worsens with fluid resuscitation; therefore, initial tidal volumes should be set between 6 and 8 ml/kg of lean body mass, with frequent adjustments made based on changes in airway pressures and tidal volumes.

Hemodynamic monitoring plays a critical role in the supportive care of these patients. Blood-pressure cuffs may be unreliable in the best settings, but with the threat of hypotension, blood pressure in this setting should be monitored continuously with an arterial line. Central venous access may also be required but can be difficult to obtain. The internal jugular route is preferred, but a lack of landmarks may make this difficult. Ultrasound guidance may be required to assist in the approach to this vein.[41] A complication with a subclavian line, such as a pneumothorax, can add significant morbidity to an unstable patient. The needle in a standard central-line kit through which the wire is passed is often not long enough to reach the subclavian vein because of the thickness of the chest wall, and longer wires should be available. These patients require large volumes of resuscitative fluids, amounts that most clinicians are not used to. Under-resuscitation is often a problem. Fluids should be replaced to support a urine output of 0.5 cc/kg based on ABW.

In the case of sepsis in the bariatric patient, a leak is not always the source. Routine blood, urine, and sputum cultures should be obtained and broad-spectrum antibiotics started. Routine radiologic studies include a chest x-ray to look for pneumonia and an abdominal CT to look for a leak or abscess.

If the patient meets criteria for severe sepsis syndrome, as defined by the American College of Chest Physicians,[42] the health care provider should consider administration of drotrecogin alfa. Dosing is strictly weight based, although maximum dosing should be based on a weight no greater that 175 kg, which balances efficacy with cost effectiveness.[43]

Death

Recent literature addresses risk factors that predispose bariatric patients to death, with the most universally recognized combination being gender, age, and BMI.[44] Male gender has been associated with death and is likely related to fat distribution. Males have a higher distribution of intra-abdominal fat than do females, which makes surgery of the abdomen more difficult. In addition, the weight-related comorbidities are more frequent and often more severe in males.

Operative approach influences death rates. The open procedure is associated with a higher death rate than is the laparoscopic (0.87% versus 0.23%),[13] despite a higher leak rate in laparoscopic surgeries. There is also a slightly higher but not significant incidence of pulmonary embolism with the open approach, and pulmonary embolism accounts for 50% of the deaths after gastric-bypass surgery.

Surgeon experience also influences death rates. In a recent study in Pennsylvania, surgeons who performed fewer than 10 gastric-bypass procedures a year had a 5% risk of death, compared to a risk of death of 0.3% for high-volume surgeons.[45]

Procedure-Specific Complications: Laparoscopic Adjustable Gastric Banding

The immediate postoperative complications of laparoscopic adjustable gastric banding (LAGB) occur less frequently than do those after other forms of obesity surgery. The advocates of this approach value the fewer postoperative complications over less excess-weight loss, although, in some series, LAGB results in long-term weight loss are similar to those of RYGB at 5 years.[46] The immediate postoperative complications of a banding procedure include all those of a surgical procedure on a patient with morbid obesity (respiratory failure, DVT, etc) but at a lower rate. This is likely because banding requires shorter operative times and leaves the GI tract in continuity. The specific immediate postoperative complications of gastric banding include perforation of the stomach, obstruction at the level of the device, and port-site infections.

Perforation

Perforation of the stomach occurs in 0.8% of LAGB procedures[47] and is associated with surgeon experience.[48] Perforation is usually discovered either at the time of surgery or via UGI series and can be repaired laparoscopically or by an open technique. When discovered on a postoperative UGI series, treatment is removal of the band (a foreign body in a contaminated field) and repair of the perforation. A decision to convert to an alternative operation for obesity is then considered, although a safe approach is to consider this for a later surgery.

Obstruction

Obstruction at the level of the band has become a more frequent occurrence with the adoption of the pars flaccida technique of band placement. Although this technique is easier and has resulted in a marked decrease in band slippage rates, it leads to incorporation of more posterior gastric fat, which can lead to obstruction.[49] Diagnosis is made during an esophogram done routinely on the first postoperative day. Abnormal esophograms can reveal either complete esophageal obstruction or significantly delayed emptying. Patients with complete obstruction present with retching and inability to tolerate their own saliva. Return to the operating room is recommended for removal of the perigastric fat pads. Resolution of the occlusion is demonstrated during the operation by passage of an NG tube into the distal stomach. Delayed emptying can be treated by enteral or intravenous (no oral) nutrition, drainage with an NG tube, anti-inflammatory medications, and expectant management. Resolution of symptoms occurs usually within a few days. Obstruction can be avoided by the routine removal of the perigastric fat pads or the use of the larger Bioenterics Lap-Band VG System (Inamed Health; Santa Barbara, Calif). This band has a larger stomal area and is designed for patients of larger BMI who have substantial amount of visceral obesity or thicker stomach walls.

Port Infection

Because of the presence of a foreign body, port-site infection after gastric banding poses a unique problem. Incidence of this is much lower than is the wound-infection rate after RYGB, most likely because the GI tract is not entered. The diagnosis of a port infection is made by clinical evaluation for infection—pain, swelling, warmth, and erythema. Antibiotics should be the first line of therapy; if the infection does not clear, however, the port must be removed. This can be done under local anesthesia with placement of the tubing into the abdominal cavity to be reconnected after a suitable time has elapsed for the infection to clear (usually 3 months).

Summary

Surgery for obesity should be considered a high-risk procedure in a high-risk patient population. It carries with it the potential for significant perioperative complications, including death. Having surgery performed by well-trained surgical teams, with knowledge of the potential complications and methods to prevent them, is essential. In dealing with the immediate postoperative complications in a bariatric surgical patient, it is important to have early recognition and early aggressive management. These principles coupled with an experienced health care provider and a medical center that is a center of excellence for bariatric surgery will reduce the morbidities and the mortality.

References

1. Nguyen NT, Perez RV, Fleming N, Rivers R, Wolfe BM. Effect of prolonged pneumoperitoneum on intraoperative urine output during laparoscopic gastric bypass. *J Am Coll Surg.* 2002;195(4):476-483.
2. Chang DT, Kirsch AJ, Sawczuk IS. Oliguria during laparoscopic surgery. *J Endourol.* 1994;8(5):349-352.
3. Livingston E, Procedure incidence and in-hospital complication rates of bariatric surgery in the United States. *Am J Surg.* 2004;188:105-110.
4. Schauer PR, Ikramuddin S, Gourash W, Ramanathan R, Luketich J. Outcomes after laparoscopic Roux-en-Y gastric bypass for morbid obesity. *Ann Surg.* 2000;232:515-529.
5. Ray CS, Sue DY, Bray G, Hansen JE, Wasserman K. Effects of obesity on respiratory function. *Am Rev Respir Dis.* 1983;128(3):501-506.
6. Vaughn RW. Anesthesia and the obese patient. In: Brown BR, ed. *Contemporary Anesthesia Practice.* Philadelphia, Pa: FA Davis Co.; 1982(5): 26.
7. Brooks-Brunn JA. Predictors of postoperative complications following abdominal surgery. *Chest.* 1997;111:564-571.
8. Winslow ER, Brunt LM. Perioperative outcomes of laparoscopic versus open splenectomy: a meta-analysis with an emphasis on complications. *Surgery.* 2003;134(4):647-653.
9. Anand PK, Ralph-Edwards A, Deitel M. Pulmonary complications in obesity surgery. *Obes Surg.* 1992;2:327-331.
10. Papagiannopoulou P, Argiriadou H, Georgiou M, Papaziogas B, Sfyra E, Kanakoudis F. Preincisional local infiltration of levobupivacaine vs ropivacaine for pain control after laparoscopic cholecystectomy. *Surg Endosc.* 2003;17(12):1961-1964.
11. McClain DA, Hug CC Jr. Intravenous fentanyl kinetics. *Clin Pharmacol Ther.* 1980;28(1):106-114.
12. Helling TS, Willoughby TL, Maxfield DM, Ryan P. Determinants of the need for intensive care and prolonged mechanical ventilation in patients undergoing bariatric surgery. *Obes Surg.* 2004;14(8):1036-1041.

13. Podnos YD, Jimenez JC, Wilson SE, Stevens CM, Nguyen NT. Complications after laparoscopic gastric bypass: a review of 3464 cases. *Arch Surg.* 2003;138:957-961.

14. Livingston EH, Ko CY. Assessing the relative contribution of individual risk factors on surgical outcome for gastric bypass surgery: a baseline probability analysis. *J Surg Res.* 2002;105:48-52.

15. Chousleb E, Szomstein S, Podkameni D, et al. Routine abdominal drains after laparoscopic Roux-en-Y gastric bypass: a retrospective review of 593 patients. *Obes Surg.* 2004;14(9):1203-1207.

16. Hamilton EC, Sims TL, Hamilton TT, Mullican MA, Jones DB, Provost DA. Clinical predictors of leak after laparoscopic Roux-en-Y gastric bypass for morbid obesity. *Surg Endosc.* 2003;17(5):679-684.

17. Yu J, Turner MA, Cho SR, et al. Normal anatomy and complications after gastric bypass surgery: helical CT findings. *Radiology.* 2004;231(3):753-760.

18. Sanchez NC, Tenofsky PL, Dort JM, Shen LY, Helmer SD, Smith RS. What is normal intra-abdominal pressure? *Am Surg.* 2001;67(3):243-248.

19. Geerts WH, Pineo GF, Heit JA, et al. Prevention of venous thromboembolism: the Seventh ACCP Conference on Antithrombotic and Thrombolytic Therapy. *Chest.* 2004;126(Suppl 3):338S-400S.

20. Nguyen NT, Owings JT, Gosselin R, et al. Systemic coagulation and fibrinolysis after laparoscopic and open gastric bypass. *Arch Surg.* 2001;136(8):909-916.

21. Fedullo PF, Tapson VF. Clinical practice. The evaluation of suspected pulmonary embolism. *N Engl J Med.* 2003;349:1247-1256.

22. Hirsh J, Warkentin TE, Shaughnessy SG, et al. Heparin and low-molecular-weight heparin: mechanisms of action, pharmacokinetics, dosing, monitoring, efficacy, and safety. *Chest.* 2001;119(Suppl 1):64S-94S.

23. Wu EC, Barba CA. Current practices in the prophylaxis of venous thromboembolism in bariatric surgery. *Obes Surg.* 2000;10:7-14.

24. Scholten DJ, Hoedema RM, Scholten SE. A comparison of two different prophylactic dose regimens of low molecular weight heparin in bariatric surgery. *Obes Surg.* 2002;12(1):19-24.

25. Sapala JA, Wood Mh, Schuhknecht MP, Sapala MA. Fatal pulmonary embolism after bariatric operations for morbid obesity: a 24-year retrospective analysis. *Obes Surg.* 2003;13(6):819-825.

26. Mehran A, Szomstein S, Zundel N, Rosenthal R. Management of acute bleeding after laparoscopic Roux-en-Y gastric bypass. *Obes Surg.* 2003;13(6):842-847.

27. Nguyen NT, Longoria M, Chalifoux S, Wilson SE. Gastrointestinal hemorrhage after laparoscopic gastric bypass. *Obes Surg.* 2004;14(10):1308-1312.

28. Nguyen NT, Rivers R, Wolfe BM. Early gastrointestinal hemorrhage after laparoscopic gastric bypass. *Obes Surg.* 2003;13(1):62-65.

29. Higa KD, Ho T, Boone KB. Laparoscopic Roux-en-Y gastric bypass: technique and 3-year follow-up. *J Laparoendosc Adv Surg Tech A.* 2001;11:377-382.

30. Christou NV, Jarand J, Sylvestre JL, McLean AP. Analysis of the incidence and risk factors for wound infections in open bariatric surgery. *Obes Surg.* 2004;14(1):16-22.

31. Kabon B, Nagele A, Reddy D, et al. Obesity decreases perioperative tissue oxygenation. *Anesthesiology.* 2004;100(2):274-280.

32. Forse RA, Karam B, MacLean LD, Christou NV. Antibiotic prophylaxis for surgery in morbidly obese patients. *Surgery.* 1989;106(4):750-756.

33. Lachiewicz PF, Latimer HA. Rhabdomyoslysis following total hip arthroplasty. *J Bone Joint Surg Br.* 1991;73(4):576-579.

34. Khurana RN, Baudendistell TE, Morgan EF, Rabkin RA, Elkin RB, Aalami OO. Postoperative rhabdomyolysis following laparoscopic gastric bypass in the morbidly obese. *Arch Surg.* 2004;139(1):73-76.

35. Mognol P, Vignes S, Chosidow D, Marmuse JP. Rhabdomyolysis after laparoscopic bariatric surgery. *Obes Surg.* 2004;14(1):91-94.

36. Wiltshire JP, Custer T. Lumbar muscle rhabdomyolysis as a cause of acute renal failure after Roux-en-Y gastric bypass. *Obes Surg.* 2003;13:306-313.

37. Eneas JF, Schoenfeld PY, Humphreys MH. The effect of infusion of mannitol-sodium bicarbonate on the clinical course of myoglobinuria. *Arch Intern Med.* 1979;139:801-805.

38. Gawande AA, Studdert DM, Orav EJ, Brennan TA, Zinner MJ. Risk factors for retained instruments and sponges after surgery. *N Engl J Med.* 2003;348(3):229-235.

39. Oliak D, Ballantyne GH, Davies RJ, Wasielewski A, Schmidt HJ. Short-term results of laparoscopic gastric bypass in patients with BMI > or = 60. *Obes Surg.* 2002;12(5):643-647.

40. Papasavas PK, Caushaj PF, McCormick JT, et al. Laparoscopic management of complications following laparoscopic Roux-en-Y gastric bypass for morbid obesity. *Surg Endosc.* 2003;17:610-614.

41. Miller AH, Roth BA, Mills TJ, Woody JR, Longmoor CE, Foster B. Ultrasound guidance versus the landmark technique for the placement of central venous catheters in the emergency department. *Acad Emerg Med.* 2002;9(8):800-805.

42. Bone RC, Balk RA, Cerra FB, et al. Definitions for sepsis and organ failure guidelines for the use of innovative therapies in sepsis. The ACCP/SCCM Consensus Conference Committee. American College of Chest Physicians/Society of Critical Care Medicine. *Chest.* 1992;101:1644-1655.

43. Savel RH, Pulipati RC, Mangone-Cholewczynski C, Lazzaro RS, Macura JM, Lehman HE. Use of drotrecogin alfa (activated) in bariatric surgery patients with severe sepsis syndrome: experience in an urban community teaching hospital. *Obes Surg.* 2004;14:107-115.

44. Fernandez AZ Jr, DeMaria EJ, Tichansky DS, et al. Experience with over 3,000 open and laparoscopic bariatric procedures: multivariate analysis of factors related to leak and resultant mortality. *Surg Endosc.* 2004;18(2):193-197.

45. Courcoulas A, Schuchert M, Gatti G, Luketich J. The relationship of surgeon and hospital volume to outcome after gastric bypass surgery in Pennsylvania: a 3-year summary. *Surgery.* 2003;134(4):613-621.

46. O'Brien PE, Dixon JB. Lap-band: outcomes and results. *J Laparoendosc Adv Surg Tech A.* 2003;13(4):265-270.

47. Chapman AE, Kiroff G, Game P, et al. Laparoscopic adjustable gastric banding in the treatment of obesity: a systematic literature review. *Surgery.* 2004;135(3):326-351.

48. Chevallier JM, Zinzindohoue F, Douard R, et al. Complications after laparoscopic adjustable gastric banding for morbid obesity: experience with 1,000 patients over 7 years. *Obes Surg.* 2004;14(3):407-414.

49. Shen R, Ren CJ. Removal of peri-gastric fat prevents acute obstruction after lap-band surgery. *Obes Surg.* 2004 Feb;14(2):224-229.

Color Atlas

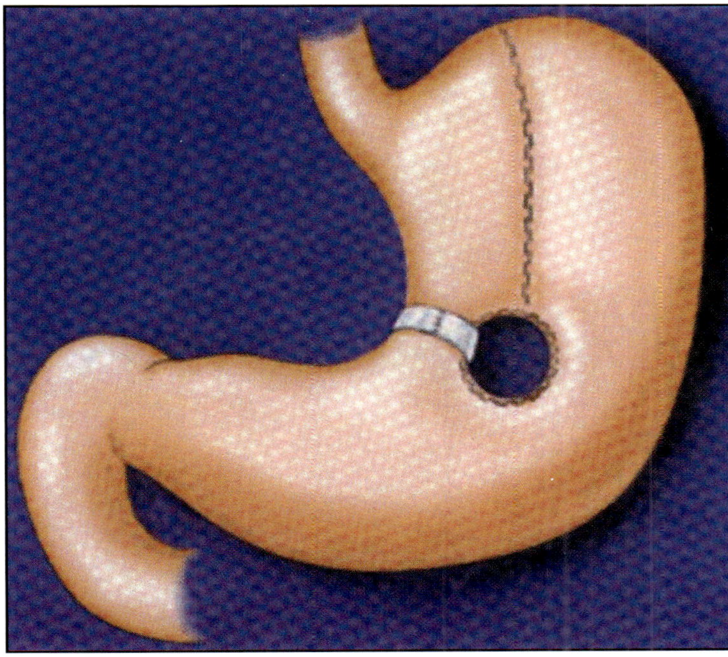

Figure 3-1. Diagram of VBG. (Reprinted, with permission of Dr. Michel Gagner and Springer-Verlag, from Gentileschi P, Kini S, Catarci M, Gagner M. Evidence-based medicine: open and laparoscopic bariatric surgery. *Surg Endosc*. 2002;16:736-744.) *Also shown on page 49.*

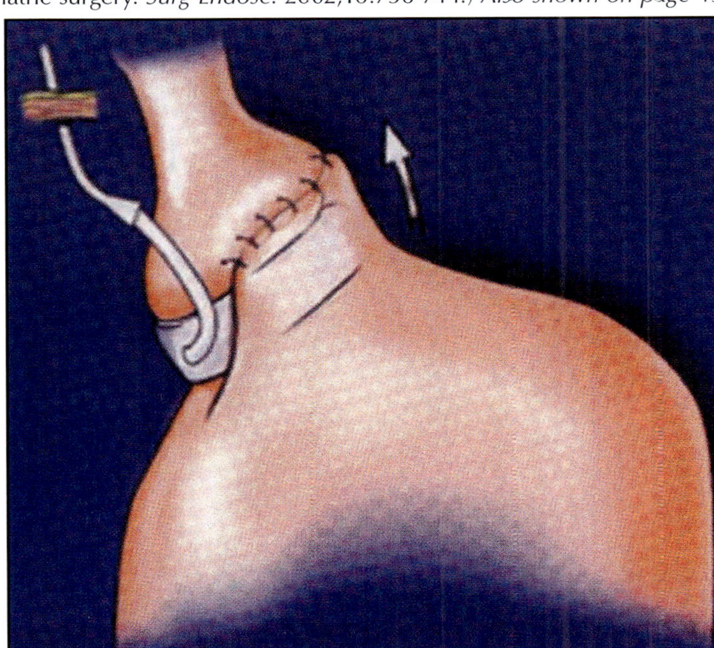

Figure 3-2. Diagram of LAGB. (Reproduced, with permission of Dr. Michel Gagner and Springer-Verlag, from Gentileschi P, Kini S, Catarci M, Gagner M. Evidence-based medicine: open and laparoscopic bariatric surgery. *Surg Endosc*. 2002;16:736-744.) *Also shown on page 50.*

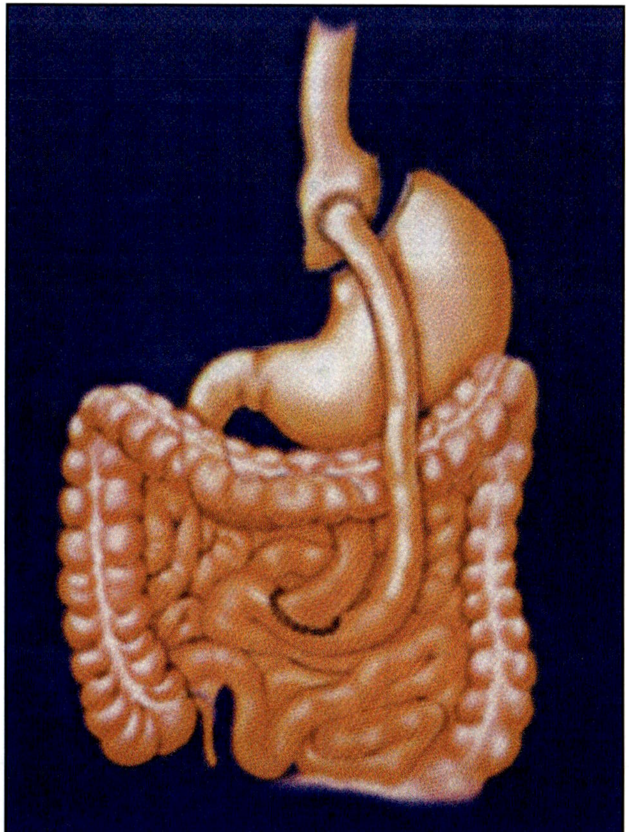

Figure 3-3. Diagram of RYGB. (Reproduced, with permission of Dr. Michel Gagner and Springer-Verlag, from Gentileschi P, Kini S, Catarci M, Gagner M. Evidence-based medicine: open and laparoscopic bariatric surgery. *Surg Endosc.* 2002;16:736-744.) *Also shown on page 52.*

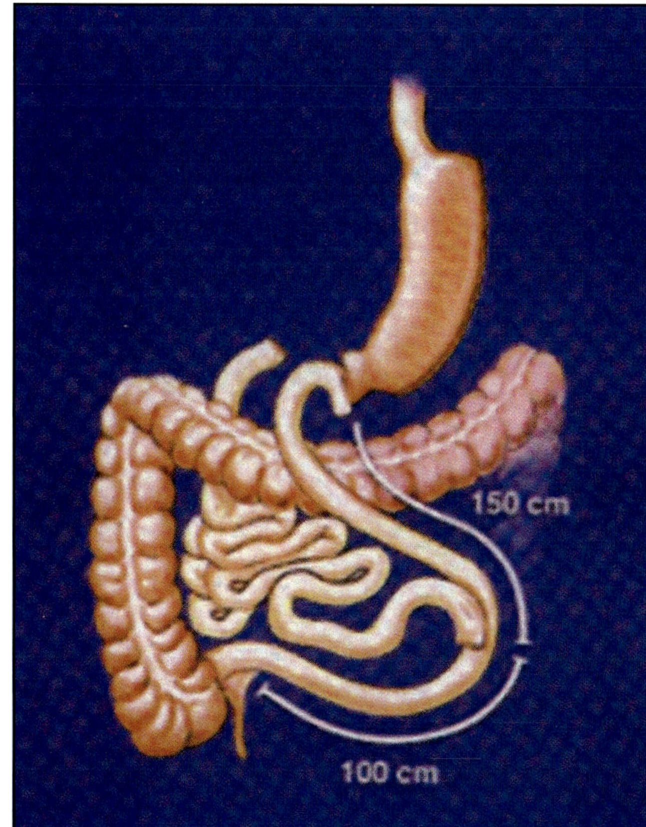

Figure 3-4. Diagram of BPD/DS. (Reproduced, with permission of Dr. Michel Gagner and Springer-Verlag, from Gentileschi P, Kini S, Catarci M, Gagner M. Evidence-based medicine: open and laparoscopic bariatric surgery. *Surg Endosc.* 2002;16:736-744.) *Also shown on page 53.*

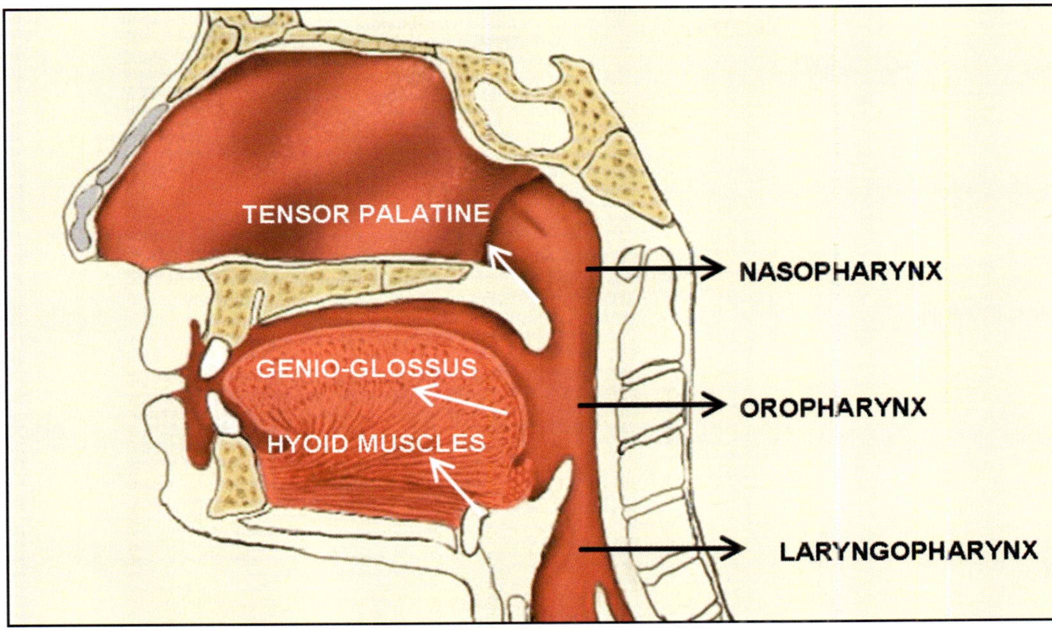

Figure 5-1. Upper airway dilator muscles. *Also shown on page 87.*

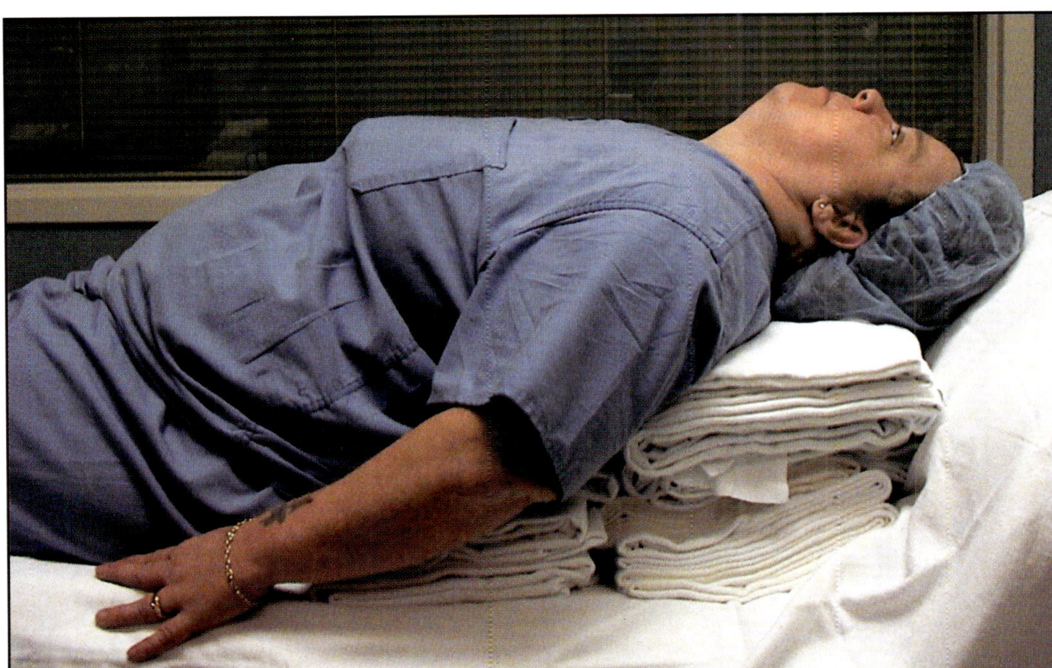

Figure 5-2. Positioning for intubation. The head, neck, and shoulders should be properly elevated with the external auditory canal—at the same level as the top of the sternum—to facilitate intubation. *Also shown on page 89.*

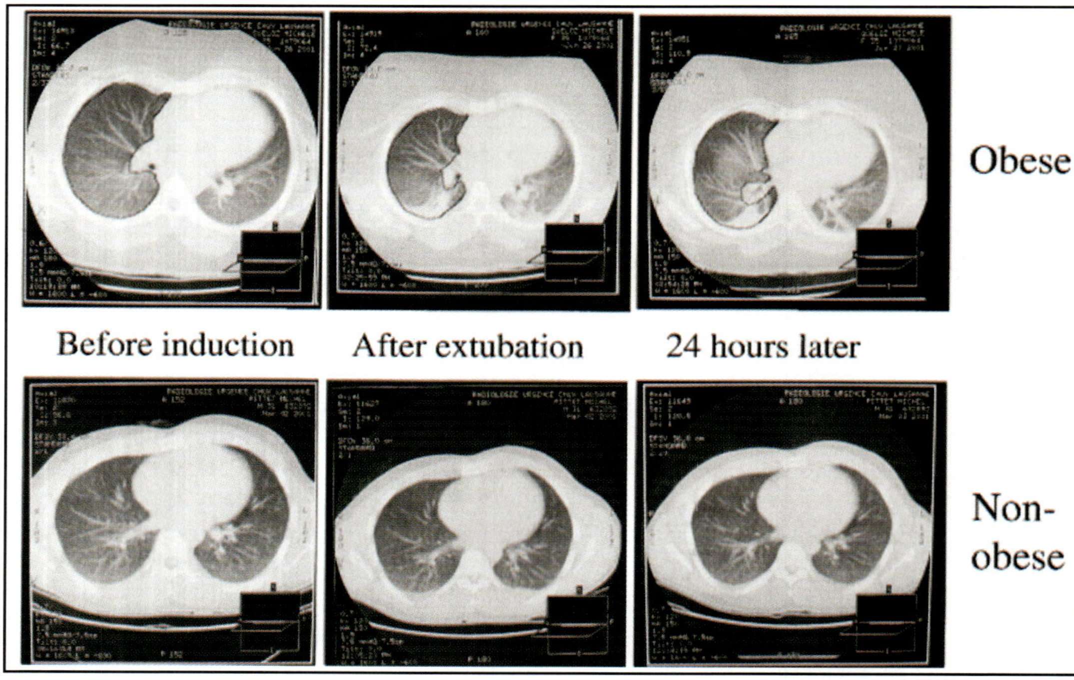

Figure 5-3. Atelectasis following surgery in obese and nonobese patients. Computerized tomography scans in one nonobese patient and in one morbidly obese patient before anesthesia induction, after extubation, and 24 hours post-surgery. The slices are at the level of the interventricular septum. (Reproduced, with permission of Dr. L. Magnusson and Lippincott Williams & Wilkins, from Eichenberger A, Proietti S, Wicky S, et al.[71]) *Also shown on page 98.*

Figure 9-1. Example sketch of a RYGB. A=gastric pouch formed after stomach is stapled and separated into two sections. B=stoma (also "outlet" or "anastomosis") where a limb of separated jejunum is brought up and stapled to the pouch to form the gastrojejunostomy; C=gastric remnant/antrum; and D (blue line with arrow)=alimentary canal. *Also shown on page 159.*

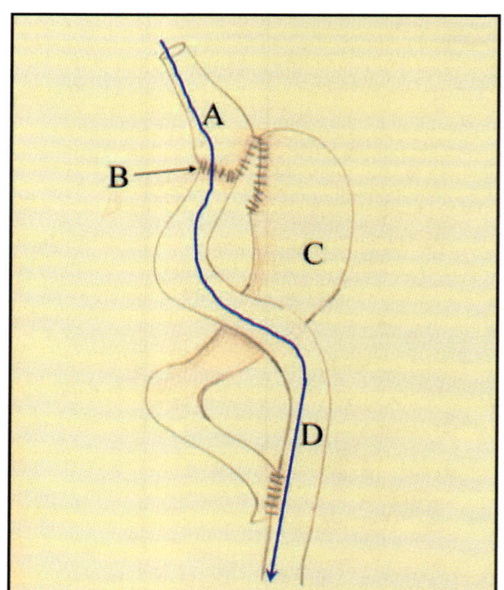

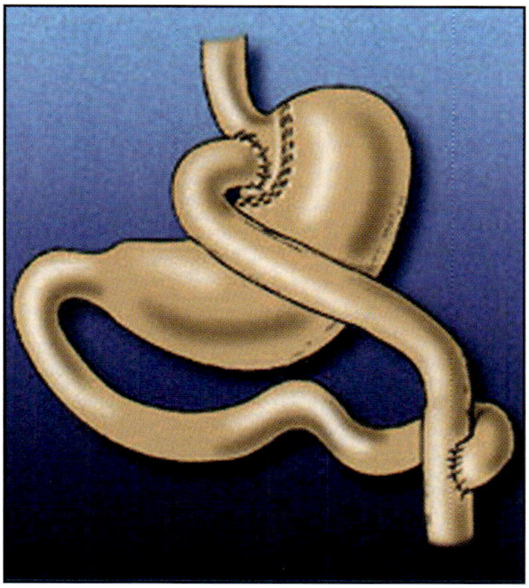

Figure 10-1. Illustration of the RYGB. (Courtesy of the American Society for Bariatric Surgery [ASBS]; Gainesville, FL.) *Also shown on page 185.*

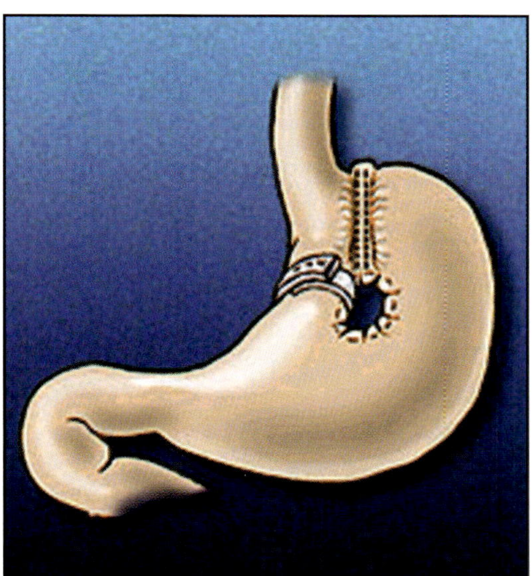

Figure 10-2. Illustration of the VBG. (Courtesy of the ASBS; Gainesville, FL.) *Also shown on page 186.*

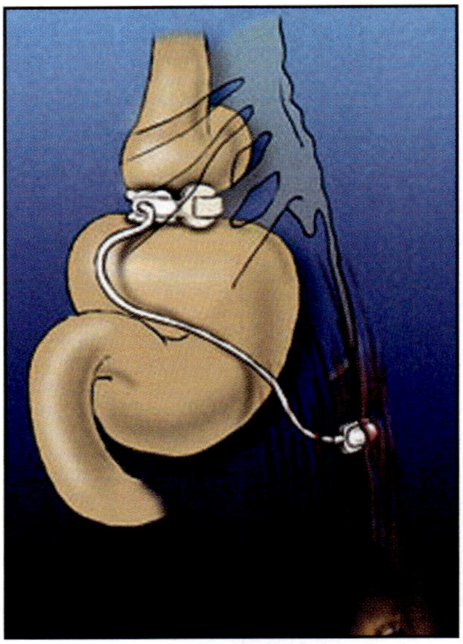

Figure 10-3. Illustration of the LAGB. (Courtesy of the ASBS; Gainesville, FL.) *Also shown on page 187.*

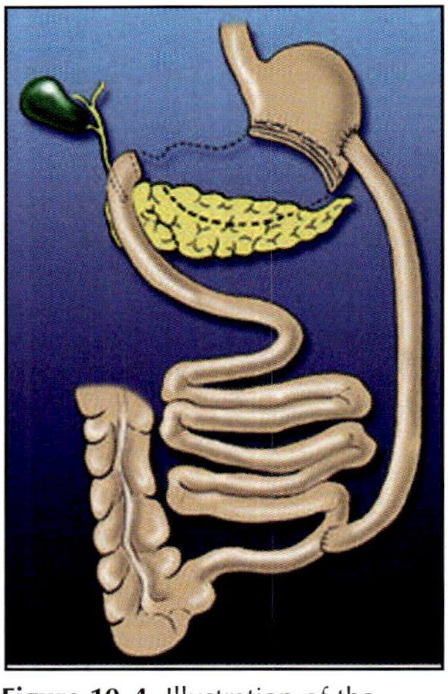

Figure 10-4. Illustration of the BPD. (Courtesy of the ASBS; Gainesville, FL.) *Also shown on page 188.*

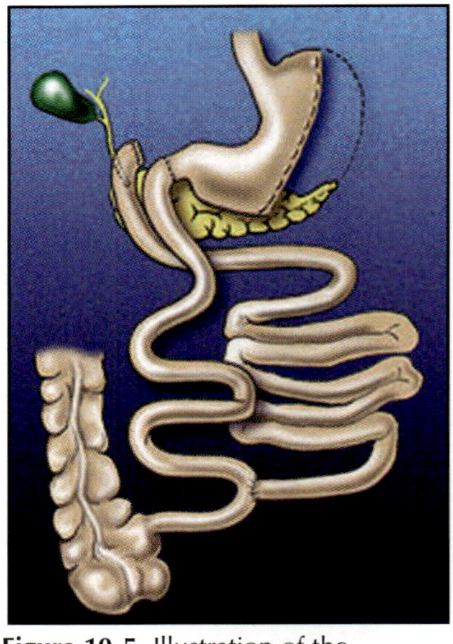

Figure 10-5. Illustration of the BPD/DS. (Courtesy of the ASBS; Gainesville, FL.) *Also shown on page 188.*

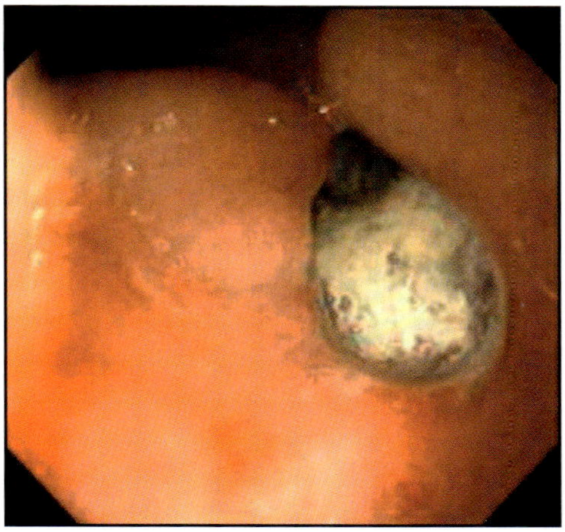

Figure 10-6. Endoscopic appearance of a marginal ulcer following RYGB. *Also shown on page 189.*

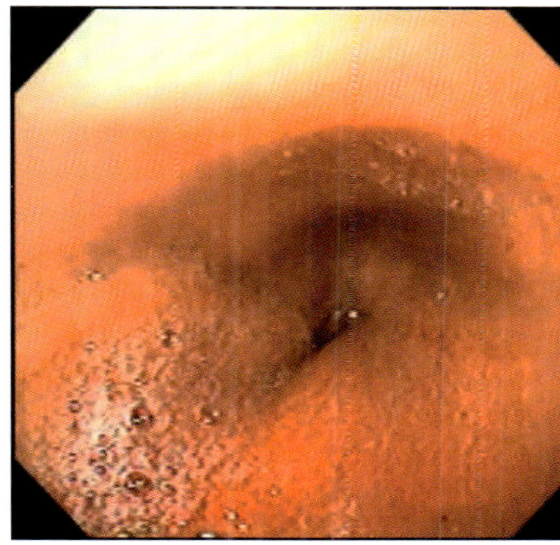

Figure 10-7. Endoscopic appearance of stomal stenosis, characterized by a pinhole orifice in the distal pouch. *Also shown on page 189.*

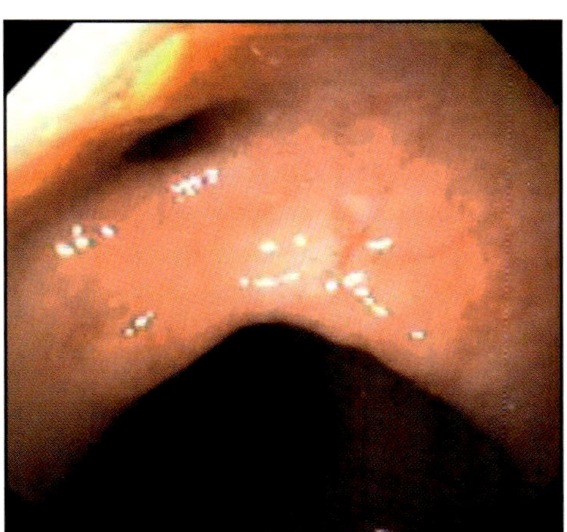

Figure 10-8. Endoscopic appearance of a small staple-line dehiscence within the gastric pouch following RYGB. *Also shown on page 190.*

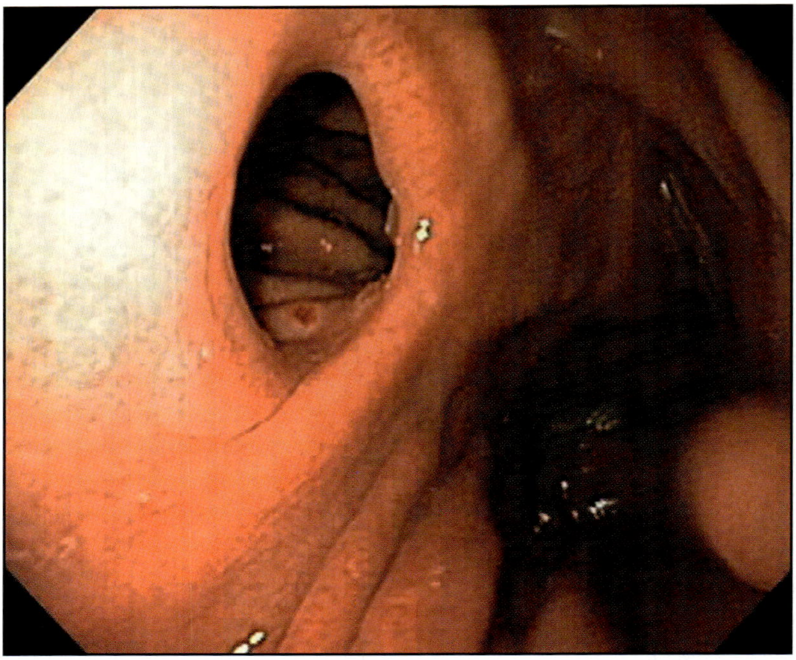

Figure 10-9A. Endoscopic appearance of staple-line dehiscence prior to closure. (Courtesy of Christopher Thompson, MD; Boston, MA.) *Also shown on page 191.*

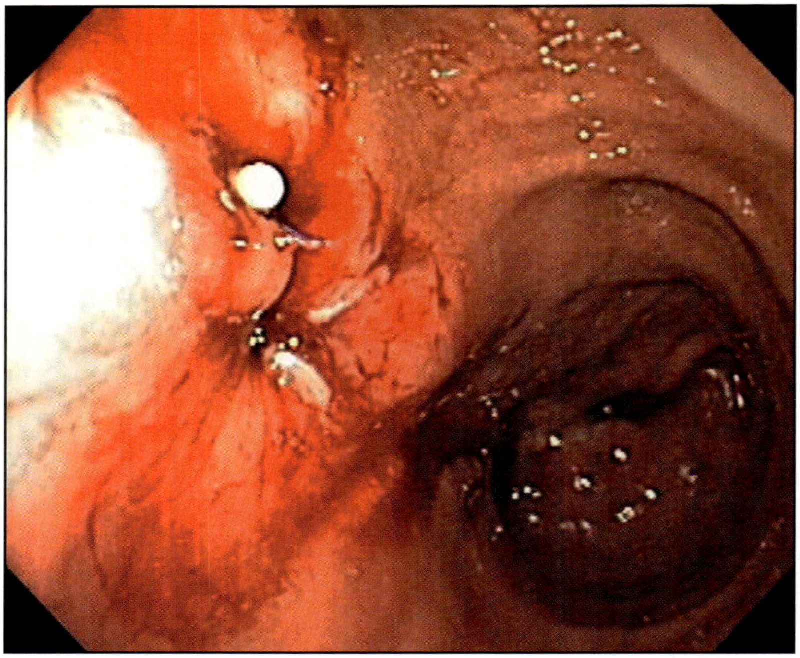

Figure 10-9B. (B) Staple-line dehiscence successfully closed using combination of endoscopic suturing, argon plasma coagulation, and endoscopic clips. (Courtesy of Christopher Thompson, MD; Boston, MA.) *Also shown on page 191.*

8

Nutritional Consequences Following Bariatric Surgery

Wendy A. Anderson, MS, RD, LDN and Laura Foresta, RD, LDN

Introduction

Bariatric surgeries have proven to be efficacious for long-term weight loss, with the Roux-en-Y gastric bypass procedure (RYGBP) yielding the greatest benefit with the fewest complications.[1] These surgeries predispose patients to maldigestion and malabsorption due to the anatomical changes of the stomach and small bowel and the potential for inappropriate dietary and eating behaviors. It is critical that patients fully comprehend the dietary and eating behavior restrictions following bariatric surgery necessitating comprehensive preoperative nutrition education and behavior modification counseling.

The postoperative care of bariatric surgery patients should include a multidisciplinary approach. The dietitian plays a pivotal role in this team approach, in the prevention and treatment of disordered eating behaviors and nutritional deficiencies. Patients with preoperative active eating disorders should not be considered candidates for bariatric surgery unless they undergo treatment with documented resolution of this behavior prior to surgery. However, disordered eating behavior might develop postoperatively, requiring judicious monitoring by the team. Nutrition support following bariatric surgery aims to promote adequate nutrition and hydration to ensure homeostatic support of bodily functions, promote wound healing, and spare lean body mass. The post-bariatric surgery diet should be advanced in stages to achieve adequate nutrition support and food tolerance.[2] The following chapter will delineate the primary nutritional considerations following bariatric surgeries including short- and long-term medical nutrition therapy.

Energy and Macronutrient Needs

Energy

Insufficient data is available to provide evidence-based recommendations for daily energy, protein, carbohydrate, and fat intake following bariatric surgery. Energy intake during the first few months postoperatively might be fewer than 1000 kilocalories daily with a moderate increase during the first year.[2-5] Due to limited data, many programs use the standard recommendations for energy intake and the National Academy of Sciences' Institute of Medicine Daily Reference Intakes (DRIs)[6] for continued weight reduction after the first three months following surgery and for weight maintenance. As dietary intake increases after surgery, energy provided varies with the volume of food and fluid that is tolerated. Daily energy intake usually approaches 400 kilocalories for the first 4 weeks postoperatively. Intake can be expected to increase to 800 to 1000 kilocalories daily by the end of the third postoperative month, with weight loss being most rapid during this time period.

Protein

Protein-kilocalorie malnutrition is uncommon in patients who have had gastric restrictive surgeries such as the RYGBP and vertical banded gastroplasty (VBG) unless an anatomical problem such as stomal stenosis is present leading to food intolerances and poor dietary intake.[7] Adequate protein intake is encouraged postoperatively for improved healing and to maintain adequate visceral protein stores and to decrease loss of lean body mass. Due to the small capacity of the gastric pouch following restrictive surgeries, an increased intolerance to meats might occur. Modular and liquid protein supplements might be necessary to promote adequate daily protein intake. The recommendation for protein intake as indicated by the Betsy Lehman Center Weight Loss Surgery Expert Panel is 1 to 1.5 g/kg ideal body weight (IBW) daily.[2,3,8] High biological value protein sources such as meats (ie, chicken, fish) and dairy (ie, milk, cheese) are encouraged to ensure intake of all essential amino acids for the promotion of wound healing.

As patients become more weight stable, adequate protein intake continues to be encouraged for the preservation and restoration of lean body mass and increased satiety. As is widely accepted, adequate energy intake is required for positive nitrogen balance. It has been noted that protein intake and absorption are compromised due to gastric restriction and intestinal bypass. Decreased availability of pepsin, rennin, and hydrochloric acid might inhibit optimal protein digestion with subsequent intolerances.[3]

Protein malnutrition, particularly the hypoalbuminemic form, is of greatest concern following highly malabsorptive surgeries. Therefore, postoperative protein requirements have been estimated at 90 grams per day from high biological value sources.[9]

Carbohydrate

Carbohydrate intake is gradually increased postoperatively, as outlined in the dietary advancement discussion later in this chapter. Patients should be educated on the types and amounts of carbohydrate to consume using resources such as the ADA Exchange System.[10] Due to limited evidence-based data on macronutrient needs following bariatric surgery, recommendations can be based on the DRIs of 2002 and modified to individual need.

Nutrition education focusing on reading food labels is useful to help patients avoid foods containing large amounts of sugar. Consumption of such foods might lead to the rapid gastric emptying, diarrhea, and gastrointestinal discomfort associated with dumping syndrome, discussed in greater detail later in this chapter. Patients should choose foods with 7 grams or less of sugar per 100-kilocalorie serving. Furthermore, patients should be counseled on avoiding foods containing elevated levels of sugar alcohols due to their laxative effect.[2]

Fat

Significant decreases in dietary intake usually occur up to 1 year postoperatively as a result of gastric restriction, potential food intolerances, and anatomic anomalies. After the first year, the percentage of kilocalories from fat and carbohydrate usually increase while that of protein decreases, as patients begin to tolerate a greater variety of foods. Those patients who maintain higher protein intake and lower fat intake tend to consume fewer kilocalories rendering a better weight loss. This suggests that weight loss efficiency following bariatric surgery might be, in part, associated with a decreased percentage of total kilocalories from fat. Based on these results, dietary recommendations following bariatric surgery should not only focus on total energy intake but also on the distribution of kilocalories from protein, carbohydrate, and fat.[5]

Literature suggests that no more than 25% of total kilocalories should come from fat for a healthy diet following bariatric surgery to promote better weight loss and weight maintenance.[11] Small amounts of fat (approximately 10 grams) at each meal should be encouraged to assist with maintaining gallbladder emptying and minimizing the risk of cholelithiasis, especially during rapid weight loss. This is also recommended in patients who have had a cholecystectomy, to limit symptoms associated with fat malabsorption.

Summary of Macronutrient Needs

Adequate carbohydrate and fat are recommended with an emphasis on protein intake to provide a balanced diet.[4] However, insufficient data is available to provide specific evidence-based recommendations for energy and macronutrient intake. It is prudent that future research focus on long-term nutritional needs following bariatric surgeries to help prevent weight recidivism and nutritional deficiencies.

Micronutrient Considerations

Micronutrient deficiencies might occur in all weight-loss surgery patients regardless of procedure. This is due to reduction in overall food intake and decreased consumption of specific foods or classes of foods such as dairy and red meat. Because of the limited quantity of food consumed, nutritional support is focused on maximizing the quality of these foods. Bariatric surgeries, especially malabsorptive procedures, compromise micronutrient absorption as a result of the relatively low-acid environment of the gastric pouch, impaired binding to carrier proteins, insufficient capacity to liberate food-bound micronutrients, and decreased absorptive surfaces of the small bowel. For these reasons, weight-loss surgery patients are at risk for several deficiencies including vitamin B12, folic acid, vitamin D and other fat-soluble vitamins, calcium, and iron. All preoperative bariatric patients should undergo assessment of micronutrient status with repletion of any deficiencies. Since obesity is generally associated with normal or supranormal bone mineral density, routine preoperative bone density assessment does not appear to be needed; however, assessment might be advisable for postmenopausal women or others at high risk for osteoporosis. The following pages will discuss the primary micronutrient deficiencies with guidelines for prevention and treatment.

Iron

Iron is a trace mineral that is involved in the oxidation and reduction activities of cellular respiration. Iron plays a primary role in red blood cell function, myoglobin activity, and the utilization of multiple heme and nonheme enzymes.[12] The average adult stores approximately 1 to 3 grams of iron with a depletion of about 1 milligram daily, primarily through the shedding of cells from the skin and lining of the intestinal mucosa. However, menstruating women lose an average of 1.5 milligrams daily, increasing their risk for iron-deficiency anemia.[13]

Bariatric surgeries that alter the gut physiology and bypass portions of the small intestine compromise digestion and absorption of iron leading to possible iron deficiency. Iron absorption occurs in the duodenum and proximal jejunum, which are bypassed in the RYGBP and other malabsorptive procedures. Iron requires gastric acid, primarily hydrochloric acid of the stomach, for conversion to its soluble form. Following gastric restrictive intestinal bypass surgeries, both the acid environment of the stomach and available mucosal surface of the small intestine are altered, increasing the risk for iron deficiency with or without anemia.[14,15] Due to the small size of the gastric pouch and decreased acid production, many patients have difficulty tolerating meats containing heme iron, the most bioavailable form. [3]

Iron and ferritin should be measured and deficiencies corrected pre- and postoperatively for the prevention of iron deficiency and subsequent anemias. Serum iron levels tend to decline within the first year after surgery. Supplementation is recommended with a downward trend in serum iron levels to prevent the onset of iron-deficiency anemia.[16] Due to declining iron storage over the long-term, lifelong monitoring is recommended. Patients presenting with iron deficiency should be instructed to take oral iron supplementation within a range of 180 to 220 milligrams of elemental iron daily for repletion of iron stores.[17] Women who menstruate should receive 40 to 65 milligrams of elemental iron prophylactically after gastric restrictive and intestinal bypass surgery. Iron sources such as ferrous sulfate, gluconate, or fumarate are usually recommended daily along with added vitamin C.[14,18] Vitamin C enhances iron absorption due to its role in the conversion from the ferric to the absorbable ferrous form. Iron supplements containing vitamin C are ideal for patients to prevent having to take additional supplements.[18]

Vitamin B12

The primary function of vitamin B12 is to promote normal metabolism of cells, particularly from the nervous system, gastrointestinal tract, and bone marrow.[12] Vitamin B12 deficiency is common following gastric restrictive intestinal bypass surgery.

Contributing factors to vitamin B12 deficiency include food restriction and reduced gastric hydrochloric acid, pepsin, and pancreatic enzymes leading to impaired release of protein-bound vitamin B12 from foods. Vitamin B12 eficiency might be, in part, a result of impaired secretion of intrinsic factor, impaired binding capacity of intrinsic factor with vitamin B12, and bacterial overgrowth as a result of reduced motility of the bypassed small intestine.[19] The onset of this deficiency is usually after the first postoperative year because of enterohepatic recycling of vitamin B12 and the release of hepatic stores. Serum vitamin B12 levels will deplete rapidly without daily multivitamin supplementation and adequate dietary intake of vitamin B12. Patients should be counseled on increasing dietary sources of vitamin B12 such as dairy, meat, and eggs. Supplementation with crystalline vitamin B12 found in multivitamins might prevent deficiency in some patients, and should be prescribed for all postoperative patients not identified as deficient. Vitamin B12 supplementation should be initiated in patients presenting with suboptimal serum vitamin B12 levels. Oral vitamin B12 supplementation of at least 350 micrograms per day is usually adequate; however, with severe deficiency, intramuscular vitamin B12 is recommended.[15,20]

Folate

Folate, a B vitamin, is a coenzyme involved in the metabolism of nucleotides and amino acids,[12] and plays a primary role in the prevention of megaloblastic anemia. The jejunum is the primary site of folate absorption; however, some absorption occurs throughout the small bowel.[21] Approximately 20% of patients develop folate deficiency following gastric restrictive intestinal bypass surgery. Bacterial production of folate in the proximal large bowel might compensate for some of the decreased folate absorption.[21] Intake of high folate-containing food sources such as fortified grains and dark green leafy vegetables should be encouraged, when these foods are reintroduced into the diet. Prevention of deficiency usually can be achieved with daily multivitamin supplementation containing 200 to 400 micrograms of folate.[22]

Thiamin

Thiamin (vitamin B1) deficiency is rare but has been reported following gastric restrictive intestinal bypass surgery.[23] Thiamin plays an important role in energy transformation and neural function. Primary absorption occurs in the jejunum, but thiamin can also be absorbed throughout the small intestine. Excessive vomiting, malnutrition, and alcoholism are contributors to thiamin deficiency, potentially resulting in cranial nerve palsy, peripheral neuropathies, and the encephalopathy associated with Wernicke-Korsakoff Syndrome.[12] As with folate, thiamin deficiency is most often prevented by daily multivitamin supplementation. Oral thiamin supplementation of approximately 10 milligrams daily is usually effective in correcting mild deficiency; however, severe deficiencies require intravenous infusion of 100 milligrams for 7 to 14 days followed by 10 milligrams daily until symptoms resolve.[14] All patients should be monitored for thiamin deficiency, as patients without preoperative risk factors or concurrent alcohol abuse are at risk for deficiencies.

Calcium

Calcium is a mineral essential for the health of bones and teeth, clotting of blood, hormone secretion, nerve function, and cardiac and skeletal muscle contraction.[21] Calcium absorption and utilization is affected by many factors. Reduced exposure to sunlight and diets high in oxalates found in some leafy green vegetables might result in compromised calcium absorption. Diets high in fat, protein, alcohol, and high doses of vitamin A decrease the bioavailability of dietary calcium. Caffeine and sodium, in large quantities, might increase urinary excretion of calcium.[24]

Patients undergoing weight-loss surgeries are at increased risk for developing calcium deficiencies, potentially leading to metabolic bone disease. Contributing factors include:

decreased consumption of foods containing calcium and vitamin D; bypassing the duodenum and proximal jejunum, the primary sites for calcium absorption via active transport; and malabsorption of vitamin D.[15]

Most obese patients have a decreased risk for osteoporosis; however, bone mineral density tends to lessen with weight loss and is usually proportionate to the rate and degree of weight loss and dietary intake of calcium.[25,26] Gastric secretions are more acidic prior to surgery, facilitating optimal calcium absorption. Following gastric restrictive surgery, the acidic environment lessens due to the decreased volume of the gastric pouch, resulting in impaired calcium absorption. Calcium absorption can occur throughout the bowel via passive diffusion; however, the amount of dietary calcium must increase above the recommended allowances to achieve adequate absorption.[14]

Calcium deficiency is more difficult to detect than vitamin and iron deficiencies. Serum levels are not necessarily indicative of calcium status, as multiple mechanisms, such as bone demineralization, exist to maintain serum calcium.[14,19] Serum calcium is bound to albumin and is found free-floating as ionized calcium. Calcium levels may be falsely depleted if serum protein levels are low. It is prudent to obtain ionized calcium levels in these circumstances.[14]

Markers for metabolic bone diseases have been observed as early as three months after surgery, and include increased alkaline phosphatase levels, reduced serum calcium levels, and decreased 25 (OH) vitamin D levels.[27] Hypocalcemia occurs more frequently with procedures inducing a greater degree of malabsorption. Serum calcium, phosphorus, alkaline phosphatase, and 25 (OH) vitamin D levels should be periodically monitored postoperatively. Long-term consequences of altered calcium metabolism have not been well defined.[28] More research is needed to establish conclusive evidence with regard to bone health.

As a result of the potential for metabolic bone disease, the literature suggests lifelong daily supplementation of 1200 to 1500 milligrams of calcium citrate with vitamin D in divided doses, as calcium citrate is the most soluble form in the absence of gastric acid production.[14] Supplemental calcium absorption is most often increased when taken with meals. Calcium and iron tend to compete for absorption, and therefore should be taken at least 1 hour apart.

Vitamin D

Vitamin D is essential for the regulation of normal serum calcium levels and bone health. It is rapidly absorbed in the duodenum, but a greater amount is absorbed in the ileum with the aid of pancreatic and biliary secretions. Due to the bypassing of the duodenum and upper jejunum in gastric restrictive intestinal bypass surgeries, these secretions have less contact with food leading to malabsorption of vitamin D.[19,21] This is generally not seen in solely restrictive bariatric surgeries. Due to the decreased volume capacity of the gastric pouch and variable tolerances to milk-based products, dietary intake is usually inadequate. Compliance with taking multivitamins and calcium with vitamin D, providing approximately 800 International Units (IUs), protects against this deficiency.[23] Supplementation for vitamin D deficiency ranges from 10,000 to 50,000 IUs weekly, tapering as indicated by laboratory indices. In highly malabsorptive surgeries, vitamin D supplementation of 400,000 IUs intramuscularly per month is usually recommended.[9]

Hydration

Hydration guidelines are not well documented in the literature for bariatric surgeries. Hydration requirements are most often estimated by using energy expenditure, age,

Table 8-1
Estimation of Fluid Needs After Bariatric Surgery

Based on Energy Expenditure	
1 mL/kcal estimated energy expenditure	
Based on Age	
30 to 40 mL/kg ABW: 18 to 64 years of age	
30 mL/kg ABW: 55 to 65 years of age	
Based on ABW	
1st 10 kg	**100 mL/kg**
2nd 10 kg	**50 mL/kg**
Each additional kg	**20 mL/kg (≤50 y)**
	15 mL/kg (>50 y)

Adapted from *The Science and Practice of Nutrition Support: A Case-Based Core Curriculum.* Kendall/Hunt Publishing Company; 2001.[29]

and body weight. These calculations are detailed in Table 8-1. As an estimated 25 to 50% of excess weight is metabolically active tissue, it is prudent to use adjusted body weight when calculating daily fluid requirements as follows: (ABW = [actual + (actual-ideal)/4 (or 2 for 50%)]). Generally, an estimate of 50% is used for those patients presenting with a BMI greater than 50 kg/m^2.[29]

Dehydration is commonly seen after gastric restrictive intestinal bypass surgeries. Obese patients require greater amounts of fluid than their nonobese counterparts to maintain normal fluid balance and homeostasis.[30] It is recommended that patients drink no more than 8 fluid ounces of liquid per hour, at least during the first 2 months following bariatric surgery due to increased gastric pouch swelling. While on soft solid food, patients should wait approximately 30 minutes before and after eating 3 ounces of solid food to consume fluids. After beginning a low-fat diet consisting of added fruits, vegetables, and starches, patients should wait approximately 1 hour after meals to drink fluids. Following this fluid intake schedule helps prevent dumping syndrome and vomiting. Noncompliance resulting in dumping syndrome might lead to increased hunger and grazing between meals with decreased weight loss.[15] It is imperative that clinicians promote and monitor for adequate hydration.

Following gastric restrictive procedures, consumption of carbonated beverages tends to result in gastric sequelae[15] such as cramping, bloating, nausea, and vomiting. It is recommended that patients abstain from the consumption of carbonated beverages, especially during the first 6 postoperative months. Caffeinated beverages such as coffee and tea should be avoided in the short-term following most procedures, especially restrictive procedures, due to the potential for increased gastric acid secretion with resulting gastroesophageal reflux.[31,32] Caffeine also induces increased urine output, which can increase risk for dehydration, particularly during rapid weight loss. Caffeinated beverages in moderation may be resumed if hydration is adequate, and the risk for dehydration minimal, as determined by laboratory indices and clinical symptoms such as nausea and faintness.

Dietary Advancement and Eating Behaviors After Bariatric Surgery

The importance of thorough nutrition education for bariatric surgery patients has been indicated at the beginning of this chapter and cannot be overstated. Evidence-based guidelines for dietary advancement have not been established for all of the bariatric procedures currently in use. Recommendations for dietary advancement following bariatric surgery have been compiled based on postgastrectomy nutritional guidelines. Close monitoring of dietary advancement and tolerance by a bariatric dietitian is recommended to avoid potential complications.[2,33]

Short-term postoperative nutritional considerations include adequate intake of protein and fluid and the prevention of vomiting and dumping syndrome. Dumping syndrome is characterized by rapid emptying of food into the jejunum increasing the osmolarity of intestinal contents with a subsequent influx of fluid into the small intestine. It is most common in the early postoperative period and becomes less prominent after the first postoperative year.[19] There is great individual variability in the degree and severity of symptoms. This syndrome is most often precipitated by ingestion of food and beverages with high sugar content, and is prominent in gastric restrictive malabsorptive procedures such as the RYGBP. To avoid symptoms, patients should be instructed to avoid juices, soda, and other high sugar-containing beverages.[15,19] Sensitive individuals should avoid large doses of sugar alcohols; less than 5 grams per serving can be used as a guideline to avoid a laxative effect.

Several stages of dumping syndrome have been observed. The first stage occurs within 10 to 20 minutes after eating and may include abdominal bloating, tachycardia, diaphoresis, flushing, and lightheadedness. The intermediate stage occurs approximately 20 to more than 60 minutes following a meal and presents as abdominal bloating, cramping, flatulence, and diarrhea. Finally, late stage dumping occurs 1 to 3 hours following a meal and is more often a consequence of reactive or alimentary hypoglycemia. Symptoms of this stage most often include diaphoresis, nervousness, lethargy, shakiness, decreased concentration, and increased hunger.[12]

Following gastric restrictive intestinal bypass surgeries, food and liquid intake is minimized due to the small size of the gastric pouch. Immediately postoperatively, the pouch has a capacity of approximately 2 ounces but can increase anywhere from 2 ½ to 9 ounces over time.[33] Due to the small pouch size, it is important for the patient and dietitian to focus on incorporating high-quality, nutrient-dense foods. Fluid and protein goals must be established in achievable, realistic amounts based on the reduced gastric capacity and early satiety of the bariatric surgery patient.

The bariatric surgery diet progresses in a series of stages beginning with liquids and progressively increases in texture. There is great variation among programs in the rate of diet advancement due, in large part, to individual differences in tolerance and readiness to advance.[15,34] The standard postoperative diet consists of 5 to 6 stages, progressing over a 2-month period.

In the immediate postoperative period, patients consume no food or fluid by mouth for approximately 24 hours and are supported with intravenous solutions of dextrose, saline, or lactated ringers to provide adequate hydration. It is recommended that this therapy be continued until patients tolerate a full liquid diet for a minimum of 24 hours. Amino acid/saline intravenous solutions are sometimes provided; however, there is no literature indicating this therapy will result in preservation of visceral protein given the small amount of kilocalories provided and the short duration of the therapy.[35]

Stage 1 of the diet is initiated approximately 24 hours after surgery, and consists of 30 mL per hour of water for a 24-hour period. If tolerated, patients are advanced to Stage 2, consisting of no added sugar clear liquids for another 24 hours. No-added-sugar full liquids are provided in Stage 3 for another 24 hours. In the absence of complications, patients are normally discharged after 24 hours on a Stage 3 diet. Postoperative outpatient follow-up visits are scheduled with both the surgeon and the dietitian. At this time, patients are instructed to begin the Stage 4 high-protein soft-solid diet 3 weeks after surgery, as tolerated. Patients remain on the Stage 4 diet for approximately 1 month. Advancement to the Stage 5 low-fat solid diet occurs when the patient demonstrates tolerance to soft solids. Patients should continue on the low-fat diet indefinitely with modifications made as needed.

Although not well documented in the scientific literature, there appear to be common food intolerances. Typically, patients have difficulty tolerating milk, red meat, dry or tough poultry or pork, bread or doughy starches, and vegetables high in insoluble fiber.[15,19] Over time, tolerance to these foods often improves. Tolerance to diet advancement is facilitated by eating slowly, chewing foods thoroughly, avoiding tough-textured meats, and drinking fluids a minimum of 30 minutes before or after meals. Postoperative vomiting is often subsequent to inappropriate eating behaviors. However, vomiting can also be a sign of an anatomical problem such as an anastomatic stricture or stenosis, which should be ruled out if vomiting persists. Intractable vomiting can potentially lead to serious nutritional sequalae such as protein energy malnutrition (PEM) and thiamin deficiency. PEM is more likely to occur in highly malabsorptive procedures such as biliopancreatic diversion (BPD).[34,36] Table 8-2 illustrates a series of basic recommendations for each stage of the diet following most bariatric surgeries.

There is a need for long-term studies to determine the macro- and micronutrient requirements for patients following bariatric surgery for weight loss. Current recommendations are based on requirements for weight loss and specific complications that arise from the various procedures highlighted in earlier chapters. Dietitians play an important role as members of the medical team to help prevent nutrient deficiencies and maximize nutritional intake for improved tolerance while preserving the desired rate of weight loss. Familiarity with potential complications of each procedure can help the dietitian and patient prevent and, if necessary, treat any feeding difficulties.

Restrictive Surgeries: An Overview

General nutrition recommendations for restrictive surgeries are largely mechanical in nature. Patients are encouraged to consume small amounts of food, with some variability depending on the size of the pouch created. Typically, 1 cup of food is well tolerated at each sitting. To prevent macro- and micronutrient deficiencies, small, frequent meals containing nutrient-dense foods are recommended. Patients are encouraged to chew food thoroughly, until the bolus is nearly liquefied, prior to swallowing. This will aid in digestion and help to allow the food to pass through the small outlet from the stomach into the small intestine. Generally, micronutrient deficiencies are uncommon, as absorptive capacity is unchanged. If patients are unable to consume adequate kilocalories to provide the recommended daily intake of micronutrients, however, supplementation should be considered.[37]

Nausea, vomiting, abdominal bloating, and gastroesophageal reflux are some of the complications that might result from inadequate chewing and consuming portions of food that are too large for the gastric pouch size created. These complications might compromise the integrity of the staple line and contribute to band erosion in gastric band procedures.[38] Record keeping is useful to help patients identify types and quantities of food that might cause discomfort, distress, or intolerance. Patients are encouraged to avoid high-kilocalorie liquids and concentrated sweets because these foods can displace nutrient-dense foods, slow the rate of weight loss, or even result in weight gain.

Postoperative onset of disordered eating can occur as a result of induced vomiting to relieve discomfort after overeating. Binge eating behavior can compromise the integrity of the gastric pouch and increase the volume capacity, allowing for increased kilocalorie ingestion with decreased weight loss efficiency. To avoid discomfort, patients tend to consume soft, high energy containing foods and liquids such as ice cream, creamed soups, and juices. Overeating can lead to outlet obstruction, symptoms of which include vomiting and gastric reflux.[37]

Combination Surgeries: An Overview

Biliopancreatic Diversion With and Without Duodenal Switch

Biliopancreatic Diversion (BPD) combines partial gastrectomy with intestinal bypass, with the greatest impact of weight loss resulting from malabsorption. While the weight loss is greater than that seen in RYGBP, the surgery carries an increased risk of long-term nutritional complications. It has been postulated that modification of the length of the bypassed intestinal limb might allow for desired weight loss, while minimizing malabsorptive complications.[9]

For up to 1 year postoperatively, dietary recommendations are similar to those described earlier in this chapter. Patients might return to preoperative eating habits within 1 year after BPD surgery without discomfort or impact on weight loss, due to the effect of intestinal adaptation.[9] Fewer side effects have been demonstrated with the duodenal switch procedure, although the incidence of the most troublesome side effects of abdominal bloating and malodorous stool were relatively unchanged. The degree of micronutrient deficiency appears to be decreased with the duodenal switch approach, but it is recommended that patients be monitored for these deficiencies as discussed earlier in this chapter.[39]

Special Considerations

Nutrition Support

Nutrition support guidelines following gastric restrictive intestinal bypass surgeries generally are the same as for the postoperative gastrointestinal surgery patient. Enteral nutrition may be utilized if a gastrostomy feeding tube was placed during the bariatric procedure. If enteral access is not available, and the patient is expected to be NPO more

Table 8-2

Common Dietary Stages Following Bariatric Surgery

Stage 1 (does not include fluid provided by intravenous infusion)

Food Type: Water
Duration: 0-1 day
Begin: Postoperative day 1
End: Postoperative day 1
Amount: 1-2 fl oz/hr
Fluid Goal: 14-32 fl oz/d (within 14-16 waking hours)
Protein Goal: 0 g/d

Stage 2

Food Type: Clear liquids—noncaloric, decaffeinated, and noncarbonated beverages
Duration: 1-2 days
Begin: Postoperative day 1-2
End: Postoperative day 2-3
Amount: 2-3 fl oz/hr
Fluid Goal: 32-48 oz/d (within 14-16 waking hours)
Protein Goal: 0 g/d

Stage 3

Food Type: Full liquids—liquids containing high biological value protein: Nonfat or low-fat milk, low-fat creamed soups, blended and strained sugar-free pudding and custard, blended low-fat cottage and ricotta cheese. Some protocols recommend adding additional protein to these drinks through powdered skim milk or powdered egg white.
Duration: 14-21 days/2-3 weeks
Begin: Postoperative day 2-4
End: Postoperative day 16-25/week 2.5-3.5
Amount: 3-6 servings of 4-8 fl oz
Fluid Goal: 48-72 fl oz/d, or estimated needs
Protein Goal: 60-80 g/d, or estimated needs
Other Recommendations: Sip all liquids slowly; avoid gulping fluids; limit to approximately 8 fl oz/hr.

Stage 4

Food Type: Pureed or soft (ground/diced) foods—generally foods allowed include meat, poultry, fish, tofu and dairy products. Starches, fruits, and vegetables are typically excluded from this stage although soft fruits and vegetables have been included in some protocols.
Duration: 21-42 days/3-6 weeks
Begin: Postoperative day 17-26/week 2.5-3.5
End: Postoperative day 38-68/week 5.5-10
Amount: 2-3 fl oz of pureed/ground/diced food taken 3-5 times/d
Fluid Goal: 48-72 fl oz/d, or estimated needs
8-16 fl oz/d of full liquids (Beverages containing high biological value protein)
Protein Goal: 60-80 g/d, or estimated needs
Other Recommendations: Ground beef and shellfish might be difficult to tolerate. Eat slowly: 10 minutes/oz. Chew food thoroughly. Drink fluids at least 1 hour after meals.

Stage 5

Food Type: Small meals/snacks, consisting of low-fat solids
Duration: Ongoing
Begin: Postoperative day 38-68/week 4.5-10
End: Ongoing
Amount: Typically based on the American Diabetes/Dietetic Association food exchange list. Number of servings tolerated is widely variable per individual.

Table 8-2 (continued)

Common Dietary Stages Following Bariatric Surgery

Sample Meal Plan (recommendations might vary based on individual needs)

Starch: 3-7 exchanges	Milk: 1 exchange
Fruit (soft): 2-3 exchanges	Meat: 6-9 exchanges
Vegetable: 2-4 exchanges	Fat: 1-5 exchanges

Fluid goal: 48-72 fl oz/d, or based on estimated needs
Protein goal: 60-80 g/d, or based on estimated needs

Other Recommendations:

- Make protein the priority food
- Allow a minimum of 10 minutes per oz of food, or 30 minutes per 3 oz
- Often hard starches such as toast and crackers are better tolerated than untoasted bread
- Peel fresh vegetables and fruit when beginning to add in these foods

Problematic foods typically include the following:

- Red meat, ground beef, dry meats, shellfish, cores, hard skins (such as from an apple), seeds, membranes (particularly from thick-skinned fruits and vegetables), popcorn kernels, nuts, seeds, rice, and pasta

Adapted from Betsy Lehman Center for Patient Safety and Medical Error Reduction Expert Panel on Weight Loss Surgery-Multidisciplinary Care Task Group.[2]

than 7 days, total parenteral nutrition (TPN) may be initiated. Contraindications to TPN are usually the same as for gastrointestinal surgery patients in the presence of critical illness and sepsis. Bariatric surgery patients might be at risk for refeeding syndrome if they have been NPO or on clear liquids prior to initiation of nutrition support. Judicious monitoring of electrolytes and fluid balance is recommended while advancing nutrition support. Guidelines for advancement have been established by the American Society for Parenteral and Enteral Nutrition (ASPEN) and others and are appropriate for the bariatric surgery patient as well.[29]

Pregnancy

Pregnancy following weight loss surgery is considered high risk and should be postponed for at least 1 year or until patients have reached a stable weight and nutritional status. Prepregnancy assessment and planning is prudent to identify and ameliorate micronutrient deficiencies prior to pregnancy. Prenatal vitamins are recommended in addition to prescribed vitamin and mineral supplementation as preparation for pregnancy and should continue throughout pregnancy.[40,41]

Iron requirements for women are greater in pregnancy and vary with each trimester. During the first trimester, iron needs are reduced as a result of amenorrhea. However, during the second trimester, as the plasma volume and red blood cell mass increases close to 50% and 40%, respectively, iron needs also increase. Bariatric surgery resulting in decreased intake of iron-containing foods due to intolerance and altered digestion and absorption require prudent monitoring during pregnancy to prevent the onset of iron-deficiency anemia. If patients present with iron deficiency with or without anemia, iron supplementation should be initiated. Ferrous fumarate is often tolerated and absorbed better by most patients following surgery.[40]

To prevent the onset of iron deficiency, women should exhibit iron stores of more than 300 milligrams prior to pregnancy. Iron supplementation of 30 milligrams daily during the second trimester is recommended. However, 60 milligrams is recommended for women presenting with a prepregnancy iron deficiency. Iron supplements should be taken between meals to decrease gastric irritation and to increase absorption.[42]

Summary

Medical nutrition therapy following bariatric surgery is an essential element of postoperative care. Patients must be educated on dietary advancement to ensure optimal tolerance and utilization of nutrients. Registered dietitians specializing in bariatric surgery are an important part of the multidisciplinary team in facilitating appropriate dietary and eating behaviors. Close monitoring following surgery is crucial to identify potential nutrient deficiencies and disordered eating behaviors and to support optimal weight loss.

References

1. NIH Conference Development Conference Panel: Gastrointestinal surgery for severe obesity. *Ann Intern Med.* 1991;115:956-961.
2. Saltzman E, Anderson WA, Apovian CM, et. al. Criteria for patient selection and multidisciplinary evaluation and treatment of the weight loss surgery patient. *Obes Res.* 2005;13 (2):234-243.
3. Moize V, Geliebter A, Gluck ME, Yahav E, Lorence M, Colarusso T, Drake V, Flancbaum L. Obese patients have inadequate protein intake related to protein intolerance up to 1 year following Roux-en-Y gastric bypass. *Obes Surg.* 2003;13:23-28.
4. Kenler HA, Brolin RE, Cody RP. Changes in eating behavior after horizontal gastroplasty and Roux-en-Y gastric bypass. *Am J Clin Nutr.* 1990;52:87-92.
5. Coughlin K, Bell RM, Bivins BA, Wrobel S, Griffen WO Jr. Preoperative and postoperative assessment of nutrient intakes in patients who have undergone gastric bypass surgery. *Arch Surg.* 1983;188(7):813-816.
6. National Academy of Sciences' Institute of Medicine. Dietary Reference Intakes for Energy, Carbohydrate, Fiber, Fat, Fatty Acids, Cholesterol, Protein, and Amino Acids; 2002.
7. Byrne KT. Complications of surgery for obesity. *Surg Clin North Am.* 2001;81(5):1181-1193.
8. Bobbioni-Harsch E, Huber O, Morel P, et.al. Factors influencing energy intake and body weight loss after gastric bypass. *Eur J Clin Nutr.* 2002;56:551-556.
9. Scopinaro N et al. Biliopancreatic Diversion. *World J. Surgery.* 1998;22:936-946
10. Exchange Lists for Weight Management. American Diabetes and Dietetic Association. 1995.
11. Mallory G. Maximum nutrition, minimum calories. *Obes Surg.* 1992;2:375-378.
12. Mahan K, Escott-Stump S. *Krause's Food, Nutrition, & Diet Therapy.* Philadelphia, Pa: WB Saunders Company; 2000.
13. Beard JL. Iron-deficiency anemia: Reexamining the nature and magnitude of the public health problem. *J Nutr.* 2001; 131(2S-2):568S-579S.
14. Kushner R. Managing obese patient after bariatric surgery: a case report of severe malnutrition and review of the literature. *JPEN.* 2000;24(2):126-132.
15. Elliot K. Nutritional considerations after bariatric surgery. *Critical Care Nursing Quarterly.* 2003;26(2):133-138.

16. Brolin RE, Gorman RC, Milgrim LM, Kenler HA. Multivitamin prophylaxis in prevention of post-gastric bypass vitamin and mineral deficiencies. *Int J Obes.* 1991;15:661-667.

17. Brolin RE et al. Prophylactic iron supplementation after Roux-en Y gastric bypass: a prospective, double blind, randomized study. *Arch Surg.* 1998;133(7):740-744.

18. Rhode BM, Shustik C, Christou NV, Maclean. Iron Absorption and therapy after gastric bypass. *Obes Surg.* 1999;9:17-21.

19. Collene AL, Hertzler SH. Metabolic Outcomes of Gastric Bypass. *Nutr in Clin Prac.* 2003;18:136-140.

20. Rhode BM, Arseneau, P, Cooper BA, Katz M, Gilfix BM, Maclean LD. Vitamin B-12 deficiency after gastric surgery for obesity. *Am J Clin Nutr.* 1996;63:103-109.

21. Hunt SM, Groff JG. *Advanced Nutrition and Human Metabolism.* West Publishing Company; 1990.

22. Brolin RE, Gorman JH, Gorman RC, et.al. Are vitamin B12 and folate deficiency clinically important after roux-en-Y gastric bypass? *J Gastointest Surg.* 1998;2:436-442.

23. Deitel M, Cowan GSM. *Update: Surgery for the morbidly obese patient.* Philadelphia, Pa: Lippincott Williams and Wilken; 2000.

24. Charles P. Calcium absorption and calcium bioavailability. *J Internal Med.* 2003;231:161-168.

25. Goode LR, Brolin RE, Chowdhury HA, Shapses SE. Bone and gastric bypass surgery: effects of dietary calcium and vitamin D. *Obes Res.* 2004;12(1):40-47.

26. Brano G, Rodin DA, Pazianas M, Nussey SS. Reduced bone mineral density after surgical treatment for obesity. *Int J Obes Relat Metab Disord.* 1999; 23:361-365.

27. Coates PS et al. Gastric bypass surgery for morbid obesity leads to an increase in bone turnover and a decrease in bone mass. *J Clin Endocrinol Metab.* 2004;89:1061-1065.

28. Ott MT et al. Biochemical evidence of metabolic bone disease in women following Roux-en-Y gastric bypass for morbid obesity. *Obes Surg.* 1992;2:341-348.

29. *The Science and Practice of Nutrition Support: A Case-Based Core Curriculum.* Dubuque, Iowa: Kendall/Hunt Publishing Company; 2001.

30. Kim JJ et al. Surgical treatment for extreme obesity: Evolution of a rapidly growing field. *Nutr in Clin Prac.* 2003;18:109-123.

31. Boekema PJ, et al. Coffee and gastrointestinal function: facts and fiction. A review. *Scand J Gastroenterol Suppl.* 1999;230:35-39.

32. Marotta RB, Floch MH. Diet and Nutrition in Ulcer Disease. *Med Clin North Am.* 1991; 75(4):967-979.

33. Flanagan L. Measurement of Functional Pouch Volume following the Gastric Bypass Procedure. *Obes Surg.* 1996;6:38-43.

34. Marcason W. What are the dietary guidelines following bariatric surgery? *JADA.* 2004;104(3):487-488.

35. Abbott WC, Bistrian BR, Blackburn GL. The effect of dextrose and amino acids on respiratory function and energy expenditure in morbidly obese patients following gastric bypass surgery. *J Surg Res.* 1986;41(3):225-235.

36. Knol JA. Management of the problem patient after bariatric surgery. *Gastroenterol Clin North Am.* 1994;23(2):345-369.

37. MacDonald KG Jr et al. Bariatric Surgery: A Review. *General Surgery News.* 2001;1-12.

38. Sonnanstine TE, et al. Surgical Options in the Treatment of Morbid Obesity: An Overview. *Support Line.* 2004;26(5):3-17.

39. Marceau P et al. Biliopancreatic Diversion with Duodenal Switch. *World J. Surg.* 1998;22:947-954.

40. Wittgrove A. Pregnancy following gastric bypass for morbid obesity. *Obes Surg.* 1998;8:461-464.

41. Preziosi P. Effect of iron supplementation on the iron status of pregnant women: consequence for newborns. *J Clin Nutr.* 1997;66:1178-1182.

42. Bothwell TH. Iron requirements in pregnancy and strategies to meet them. *Am J Clin Nutr.* 2000;72:257S-264S1.

Selected Readings

Andrews, G, LeMont, D, Myers, S, Nelson, E, Smiertka, J. *Caring for the Surgical Weight Loss Patient.* Sierra Madre, Calif: Wheat Field Publications; 2004.

Betsy Lehman Center for Patient Safety and Medical Error Reduction-Expert Panel on Weight Loss Surgery (2004), from http://www.mass.gov/dph/betsylehman/index.htm.

Deitel, M, Cowan, G S.M. *Update: Surgery for the morbidly obese patient.* Philadelphia, Pa: Lippincott Williams and Wilken; 2000.

Elliot K. Nutritional considerations after bariatric surgery. *Critical Care Nursing Quarterly.* 2003; 26(2):133-8.

Marcason, W. What are the dietary guidelines following bariatric surgery? *Journal of the American Dietetic Association.* 2004;104(3):487-488.

Saltzman E, Anderson W, Apovian CM, et. al. Criteria for patient selection and multidisciplinary evaluation and treatment of the weight loss surgery patient. *Obes Res.* 2004;13(2):234-43.

Stocker, DJ. *Management of the bariatric surgery patient.* Endocrinolgy and Metabolism Clinics. Philadelphia, Pa: WB Saunders Company; 2003.

9

Medical Management of the Patient After Gastric-Bypass Surgery

Marie E. McDonnell, MD; Caroline M. Apovian, MD; and Donald T. Hess, Jr, MD

Introduction

During the year 2000, approximately 40,000 bariatric procedures were performed in the United States, and in 2004, this number exceeded 140,000. Despite better understanding of postoperative complications, only 5% of bariatric patients participated in surgical follow-up in the early 1990s.[1] Thousands of patients have undergone bariatric surgery in the US in the past 20 years but do not participate in a multidisciplinary follow-up program to address ongoing nutritional and behavioral needs. To meet the needs of the increasing population of bariatric patients, primary care providers (PCPs) will have to assume the majority of their care.

The Role of the Primary Care Provider

The PCP undoubtedly plays a key role in the management of patients who have undergone bariatric procedures. After surgery, most patients have significant, and at times very rapid, improvement of obesity-related conditions—eg, diabetes, hypertension (HTN), peripheral edema, obstructive sleep apnea (OSA), urinary incontinence, and osteoarthritis. Generally, within 2 to 3 postoperative months, a patient will feel better than he or she did before surgery. There are also conditions that may develop after surgery, such as alopecia due to rapid weight loss. The degree and timing of these changes vary per individual; this chapter provides basic guidelines for the PCP to follow.

Identifying signs and symptoms of early, delayed, and late complications related to the surgery, including nutritional deficiencies, is an essential task of the PCP. Identification of complications requires a methodical and informed approach to differential diagnosis. Many complications that occur following bariatric procedures, particularly those that are nutrition related (Chapter 8), can be predicted before surgery.[2,3] Some of these are often treated prophylactically in the early postoperative period (eg, iron supplementation to prevent iron-deficiency anemia). There are, however, complications that are not predict-

Table 9-1
Members of the Bariatric Team

Bariatric surgeon
Bariatric nurse specialist
Medical obesity specialist (internist, endocrinologist, or nutrition specialist)
Registered dietician
Psychologist
Gastroenterologist

able; therefore, the PCP must recognize the connection between subtle symptoms and diseases. An understanding of the natural history of such complications—such as when they occur (early, within the first 6 postoperative months, or late)—is a tool that can aid the clinician in directing treatment and, when necessary, referring the patient to a specialist.

Perhaps one of the most important roles of the PCP is to provide ongoing support of behavior modification. In choosing bariatric surgery as a treatment for obesity, patients do not eliminate the need for careful dietary restriction; rather, they face a set of new limitations with potentially serious consequences should they not adhere. The patient who does not comply with postoperative instructions may not follow-up with the bariatric team, which makes his or her PCP the first to assess the patient who requires chronic medication adjustments, the symptomatic patient, and the patient who is at risk for weight regain.

Postoperative Medical Management

The PCP must follow 4 key steps to provide the best care possible for the bariatric patient. Understanding the patient's procedure and remaining in contact with his or her referral team is the first tool in postoperative care. The second is to have rational expectations and allow both the clinician and patient to predict the usual changes in comorbid conditions (eg, improvement of diabetes, withdrawal of antihypertensive medications). Third, a comprehensive understanding of common nutritional deficiencies serves as a guide for monitoring and prescribing appropriate treatment. (While nutritional issues are briefly outlined here, they are fully discussed in Chapter 8.) The fourth tool is an organized approach in the evaluation of the symptomatic patient who has undergone bariatric surgery.

Important Details

Know the Team

The multidisciplinary approach to the care of the bariatric patient is crucial for successful overall management. Bariatric-care teams have members from diverse specialties, and patients may meet with each member as part of their care. Some teams include a surgeon and specialized dietician, and others include a dedicated medical internist, a psychologist, and a gastroenterologist (Table 9-1). Because these providers are committed to an

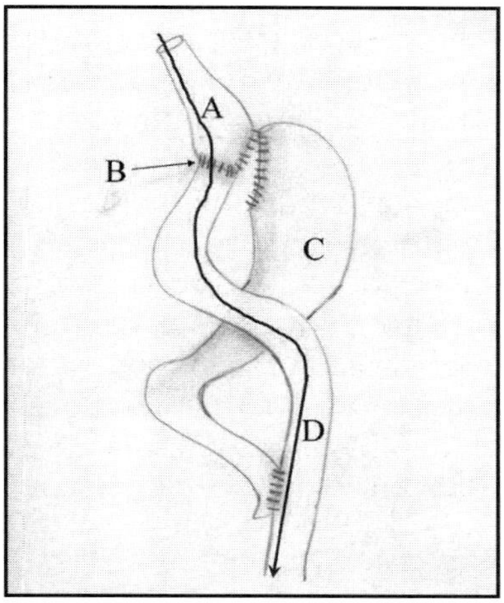

Figure 9-1. Example sketch of a RYGB. (A) Gastric pouch formed after stomach is stapled and separated into two sections. (B) Stoma (also "outlet" or "anastomosis") where a limb of separated jejunum is brought up and stapled to the pouch to form the gastrojejunostomy. (C) Gastric remnant/antrum. (D) (line with arrow) Alimentary canal. *For a full-color version, see page CA-IV of the Color Atlas.*

uncomplicated recovery and successful postoperative course for their patients, they serve as excellent referral sources for their patients, both in the short and long term. It is a good idea to have a list of their names and contact information in the patient's chart.

Know the Procedure

It is beneficial for the PCP to learn to draw the patient's procedure and to identify the gastric pouch, the bypassed stomach, the outlet or anastomosis, the alimentary limb, and the bypassed limb. The patient will benefit from a drawing with a line from the pouch to the colon to indicate the path of food (Figure 9-1). This is a basic yet invaluable tool for a medical provider who is evaluating either the postoperative patient or the patient with obesity who meets criteria for bariatric surgery (Chapter 3). When a bariatric patient has symptoms, the ability to draw the postoperative anatomy aids greatly in the PCP's ability to construct a differential diagnosis as well as to describe the problem or diagnostic possibilities to the patient. This visual understanding can be comforting and may alleviate a common underlying concern of bariatric patients: ie, the procedure has failed or requires revision, with the dreaded result of weight gain.

Every bariatric procedure is designed with 1 or both of 2 key features—(1) gastric restriction and (2) malabsorption—each to varying degrees, depending both on the procedure itself and on the individual patient. Most symptoms and complications arise because of the relative presence of these 2 elements. A procedure is chosen after careful consideration of an individual's weight, eating habits, and cardiovascular risk, in addition to the surgeon's experience.

As described in detail in Chapter 3, the 2 most commonly performed procedures are the Roux-en-Y gastric bypass (RYGB), which combines gastric restriction and malabsorption, and the vertical banded gastroplasty (VBG), which has been largely supplanted by the laparoscopic adjustable gastric banding (LAGB). The biliopancreatic diversion (BPD) and its variation—the biliopancreatic diversion with duodenal switch (BPD/DS)—are also performed yet generally less often because of increased malabsorptive complications. The BPD may have an increased risk of late sequelae related to protein– and vitamin D–malabsorption risks theoretically reduced with the BPD/DS.[4] The larger pouch of the BPD (300 ml versus 30 ml) reduces solid-food intolerance but increases the risk of marginal ulcers that form at the gastric outlet, where the intestine is anastomosed to the pouch.

The BPD/DS theoretically protects against marginal ulcers by preserving the pylorus and starting the anastomosis with a small segment of proximal duodenum. The jejunoileal bypass (JIB) is no longer performed, although there are a small number of patients who have had this procedure.

Aside from the elements of gastric restriction and malabsorption, it is useful for the PCP to know if a patient's procedure was done with an open laparotomy or laparoscopically. Both restrictive as well as malabsorptive procedures may be performed laparoscopically; that is becoming the preferred method because it is less invasive and shortens recovery time. In the case of the RYGB, most available data from experienced surgeons show that the laparoscopic approach affords improved short-term recovery from surgery, reduced rate of cardiopulmonary complications, and a lower incidence of incisional hernias than does open RYGB.[5] A recent meta-analysis that combined data on both laparoscopic and open procedures performed in experienced US institutions reported mortality rates of 0.1% for the purely restrictive procedures and 0.5% for gastric bypass.[6]

RYGB is the most common bypass procedure performed today. There is no standard technique for RYGB; for example, some patients may have a longer limb while others may have a smaller pouch. Pouch size, in particular, varies widely, because there is no standard method to evaluate the pouch size. It is difficult to compare widely varying approaches for the same operation; therefore, broad evaluation of efficacy and safety of bariatric procedures has been challenging. This is especially important because certain procedural differences are likely to be important. Long-limb (100 to 150 cm) RYGB procedures, for example, may produce superior weight loss in the short term in patients with BMI >50 or who are >200 pounds overweight.[7] However, it is not clear that these differences affect either the long-term success or complication rate in a given patient. A long-limb RYGB (up to 150 cm) is unlikely to increase the risk of nutritional deficiencies beyond that of standard gastric bypass.

Know the Perioperative Course

The patient and his or her providers should have on file a consultation letter from the bariatric surgeon or team as well as description of the postoperative course. PCPs may find it useful to include an information form (Figure 9-2), which includes the name of the procedure performed, the bariatric-team contact information, the early postoperative complications, and any particular issues that indicate an increased risk of delayed postoperative complications. Because symptomatic cholelithiasis is more common during rapid weight loss,[8] there is general acceptance that patients with cholelithiasis discovered during the screening evaluation should undergo a cholecystectomy at the time of surgery.[9] It is important that the PCP document this particular detail to form reasonable differential diagnoses in the future should a patient have gastrointestinal (GI) symptoms.

The patient will have a complete guideline as to postoperative diet, which is typically advanced in a stepwise fashion from liquids to solids (Chapter 8). Patients with diabetes mellitus may have diabetic-related complications, including hypoglycemia and hyperglycemia, which should be clearly described in the postoperative course. Because many patients have early (almost immediate) improvement of diabetes, patients may be withdrawn from some or all antihyperglycemic medications by the time they arrive home.

Re-evaluating Chronic Disease

The PCPs first postoperative visit with the patient should be devoted to making important predictions and defining reasonable expectations. Most cardiovascular risk factors,

Date of Procedure:__________ Institution __________	
Bariatric Providers (name/contact information):	
Procedure (circle one): RYGB BPD BPDDS	VBG SGB LASGB
Cholecystectomy performed?: YES NO	Cholecystectomy performed?: YES NO
Prescribed supplements/dose: B12 ______ Fe ______ Vit D ______ Calcium ______ Folate ______ Other ______	# Band Adjustments ______ Date of last Adjustment ______
Early Postoperative Complications __________ __________	
Delayed/late complications: __________ __________	

Figure 9-2. Example information form for patients who have a history of bariatric surgery.

such as elevated lipids and impaired glucose tolerance, are likely to improve postoperatively, with a lower incidence rate of comorbid conditions such as diabetes over both the short and the long term.[10,11] For the usual patient who is being treated for obesity-related conditions, alterations in metabolic parameters can be dramatic after bariatric surgery. It is crucial to be prepared for some early changes (eg, improved glucose tolerance), whereas others will be more gradual (eg, improved blood pressure, lower lipids) or may not change significantly.

While the expected degrees of weight loss should be reviewed with the patient, this should be done only to reiterate what has been discussed in detail during visits with the bariatric-team members. Most patients reach their maximum weight loss at year 1, and patients receiving care in experienced institutions will experience an average 60% loss of excess weight for all procedures.[11,12] The rates of recidivism, however, vary per procedure, with RYGB having the lowest weight regain up to 10 years after the procedure.[11]

As discussed in the following sections, there are 5 chronic conditions that often require careful reassessment for months to years following bariatric surgery: diabetes mellitus, HTN, hyperlypidemia, liver dysfunction, and OSA.

Type 2 Diabetes Mellitus

There is constantly expanding literature on the changes in insulin sensitivity and glucose tolerance that occur after bariatric surgery, particularly with bypass, or malabsorptive, procedures. With weight loss in general, one can expect a significant improvement in insulin sensitivity, which has been shown in several studies. For example, one study of females showed that weight loss of at least 5 kg led to a 50% reduction in the incidence of type 2 diabetes.[13] With a weight loss of 50 kg, which is common after bariatric procedures, such a reduction in risk is amplified.

Data from the largest bariatric cohorts to date have shown that 72% to 83% of patients with type 2 diabetes are normoglycemic within 2 years after a gastric-bypass operation.[11,14] Despite this dramatic early improvement, up to 50% of these patients revert to hyperglycemia in the future, even if substantial weight loss is maintained, thus underscoring the fact that most type 2 diabetes is caused by an underlying acquired or genetic metabolic defect. For this reason, it is wise not to suggest to patients that surgery will likely "cure" diabetes, which is a complex disorder with multiple compounding etiologies. Instead, bariatric patients previously on antihyperglycemic medications should be told that they have become "diet-controlled" type 2 diabetics, and lifelong periodic monitoring of plasma glucose levels is indicated.

Most providers who care for bariatric patients have noted that some patients who required insulin therapy for control of their diabetes became diet-controlled without difficulty postoperatively. Bariatric surgeons report early "hypoglycemic" effects soon (before significant weight loss has occurred) after procedures with significant malabsorptive components (eg, RYGB and BPD). Such changes may occur because of dramatic reduction in caloric intake, which has been shown to improve insulin sensitivity, possibly by reducing plasma-free fatty-acid levels and depleting intramuscularly-stored fat. However, several uncontrolled investigations suggest that there is a hormonal component to the improved insulin sensitivity and perhaps to the weight loss, which is induced by alteration of the gut and the route of food. It is still unclear whether changes in gut "incretins," such as glucagon-like peptide-1 (GLP-1) and glucose-dependent insulinotropic peptide (GIP) (discussed later with hypoglycemia), and hormonal appetite mediators, such as the controversial ghrelin, are major determinants of postoperative weight loss.[15-17]

Some publications advise the surgical team, as a rule, to reduce patients' diabetes-medication regimens by one-half when they discharge patients from the hospital postoperatively; however, this advice is not adequate for some patients. Most patients with type 2 diabetes have severe insulin resistance in addition to mild to moderate beta-cell dysfunction, which eventually requires them to take either insulin or insulin secretogogues (eg, sulfonylurea medications). A sudden reduction in caloric intake—to <1,000 kcal/day—in addition to hormonal changes usually improve a patient's insulin resistance enough to eliminate the need for extra insulin. Such patients may be at risk for hypoglycemia if discharged on insulin or sulfonylurea therapy. On the contrary, patients who do not require hypoglycemic agents on the day of discharge and who are advised to stop them may become hyperglycemic as their caloric intake increases. With the advent of evidence-based recommendations for tight glycemic control to reduce infection risk, hyperglycemia should be treated, albeit cautiously.[18] In addition, there is a growing number of type 1 diabetics with obesity who require insulin for survival. In many, the diagnosis may not be clear (type 1 versus type 2); for this reason, insulin should be withdrawn with caution and never abruptly stopped unless the patient has developed relative hypoglycemia (random <90 ng/dl). Upon discharge, it is wise for diabetic patients to be instructed to report their finger-stick glucoses frequently (every other day) to a nurse or the PCP so appropriate adjustments can be made (Table 9-2).

In addition to re-evaluating a patient's diabetes medication, the PCP must also consider the minor risks to bariatric patients who are taking oral agents that can cause toxicity. Because the bariatric patient is at risk for both hypovolemia and liver dysfunction following surgery (Chapter 7), agents such as metformin and the thiazolidinediones (TZDs) should be discontinued. These agents, which mainly work to improve insulin sensitivity, have a minimal role after bariatric surgery in the short term because a dramatic reduction in caloric intake will naturally increase glucose tolerance. The safest option is to initially discontinue the patient's use of these drugs and re-evaluate his or her need for the medication as postoperative weight loss proceeds.

Table 9-2

Tips for Managing Diabetes After Bariatric Surgery

For Patients on Oral Agents
For patients on sulfonylureas (glipizide, glyburide, repaglinide), continue at ½ preoperative dose QD, in the morning only. Discontinue if fasting glucose is <90 ng/dl and/or bedtime glucose is <110 ng/dl.
Discontinue thiazolidinediones (rosiglitazone, pioglitazone) and metformin.
For Patients on Insulin
Discontinue all rapid-acting insulins (Humalog, Regular, Novolog) unless glucose 2 h after meals is >150 ng/dl.
Continue basal insulins (NPH, Lantus, Lente, Ultralente) at ½ preoperative dose. Discontinue if fasting glucose is <90 ng/dl and/or bedtime glucose is <110 ng/dl.
Instructions for Patients to Follow for 2 Weeks Postoperatively
Check finger sticks 2 to 3 times daily and keep a record.
Call in glucose values every other day to PCP's office for 2 wk.

Hypertension

Medical weight loss, which often includes lifestyle modification and pharmacotherapy, has been proven to lower blood pressure.[19,20] Several trials show that weight loss reduces blood pressure,[21] and blood pressure has been shown to normalize during weight loss after RYGB. A group of 275 patients was followed for outcomes after laparoscopic RYGB and had an average excess weight loss at 24 months of 83%. Remarkably, 70% of the patients with HTN had normal blood pressure at the end of the follow-up period.[22]

In the early postoperative period, patients are at significant risk for hypotension for a variable amount of time. Patients are generally mildly hypovolemic, with a limited ability to rehydrate orally and naturally reduce their salt intake. When occurring concomitantly, these factors can dramatically alter hemodynamics. Moreover, in the following weeks, weight loss will be rapid, an occurrence that improves endothelial function and lowers blood pressure.[23] For these reasons, most patients will appropriately have both antihypertensive and diuretic medications withheld after bariatric surgery.

HTN, especially longstanding HTN, however, does not typically "disappear" for the remainder of the individual's life. HTN may improve but return as the patient ages, even when weight loss is mostly maintained.[11] This is likely because of the multifactorial etiology of essential HTN. While a large proportion of patients require a reduction in their antihypertensive medications, the PCP can expect that 50% to 80% of patients treated for HTN preoperatively will become normotensive without medications in the first 2 years following bariatric surgery.[24]

If blood pressure does not improve with weight loss, the patient may not have essential HTN but rather a secondary cause of HTN that was incorrectly attributed to obesity. Causes of secondary HTN in this population may be generally categorized under endocrine or renovascular disease. Endocrine causes include hyperaldosteronism from adrenal adenoma or bilateral adrenal hyperplasia; the rare Cushing's syndrome from excess cortisol production; and pheochromocytoma, which produces excess catecholamines. Generally speaking, endocrine causes explain less than 1% of HTN, although aldosterone excess may be substantially more common.[25] Renovascular disease is estimated to occur in less than 5% of all hypertensive patients: it is usually a result of atherosclerotic plaques in renal arteries and should be considered in patients with known cardiovascular disease or risk factors. For persistent HTN that requires 3 or more medications despite weight loss, screening for secondary cause is indicated (Table 9-3).

Hyperlipidemia

According to NIH consensus, weight loss effectively lowers elevated levels of total cholesterol, low-density lipid cholesterol, and triglycerides and raises high-density lipid cholesterol in persons with obesity.[19] Several studies have demonstrated that up to 63% of patients who have lost >60% of their excess weight after bariatric surgery will have normal lipid parameters without medications within 1 postoperative year.[21] In patients who undergo bypass procedures, lipid malabsorption may play a major role in lowering lipids, as some patients tend to have the same serum lipid pattern as do patients with congenital lipid malabsorption.[26] Given the variability of procedures, the timing of the lipid-lowering effect may differ from patient to patient. Some cholesterol-lowering medications, such as HMG-CoA reductase inhibitors, can have other potentially beneficial vascular effects in those patients with cardiovascular disease. It is thus generally advisable for patients to continue statin medications at a lower dose upon discharge following surgery. Other medications, such as fibrate drugs (eg, gemfibrozil) for hypertriglyceridemia, may be safely discontinued until the 3-month follow-up appointment, when serum lipid levels can be measured.

Liver Dysfunction

It is estimated, based on small cohorts, that up to 90% of patients with morbid obesity have steatosis and as many as 42% have steatohepatitis.[27] Patients with presumed or biopsy-proven nonalcoholic fatty liver disease generally experience improvement in liver-function tests and steatosis following bariatric surgery.[28,29] Interestingly, however, biopsies performed months to years after surgery in a small number of patients have shown increased inflammation, progression of fibrosis, and cirrhosis.[30,31] Progression to end-stage liver disease, need for transplantation, and mortality secondary to cirrhosis have been reported but in numbers too small to allow generalization. At present, because it is not yet clear how to predict either result (ie, improvement or exacerbation), medications known to be hepatotoxic should be used with caution in patients for at least 6 months following bariatric surgery.

Obstructive Sleep Apnea

More than 80% of patients with obesity and OSA will experience either improvement or resolution of OSA, which allows for withdrawal of nocturnal continuous positive airway pressure (CPAP) ventilation within a year of bariatric surgery. In an observational study of 15 patients, surgically-induced weight loss (ranging from 27 kg to 100 kg) reduced the mean apnea-hypopnea index on polysomnography from 97 to 11.[32] However, it is important not to overestimate the contribution of obesity to the development of OSA. Obesity does not always explain the entire syndrome, and apneic episodes may continue, even after massive weight reduction.[33] Some surgeons recommend discontinuation of CPAP during the immediate postoperative period. This practice is thought to reduce the theoretical risk of increased pressure placed on the newly constructed gastric pouch, although recent data suggest that this practice may be unnecessary.[34] The majority of patients will be restarted on CPAP during the early postoperative period. Following significant weight loss (>30% excess body weight), a referral for repeated polysomnography with oximetry is indicated to re-evaluate the need for CPAP.

Nutritional Consequences

All patients undergoing bariatric surgery require nutrition support both before and after surgery. Although the specific recommendations may vary slightly among bariatric programs, the general idea is the same. Before surgery, the focus is to change the patient's lifelong eating behaviors (eg, drinking fluids with food is no longer allowed). After surgery, the focus is multifold to achieve specific early goals: adequate hydration, normal electrolytes, normal wound healing, and maintenance of lean body mass during rapid weight loss. As outlined in detail in Chapter 8, the diet after bariatric surgery is provided in stages to achieve these goals.

Just as the diabetic patient is required to bring his or her glucose record to medical visits, the bariatric patient should be encouraged to share his or her food and supplementation diary with their PCP. Patients are placed on multivitamins and chewable calcium because data from bariatric cohorts have identified common nutritional needs.[35] Iron supplementation may or may not be recommended prophylactically, as iron pills are common GI irritants, and vitamins B12 and D may be prescribed. In the year following surgery, most programs require patients to return every 3 months for laboratory evaluation to assess for iron-deficiency anemia and other deficiencies. Deficiencies of the following nutrients occur in >10% of patients at some point following gastric-bypass procedures: vitamin B12 (appears 6 to 10 months postoperatively), iron, vitamin D (hypocalcemia is uncommon), and hypomagnesemia. Vitamin-D deficiency is likely overlooked in most patients, and all bariatric patients should undergo routine measurements of 25-hydroxy vitamin D [25(OH)D] levels and calcium plus vitamin-D supplementation after gastric bypass. Only rarely do patients suffer from protein energy malnutrition. Clinical syndromes due to nutritional deficiencies, their evaluation, and appropriate therapies are included in Table 9-3. Chapter 8 provides a full review of the nutritional consequences of bariatric surgery.

For the woman of childbearing age, the PCP also plays an important role in fertility counseling. Pregnancy should be avoided in at least the first 12 months following surgery—until weight loss stabilizes, which usually occurs in the first 12 to 18 postoperative months—because rapid weight loss, dehydration, and vitamin deficiency have potentially deleterious effects on the fetus. Folate deficiency, for example, is associated with a higher than normal risk of fetal neural tube defects.[36]

Evaluating the Symptomatic Patient

Depending on the operation, postoperative complications occur in 10% to 50% of patients and largely depend on patient compliance.[37] When faced with the symptomatic bariatric patient, the PCP should categorize a patient according to perioperative stage to form a working diagnosis. Surgeons define the early postoperative period as <30 days after surgery. Symptoms occurring during this time—such as wound infections, deep vein thrombosis, nausea, and vomiting—are more likely to be directly related to surgery

Table 9-3

*Symptom-Based Approach to Postoperative Complications of Bariatric Surgery**

Symptom	Differential Diagnosis†	Initial Work-Up¶	Appropriate Initial Therapy¶
Weight regain (L) ‡	Diet noncompliance Pouch staple-line disruption or gastro-gastric fistula Anastomotic leak Hypothyroidism Undiagnosed Cushing's syndrome§	Food diary LAB: TSH level, overnight dexamethasone suppression test	Change diet as needed; increase exercise; advise counseling through bariatric team*
Constipation	Inadequate hydration Low fiber intake Bacterial overgrowth Small-bowel obstruction	Food diary RAD: upright, flat x-rays if >4 d, diminished flatus	Food diary; increase fluids and dietary fiber (if no effect: increase dietary active yogurt cultures or add acidophilus tablets) RX: milk of magnesia at bedtime; mineral oil by mouth
Diarrhea	Dumping Lactose intolerance Bacterial overgrowth	LAB: Electrolytes if >4 d; stool hemoccult	Evaluate/RX for GIB as necessary RX: replace milk with fat-free Lactaid; replete electrolytes as necessary (if no effect: increase dietary active yogurt cultures or add acidophilus tablets)
Abdominal bloating; increased flatus	Lactose intolerance Bacterial overgrowth Early/partial small-bowel obstruction	RAD: upright, flat x-rays if >1 wk or severe	RX: replace milk with fat-free Lactaid; replete electrolytes as necessary (if no effect: increase dietary active yogurt cultures or add acidophilus tablets)
Nausea +/- vomiting‖	Rapid eating Anastomotic stricture	Food diary RAD: upright, flat x-rays if >4 d	Dietary counseling; immediate referral to bariatric team* for severe or persistent symptoms
Reflux‖	Caffeine, carbonated drinks, spicy foods	Food diary	No eating after 6pm; avoid exacerbating foods/drinks RX: oral PPI 30 min before breakfast, dinner for 2 wk
Postprandial diaphoresis, "spells"‖	Dumping Hypoglycemia Menopause	Food diary; home glucose monitoring LAB: Fasting, postprandial glucose; consider 3-h OGTT	Reduce meal size Eliminate simple carbohydrates No drinking while eating

Symptom	Differential Diagnosis†	Initial Work-Up¶	Appropriate Initial Therapy¶
Dyspnea	Pulmonary embolism (E)‡ Deconditioning Angina	LAB: arterial blood gas; chest x-ray if abnormal exam	Admit to hospital if ventilatory or oxygenation defect or if symptoms are acute
Epigastric pain‖	Marginal ulcer Symptomatic cholelithiasis GERD	LAB: stool hemoccult; CBC	RX: Oral PPI 30 min before breakfast, dinner for 2 wk Immediate referral to bariatric team* for severe or persistent symptoms
Lower abdominal pain	Anastomotic leak +/- peritonitis Constipation Intussusception	LAB: electrolytes, CBC RAD: upright, flat abdominal x-rays if >4 d	Immediate referral to bariatric team* for severe or persistent symptoms
Bone pain/Arthralgias	Vitamin-D deficiency Hypomagnesemia	EXAM: tender tibial surface +/- sternum LAB: serum 25(OH)D level, Mg, Ca, Phos	RX: If 25(OH)D level is <20, Ergocalciferol (vitamin D) 50,000 IU weekly for 8 weeks (powder or pill forms are available; reserve IM for intractable cases) If no effect, increase dietary active yogurt cultures or add acidophilus tablets
Joint pain	BADAS (see text)	EXAM: focal joint swelling, tenderness, or erythema	RX: acetaminophen
(E)‡ Paresthesias	Hypomagnesemia Hypokalemia Folate deficiency Vitamin-B12 deficiency Diabetic neuropathy Thiamine deficiency	EXAM: sensory exam LAB: B12, folate, thiamine levels; serum basic metabolic panel, Mg, Phos, HA1c if appropriate	Replete deficiencies (Chapter 8)
(D)‡ Paresthesias	Vitamin-B12 deficiency Hypomagnesemia Folate deficiency Vitamin-D deficiency Diabetic neuropathy Thiamine deficiency Hypocalcemia	EXAM: sensation and proprioception LAB: B12, folate, thiamine levels; serum basic metabolic panel, Ca, Mg, Phos, HA1c if appropriate	Replete deficiencies (Chapter 8) RX: If 25(OH)D level is <20, Ergocalciferol (vitamin D) 50,000 IU Q wk for 8 wk (powder or pill forms; reserve IM for intractable cases)
Lightheadedness +/- documented hypotension	Hypovolemia Inadequate withdrawal of antihypertensive medications	EXAM: check for orthostasis, signs of hypovolemia LAB: electrolytes	Increase fluid intake; add salt or soy sauce to foods; add soups to diet Reduce/discontinue antihypertensive medications

Table 9-3 (continued)

Symptom	Differential Diagnosis†	Initial Work-Up¶	Appropriate Initial Therapy¶
Fatigue	Deconditioning Anemia Protein-energy malnutrition	Food diary LAB: CBC, B12, folate, ferritin, TIBC; stool hemoccult as needed	RX: Iron supplement; B12, folate supplements as needed Urgent referral to bariatric dietician
Restless legs/leg cramps	Hypomagnesemia Hypokalemia Hypocalcemia	EXAM: signs of hypocalcemia (Chvostek's jaw tap) LAB: electrolytes with Ca, Mg, Phos	RX: electrolyte repletion as necessary; consider low-dose oral quinine
Persistent HTN	Essential HTN Hyperaldosteronism Cushing's syndrome§ Pheochromocytoma§	LAB: Serum aldosterone level with PRA	If ratio of aldosterone: PRA is >30, refer to clinical specialist for definitive testing, possible treatment for hyperaldosteronism
Confusion, somnolence	Dehydration Hypoglycemia Persistent OSA after CPAP withdrawal Protein-energy malnutrition Thiamine deficiency (Wernicke's encephalopathy)	EXAM: evaluate hydration status, focal neurologic signs LAB: electrolytes with CO2 level, venous blood gas, CBC, prealbumin and thiamine levels	Admit for evaluation and appropriate therapy
Visual disturbance, confusion, ataxia	Severe thiamine deficiency (Wernicke's encephalopathy)	EXAM LAB: thiamine level	Admit for neurological evaluation, treatment RX: IV thiamine, then dextrose

* Symptomatic patients should be advised to follow-up with the appropriate bariatric specialty-team member: surgeon, surgical nurse specialist, nutrition expert, gastroenterologist, internist, psychologist.

† Differential diagnosis is given in order of likelihood.

‡ (E) = early, <30 postoperative days; (D) = delayed, 30 days to 6 months after surgery; (L) = late, >6 postoperative months

§ A rare disease, work up warranted with presence of other clinical signs (see text)

|| Evaluation for cardiac ischemia may be warranted.

¶ Nonstandard abbreviations in work-up and therapy guidelines: LAB = blood tests; RAD = radiography; RX = specific treatment recommendation; GIB = GI bleeding; EXAM = physical examination; OGTT = oral glucose tolerance test; Ca = calcium; Mg = magnesium; Phos = phosphate; HA1c = glycosylated hemoglobin A1c; PRA = plasma renin activity

Table 9-4

Complications After Laparoscopic Adjustable Gastric Band

Band Complications
Gastric-band slippage
Pouch perforation (usually early)
Early pouch dilation
Erosion of band
Gastric intussusception
Defect of band tube
Incisional hernia
Infection at band site
Access-Port Complications
Infection at port site
Dislocation of port

Table 9-5

Complications From Roux-en-Y Gastric Bypass and Biliopancreatic Diversion

- Internal herniation (early or delayed)
- Strictures
- Staple-line dehiscence
- Pouch dilatation
- Partial intestinal obstruction
- Anastomotic leaks
- Incisional hernia
- Staple-line hernia
- Staple-line disruption (failure)
- Marginal ulcer (usually at the gastrojejunostomy site)
- Gastrogastric fistula (when the bypassed gastric segment is not resected)
- Intestinal bacterial overgrowth
- Urinary-tract stone disease (oxalate malabsorption)
- Cholelithiasis
- Osteomalacia

or the initial challenge of relearning how to eat, and patients should be referred immediately to the bariatric team. From a medical perspective, this period is often crucial in terms of adjusting medications (discussed previously).

Primary-care physicians are likely to see patients for symptoms after the early postoperative period. Because of the patient's altered anatomy and new nutritional demands added to risk for social and psychological challenges, it is often difficult to direct the evaluation of the symptomatic patient after bariatric surgery. While the list of potential complications appears long (Tables 9-4 and 9-5), the PCP can form rational differential diagnoses based on symptoms and timing after surgery (Table 9-3). Symptoms occurring 30 days to 6 months after surgery—a period designated as midterm or delayed—often relate to the patient adapting to new behavioral modification. However, some common postoperative complications occur during this time.

After 6 months—usually termed the late postoperative phase—patients are less likely to follow-up with their surgeon. Problems such as nutritional deficiencies and anastomotic ulcers may be identified. Importantly, many common complications—eg, dumping syndrome, nutritional deficiencies, and anastomotic ulcers—may occur at any time and occurrence of these complications depends on patient behavior. Additionally, some patients with symptoms that impair food intake may not complain for fear of compromising their weight loss and will therefore not pursue regular postoperative nutritional and psychological counseling. (Postoperative complications are discussed at length in Chapter 7.)

During every encounter with the symptomatic patient after bariatric surgery, both the patient and physician must address one or more of 3 fundamental questions: (1) Is the patient compliant with diet, eating behavior, and vitamin supplementation appropriate for his or her postoperative stage? (2) Do the patient and/or physician have reasonable expectations? (3) Was a clinical condition (eg, eating disorder, coronary disease) missed in the preoperative assessment?

Although patients with active substance abuse, noncompliance with previous medical care, eating disorders, and active peptic-ulcer disease are considered unfit for bariatric surgery, some may pass the evaluation and go on to surgery. These patients are at higher risk for complications than are patients without these clinical conditions because of their preexisting issues.

Equally concerning are patients with subclinical vascular disease. In the morbidly obese state, sedentary lifestyle may render significant coronary disease clinically silent. With weight loss, an increase in physical activity may unmask the underlying coronary-artery or peripheral arterial disease. Preoperative cardiac assessment is designed to evaluate this risk, but stress testing has not proven as good a predictor as the reported preoperative exercise tolerance, which is often difficult to assess in patients with morbid obesity.

The following sections highlight some of the complications that occur after bariatric surgery, following the early postoperative period. Symptoms occurring >30 days postoperatively often require initial assessment by a primary care provider. Please refer to Table 9-3 for a comprehensive list of symptoms, signs, and recommended initial evaluation.

Delayed Complications (30 days to 6 months)

Dumping Syndrome

"Dumping" is discomfort that occurs episodically following a meal. It is a behavior-induced syndrome that often follows bariatric procedures in which the pyloric sphincter is bypassed and the pouch is small (eg, RYGB). It occurs less commonly after BPD. Dumping is thought to result from rapid and increased stretching of the intestine that results from an undigested food bolus entering through the new gastric outlet, a path that is no longer regulated by a physiologic sphincter. In response to the combined effect of gut peptides (eg, cholecystokinin) and the rapid delivery of hypertonic gastric contents, luminal water content increases. Both intestinal stretch and gut peptides likely co-mediate a vagal response: sweats, salivation, nausea, vomiting, diarrhea, and (rarely) syncope. Other symptoms include tachycardia with and without palpitations and abdominal cramping.[38] Diarrhea may or may not occur. Hypoglycemia may accompany the syndrome as well.

Patients who tend to eat quickly and who drink fluids with meals are at high risk for dumping. Highly osmolar foods such as simple carbohydrates (candy), high-fat foods (ice cream), and alcohol are "high-risk" dumping foods. Dumping syndrome often leads to increased hunger for sugary foods later, which perpetuates the problem and further increases the risk.

Screening for causative behavior is usually revealing, and behavior modification prevents dumping in most patients. Patients should not drink carbonated beverages or high-calorie liquids, and they should not eat candy. Carbohydrate intake should be less than 40 to 50 g per meal, and proteins (a minimum of 70 g each day) must be eaten before carbohydrates at every meal. In the rare circumstance that a patient does not respond to behavioral change, octreotide administered by subcutaneous injection has been reported to be effective.[39] The PCP should note that recurrent dumping is considered a behavioral marker that suggests the patient is at higher risk for other complications, such as pouch staple-line disruption. See Chapter 8 for more information on dietary treatment and behavioral management of dumping syndrome.

Vomiting

Nausea with vomiting is a relatively common symptom that occurs after primarily restrictive, as well as malabsorptive, procedures. It is often related to variable tolerability of new gastric restriction, and it is often due to foods or pills becoming "stuck" at the gastric outlet. Patients who eat too quickly, eat too much, or advance prematurely to certain food textures and bite sizes are at high risk. The patient's pill gulping more than 1 medication is an easily identified culprit and should be excluded first. The second step in the evaluation is discussion of eating behaviors appropriate for the patient's stage. In addition to going through the 3 fundamental questions (see above) in the case of vomiting, it is key for the PCP to ask, "Did you completely tolerate the previous stage before advancing to the next one?" Regardless of the answer, patients should be advised to go back to their previous diet stage. (See Chapter 8 for dietary stages following surgery.) Any indication of dietary noncompliance should prompt rapid follow-up with the patient's bariatric team.

Stomal stenosis (ie, anastomotic stricture at the gastrojejunostomy) occurs in up to 15% of patients after gastric bypass and is higher after laparoscopic RYGP. This should be considered in the patient who continues to experience vomiting, despite counseling and dietary change, especially if it occurs at or beyond 6 months postoperatively.[40] Persistent vomiting associated with this complication uncommonly results in serious nutritional complications, such as protein energy malnutrition and thiamine deficiency, which can cause Wernicke's encephalopathy in bariatric patients. In most cases, the outlet can be endoscopically dilated to allow for better passage of food; occasionally, 2 to 3 dilations are necessary (Chapter 10). If the patient is still unable to adjust and has persistent vomiting, then surgical revision may be required.[39]

Early weight regain after gastric-restrictive procedures may occur in the first postoperative year in patients who inappropriately adjust their diet because of recurrent vomiting from food intolerance. As addressed above, certain foods (high fiber, grains, meats) and pills can become caught at the outlet and induce nausea and vomiting. Unfortunately, the best-tolerated foods for these patients tend to be milkshakes, cookies in milk, or other high-calorie liquid foods. This is much less of a problem now with the increased use of the LAGB, where patients can have their outlet size easily adjusted.

Hypoglycemia

Episodic low glucose (<50 ng/dl without symptoms or <80 with related symptoms relieved after blood glucose is raised) is sometimes seen in the early days after RYGB and may persist over some months if not identified and treated appropriately. Patients may complain of sweating, palpitations, sudden fatigue, and severe hunger during episodic low-blood-glucose levels. Since these symptoms may be nonspecific, documentation with a glucose meter or plasma glucose during symptoms is imperative to make this uncommon diagnosis. Early bariatric literature described patients with problematic hypoglycemia developing within hours of surgery, some of whom had type 2 diabetes.[14] Although often perplexing, hypoglycemia is often accompanied by 2 significant characteristics, as noted by experienced surgeons: (1) hypoglycemia usually occurs in patients who experience dumping syndrome, and (2) it resolves when the dumping syndrome resolves after behavior modification. Some investigators have linked the 2—dumping and hypoglycemia—when in fact, they may be 2 distinct consequences of similar behaviors. Most patients with dumping, for example, do not have symptoms or documentation of hypoglycemia.

The etiology of post-bypass hypoglycemia may be best explained by known alterations that occur in the "enteroinsular axis." This is the hormonal network whereby ingested nutrients trigger the release of gut peptides, or incretins, whose main role is to stimulate the pancreatic beta islet cell to release insulin. The 2 major incretins, GIP and GLP-1, probably act in concert to stimulate the release of insulin early enough during a meal to prevent hyperglycemia.[41] There are numerous studies performed on animals and humans after intestinal bypass that indicate, albeit variably, that this system is altered by surgery. Some evidence suggests that, while GIP is suppressed postoperatively, GLP-1 is over-expressed, which may promote hypoglycemia, especially because it simultaneously inhibits the hormone glucagon; this relationship remains unclear in humans who have undergone gastric bypass.[42,43]

Once hypoglycemia is clearly documented and it is clear that the patient has not been on any hypoglycemic agents (sulfonylurea or insulin), dietary advice is appropriate as long as the episodes do not cause severe symptoms (eg, altered mental status). Smaller portions of meals composed of both complex carbohydrates and proteins typically resolve symptoms. Patients should be reminded not to eat or drink simple carbohydrates and foods high in fat, which may cause delayed hypoglycemia. If episodes continue despite dietary changes, referral to an endocrinologist is indicated.

Diarrhea

Loose, watery stools may become problematic as patients increase their food intake, and, once dumping syndrome is excluded (see above), diarrhea is most often because of lactose intolerance.[44] Milk is an excellent source of protein for patients in the early postoperative period; for this reason patients are advised to mix it with meal-replacement powders as they progress through the dietary stages. The bypass may exacerbate underlying, subclinical, mild lactose intolerance, and patients can experience cramps, bloating, increased flatus, and/or diarrhea. The intolerance is usually temporary and may completely resolve over several weeks to months. Patients should be advised to replace their low-fat milk with lactase-containing low-fat milk (eg, Lactaid) or to add lactase tablets to milk. Soymilk is often a good alternative for patients who do not respond to lactase supplementation. Diarrhea that persists may be due to several possible factors, including those commonly seen in general practice, eg, viral gastroenteritis. Nosocomially acquired *Clostridium difficile* should be ruled out in the early postoperative period because most patients receive routine perioperative antibiotics, and treatment with metronidazole would be warranted. Lastly, bile-acid malabsorption after BPD is sometimes diagnosed empirically and treated with cholestyramine resin.[37]

Small-bowel bacterial overgrowth is a relatively uncommon cause of diarrhea after gastric-bypass procedures, but its true incidence is unknown. It is associated with abdominal pain, watery diarrhea (sometimes occurring at night), dyspepsia, and weight loss.[4] Some patients also experience arthralgias. While most often seen in the setting of severe gut dysmotility, small-bowel overgrowth is known to occur when proximal bowel is anastomosed to more distal bowel, as with the gastrojejunostomy in RYGB or with side-to-side anastomoses. The symptoms are thought to be due to increased number of bacteria in the upper gastrointestinal (UGI) tract. While the gold standard for the diagnosis of bacterial overgrowth has traditionally been the demonstration of excessive bacterial concentrations in a jejunal aspirate, which can be performed during endoscopy, most providers treat empirically and observe. Treatment is aimed at reducing bacterial load, the common species being streptococci, *Bacteroides, Escherichia coli,* and *Lactobacillus*.[45] Antibiotics, such as metronidazole, are the mainstay of therapy, although nutritional supplements, such as increased activeyeast culture intake (eg, yogurt) and probiotics, are increasingly accepted therapies for milder cases.[46]

Anemia

Iron deficiency is a common early complication of surgical-bypass procedures where the duodenum is completely bypassed (RYGB, some BPD).[47] A low ferritin, with accompanying symptoms, is detectable within the first few months if not prophylactically treated with iron supplementation. The cause is most frequently the malabsorption of iron, and a source of slow bleeding typically presents within the first few weeks following surgery; however, occult bleeding must be excluded by stool testing. Patients may not complain of an unusual degree of fatigue or dyspnea because they are already experiencing these symptoms because of their obesity. This is one rationale for treating with iron supplements soon after surgery as part of a prescribed multivitamin regimen. Although many providers in bariatric programs consider iron supplementation standard of care, a survey of surgeons in the US indicated that this practice varies widely.[48,49]

Abdominal Pain

GERD may cause epigastric abdominal discomfort and rarely pain after both gastric bypass and purely restrictive procedures. There are conflicting data on GERD outcomes following bariatric surgery, but most recent studies suggest that both LAGB and RYGB actually result in some improvement of reflux, both symptomatic as well as asymptomatic.[50] However, gastric-restriction procedures without bypass components may worsen reflux in some patients. Some authors have suggested measuring serum antibodies to *Helicobacter pylori* and prescribing an eradication regimen to patients before surgery.[9] This has not been prospectively studied but may be reasonable, especially for possible long-term ulcer prevention. Treatment is primarily based on behavioral modifications and proton pump inhibitors (PPI) taken once to twice daily 30 minutes before meals (Table 9-3).

Symptomatic cholelithiasis usually presents with colicky abdominal pain in the right upper quadrant after meals but may present atypically as severe GERD. A right upper-quadrant ultrasound to look for gallstones is the initial diagnostic step.

Marginal ulcers can form at the gastrojejunostomy site after RYGB in 7% to 15% of patients.[4] Patients with these ulcers often present with intermittent epigastric pain accompanied by bloating, occasional diarrhea, and rarely life-threatening hemorrhage requiring exploratory laparotomy. Gastric bypass is a natural "set up" for ulcer formation; the normal balance between the cellular production of acid and bicarbonate mucous is disturbed. For this reason, most patients are discharged with a prescription for histamine-type-2–inhibitor medications (eg, ranitidine) as a preventative measure. Patients who have a pouch that is too large (excess parietal cells) or who use nonsteroidal anti-inflammatory drugs, such as ibuprofen and aspirin, are at higher risk. As marginal ulcers are often present in the setting of gastric staple-line fistula (discussed below with other late complications), the evaluation is best performed by an experienced endoscopist (Chapter 10). Uncomplicated cases (no bleeding) are usually treated with an oral PPI.

Neuropathy

New-onset polyneuropathies have been described within months after gastric-bypass procedures. The overall incidence of neuropathy identified within 6 months of surgery is probably very low, with rough estimates of 6 cases per 10,000 operations. Originally thought to be idiopathic, the acute post-gastric reduction surgery (APGARS) neuropathy is an umbrella condition under which several etiologies lie. In general, APGARS refers to neuropathy that develops in the ill patient with persistent or recurrent vomiting, characterized by hyporeflexia and muscular weakness. One survey of bariatric surgical practices estimated that 40% of cases are due to a B-vitamin deficiency (thiamine or B12), while 60% are "idiopathic."[51] Other etiologies of what appears to be neuropathy are possibly overlooked by some practices, such as vitamin-D deficiency. Many of the cases are self-limited and resolve over a few months; therefore, other common etiologies, such as nerve entrapment in the type 2 diabetic patient, may be responsible. The diabetic patient population deserves special mention here because improved mobility with weight loss may unmask chronic neuropathic or myopathic disorders, many of which are not prevented with improved glycemic control. These can be difficult to diagnose and distinguish from one another and should not be quickly attributed to a bariatric surgery related condition.[52] Because the cause may be multifactorial, a careful neurologic exam and laboratory evaluation (which measures electrolytes, serum 25(OH)D, B12, folate, and thiamine levels) will identify treatable causes.

Bowel-Associated Dermatosis-Arthritis Syndrome

In the 1960s and 1970s, when JIB was first used to treat morbid obesity, up to 20% of patients were reported to suffer a postoperative syndrome of an influenza-like illness with increased temperature, chills, polyarthralgia, and myalgia, followed by a skin eruption. The skin findings were similar to neutrophilic dermatoses of various etiologies, with inflammatory papules that measured up to 1 cm in diameter and often with centralized vesicles or pustules that usually appeared on the extremities and the upper part of the trunk.[53] Originally called the bowel-bypass syndrome, bowel-associated dermatosis-arthritis syndrome (BADAS) has been reported in recent years to occur following BPD; but, while perhaps under-recognized, it is considered to be less common than originally thought.[54] Completing the serum sickness-like presentation, most patients have a nonerosive polyarthritis with or without tenosynovitis, which is asymmetric and episodic and affects both small and large joints. A similar syndrome was later described in patients with inflammatory bowel disease and following Billroth II procedures for peptic-ulcer disease.[55] The pathogenesis is as yet unclear, but both the clinical presentation and pathologic evaluations suggest immune complex formation and deposition in the synovium, epithelium, and endothelium, with resultant activation of the alternate pathway of complement; small-bowel overgrowth (discussed above) may be related. Treatments for BADAS shown to be effective in small numbers of patients include prednisone (10 to 60 mg/day), dapsone (100 mg/day), and antibiotics (tetracycline 1 to 2 g/day), minocycline (100 to 400 mg/day), clindamycin (600 mg/day), trimethoprim-sulfamethoxazole (160 to 800 mg/day), erythromycin (500 to 2000 mg/day), and metronidazole (500 to 1000 mg/day).[56,57] If medical therapy fails, in severe cases, surgical reanastomosis may be advised.

Hair Loss

Hair loss, or telogen effluvium, commonly occurs 3 to 6 months after surgery. Patients complain of diffuse shedding of normal hair, often reporting more hair found in their hairbrush or comb after use. Sometimes hair can be found on their pillow in the morning, which is particularly distressing for patients. While the exact mechanism is unknown, the stress of rapid weight loss (medical or surgical) disrupts the growth cycle of individual hair. As a result, many hair in the growing phase are interrupted and quickly "pushed" into the dying phase (telogen), giving the patient the appearance of "going bald." Treatment of telogen effluvium is reassurance, as it will reverse with time and weight stabilization.[58]

LATE COMPLICATIONS (>6 MONTHS)

Anemia

A low hematocrit occurring after 6 months postoperatively is usually due to vitamin-B12 deficiency from malabsorption, although a stool test for occult blood must be performed to rule out bleeding. B12 deficiency is very common after RYGB and BPD.[59,60] It is typically apparent around 10 months postoperatively with a mildly low hematocrit, elevated mean corpuscular volume, and multinucleated neutrophils similar to the pattern seen in patients after gastrectomy. A small percentage of patients do not present with anemia or macrocytosis, so screening postoperative B12 levels should be routine (Chapter 8).

Weight Regain

Weight regain after 2 years is well documented to occur in some patients, but the etiology is not always clear. It is important for the PCP to recognize that, in every case, the patient is absorbing more calories. Most of the time, this means the patient is eating more calories and is, therefore, reverting back to previous maladaptive eating behaviors. In a minority of cases, weight regain may be due to surgical complication(s) leading to a change in either the restrictive or the malabsorptive component of the procedure. Examples of potentially culprit complications are gastric staple-line disruption or dehiscence at the intestinal side-to-side anastomosis.

All patients who complain of weight regain should first have the gain measured on a regularly calibrated office scale and documented by his or her PCP. The patient should then be asked to complete a food diary as a first step in diagnosis. Behaviors such as binge eating, which usually stop but may continue in some patients, must be assessed carefully. Binge eating after weight-loss surgery is likely a poor prognostic sign for weight-loss maintenance, and patients should be referred immediately back to the bariatric nutritionist and/or psychologist.[61]

Gastric staple-line disruption (also termed "staple-line fistula" and "gastrogastric fistula") can lead to weight regain and may occur after any bariatric procedures that have a "stomach-stapling" component. The disruption results from a breakdown of the gastric partitioning staple line. When the pouch and the remnant are stapled but not divided, it is termed staple-line disruption "in continuity"; this occurs in up to 20% of VBG patients. However, most surgeons today divide the gastric pouch from the gastric remnant between the staple lines, particularly in laparoscopic procedures, which reduces the risk to <5% (Figure 9-1).[37] The average time to gastric staple-line disruption is 10 to 30 months after surgery. Patients with gastric staple-line disruption usually describe increased hunger, less satiety, and increased intake. Disruption often occurs adjacent to, and because of, a marginal ulcer, which adds epigastric pain to the clinical presentation. Empiric treatment of the ulcer with acid-reducing medications (as discussed earlier) is appropriate. Many patients with ulcer do have a small opening of the staple line, and most of them do not experience decreased satiety and weight gain. If, in fact, they have weight regain as a result, however, surgical revision is indicated. To treat this problem less invasively, many bariatric centers are exploring endoscopic repair of staple-line disruption.

For patients who have undergone purely restrictive procedures (eg, LAGB or VBG), weight regain may also result from gastric-pouch dilation or poor follow-up. Fortunately, with the adoption of the vertical staple line over the past decade, pouch dilation is now uncommon. Postoperative follow-up requires accessing the subcutaneous port to inject or remove saline from the balloon to change the outlet size. This is usually done every 2 to 6 months for the first year, then every 4 to 12 months thereafter, depending on the surgeon and the program.[62]

The most challenging issue facing providers caring for LAGB patients is that the success of the surgery largely depends on how reliably patients return for postoperative adjustments; this explains the wide variability of reported success rates. The PCP could have substantial role in motivating patients to remain strict with the program, with an emphasis on the likelihood of failure in patients who choose not to comply.

In a small subset of patients, it is worthwhile to consider endocrine diseases that may make weight loss difficult or lead to weight regain. Such conditions are routinely evaluated in preoperative medical assessments, but a denovo onset is always possible. Hypothyroidism is a common condition, particularly among women, but remains an uncommon cause of obesity. Hashimoto's thyroiditis is the most prevalent etiology. Decreased circulating thyroxine leads to decreased metabolic rate and therefore may cause excess fat storage. With weight loss, one would expect that the required replacement dose might be reduced, but for patients who take levothyroxine at the same time as calcium and iron tablets, the thyroid hormone may not be absorbed well. An elevated plasma thyroid-stimulating hormone level indicates a possible role of hypothyroidism and requires treatment with levothyroxine.

Cushing's syndrome and acromegaly, albeit exceedingly rare, should be considered in the face of weight regain in a patient who appears compliant with diet. Excess corticosteroid exposure, whether endogenous (Cushing's syndrome) or exogenous (therapeutic glucocorticoid use), often leads to excess adiposity, typically with a central distribution. Acromegaly is an extremely rare and insidious condition that results from excess growth hormone secretion by a tumor, usually in the pituitary gland. Because both of these syndromes are so rare, they should be considered only when a patient has consistent symptoms and signs: eg, easy bruising and osteoporosis in Cushing's syndrome and enlarged hands and feet in acromegaly.

In the absence of an obvious dietary, behavioral, or endocrine explanation for weight gain, a contrast-swallow study of the UGI tract may be necessary. Such a test may be useful in identifying disruptions of the staple line that divides the pouch and the excluded gastric remnant. It is usually better for the bariatric surgeon to direct the diagnostic approach to the evaluation of weight regain, as it may involve multiple members of the multidisciplinary team, particularly a radiologist who is familiar with the appearance of the post-gastric–bypass anatomy (Chapter 11). Referral to the bariatric team after conservative screening (eg, food diary) is recommended.

Abdominal Pain

Internal hernias are the most difficult complications of gastric-bypass surgery to diagnose. The incidence of internal hernia has risen with the increased popularity of the laparoscopic approach because of fewer postoperative adhesions. Fewer adhesions makes the bowel more mobile and able to slip into potential spaces such as the mesenteric defect, under the Roux limb, or through the transverse mesocolon.[63] Therefore, internal hernias occur commonly at 3 locations: through the transverse mesocolon, under the Roux limb (Petersen's space), or through the mesenteric defect. Approximately half of patients with an internal hernia will present with an obvious bowel obstruction: nausea, vomiting, and cramping abdominal pain. The other half will have only intermittent abdominal pain. Once the other common causes of abdominal pain after gastric bypass, such as gallstones and marginal ulcer, have been ruled out, evaluation commonly proceeds with a contrast UGI or CT scan (Chapter 11). Twenty percent of patients with a symptomatic internal hernia will have a normal contrast study. Unexplained abdominal pain can be an intermittent obstruction due to an internal hernia and should be referred back to the bariatric team for possible exploratory laparoscopy.[63]

Bone Pain

Osteomalacia due to vitamin-D deficiency (or hypovitaminosis D) is a condition observed in specific populations, including individuals with obesity and those with malabsorptive physiology. Not surprisingly, then, the bariatric patient who has undergone gastric-bypass surgery has been found to be at significant risk of hypovitaminosis D.[64,65] Up to 50% will have some degree of hypocalcemia and all of these patients with low vitamin-D levels will have secondary hyperparathyroidism.[66,67] This can be a clinically silent disease for many years, while the compensatory rise in parathyroid hormone slowly leads to demineralization of the skeleton in order to maintain adequate blood calcium levels. As with osteoporosis, low bone density is detected by bone densitometry, and patients are at increased risk for fracture. Unlike osteoporosis, however, this condition is unique in that it causes bone tenderness, easily elicited at sites where the bone is prominent (sternum, anterior tibia). Hypovitaminosis D may be diagnosed with a plasma 25(OH)D level of <20 mg/dl. Because it is often difficult to restore levels to normal once they are already low, prevention is important. Prevention is best done with a combination of a daily vitamin with D, milk, and orange juice with D supplementation, as well as cautious exposure to ultraviolet light, eg, sunlight. If a low 25(OH)D is detected, doses of 50,000 IU given orally once weekly for 8 weeks at a time is a safe and effective "repletion" schedule.[68] This may be repeated twice. If the 25(OH)D level remains low, referral to a bone specialist is indicated.

Sagging Abdominal Skin

After 12 to 18 months, when most of the weight loss has occurred, many patients are faced with severely sagging skin. Excess skin at the abdomen, forming a large panniculus on the abdominal wall, may cause intertriginous dermatitis and tinea corpus, which is often resistant to conservative therapies. It is not uncommon for a patient to complain of hindered mobility and lower back pain with a panniculus that sits on the upper thighs. All patients should be referred for consultation with a plastic surgeon. Unfortunately, most procedures are considered cosmetic by a majority of health-insurance companies and require substantial out-of-pocket payment by the patient. If the PCP is able to document severe complications from the panniculus to warrant a panniculectomy by a plastic surgeon, some companies may cover it in full.

Complications and the Risk/Benefit Ratio

Present and future research in the area of bariatric surgery should identify factors about an individual that could predict his or her success after bariatric surgery. Some providers utilize previously published guidelines, which have identified several factors likely to predict success: lower severity of obesity, younger age, surgical naivety, history of successful behavior modification, and excellent social support.[3,69] Many bariatric centers are collecting their own data on success and complications, which provides patients and their PCPs with more information when balancing risks with benefits of bariatric surgery. In the past, data on this topic has been sparse, but it is slowly increasing. Clinicians in the field of bariatrics therefore look forward to prospective data from the NIH program Longitudinal Assessment of Bariatric Surgery.[70] Major efforts in the areas of epidemiology and basic and clinical research are pursuing the following goals: (1) better define the risks and benefits of bariatric surgery, including gender-specific outcomes; (2) form evidence-based recommendations for patient selection and management; and (3) elucidate the mechanisms by which surgery affects obesity-related comorbid conditions, energy expenditure, nutrient partitioning, appetitive behaviors, and psychosocial factors.

Summary

Rising rates of obesity and increasing awareness of surgical treatments suggest that the primary clinician will have an increasing role in the care of the bariatric patient. Patients with obesity are typically more medically complex, with high-acuity comorbidities such as type 2 diabetes, and the addition of bariatric surgery to their medical history may be daunting for the PCP. However, a rational approach to the care of the bariatric patient can empower the clinician, allowing both the patient and provider to focus on the positive metabolic and physical changes that occur over a short period of time. Remaining in contact with the bariatric team is a good initial step that will reinforce efforts to detect and prevent complications in the short and long term. As more prospective data is published, it is increasingly clear what the PCP can anticipate with respect to weight loss, improvements in comorbid illnesses, and nutritional risks. Finally, when the bariatric patient presents with symptoms, the PCP can approach the differential diagnosis methodically and reinforce postoperative behavioral modification. A knowledgeable and caring provider will remember and remind the patient that the risks of lifelong obesity far outweigh those of bariatric surgery.

References

1. Renquist K, Jeng G, Mason EE. Calculating follow-up rates. *Obes Surg.* 1992;2(4):361-367.
2. Stocker DJ. Management of the bariatric surgery patient. *Endocrinol Metab Clin North Am.* 2003;32(2):347-357.
3. Kral JG. Selection of patients for anti-obesity surgery. *Int J Obes Relat Metab Disord.* 2001;25(suppl 1):S107-S112.
4. Marceau P, Hould FS, Lebel S, Marceau S, Biron S. Malabsorptive obesity surgery. *Surg Clin North Am.* 2001;81(5):1113-1127.
5. Schauer PR, Ikramuddin S, Gourash W, Ramanathan R, Luketich J. Outcomes after laparoscopic Roux-en-Y gastric bypass for morbid obesity. *Ann Surg.* 2000;232:515-529.
6. Buchwald H, Avidor Y, Braunwald E, et al. Bariatric surgery: a systematic review and meta-analysis. *JAMA.* 2004;292(14):1724-1737.
7. Brolin RE, Kenler HA, Gorman JH, Cody RP. Long-limb gastric bypass in the superobese. A prospective randomized study. *Ann Surg.* 1992;215(4):387-395.
8. Liddle, RA, Goldstein RB, Saxton J. Gallstone formation during weight-reduction dieting. *Arch Intern Med.* 1989;149(8):1750-1753.
9. Brolin RE. Gastric bypass. *Surg Clin North Am.* 2001;81(5):1077-1095.
10. Tuomilehto J, Lindstrom J, Eriksson JG, et al. Prevention of type 2 diabetes mellitus by changes in lifestyle among subjects with impaired glucose tolerance. *N Engl J Med.* 2001;344(18):1343-1350.
11. Sjostrom L, Lindroos AK, Peltonen M, et al. Lifestyle, diabetes, and cardiovascular risk factors 10 years after bariatric surgery. *N Engl J Med.* 2004;351(26):2683-2693.
12. Belachew M, Legrand M, Vincent V, Lismonde M, Le Docte N, Deschamps V. Laparoscopic adjustable gastric banding. *World J Surg.* 1998;22(9):955-963.
13. Colditz GA, Willett WC, Rotnitzky A, Manson JE. Weight gain as a risk factor for clinical diabetes mellitus in women. *Ann Intern Med.* 1995;122(7):481-486.
14. Pories WJ, Swanson MS, MacDonald KG, et al. Who would have thought it? An operation proves to be the most effective therapy for adult-onset diabetes mellitus. *Ann Surg.* 1995;222(3):339-350.
15. Rubino F, Marescaux J. Letter to the editor: in reply. *Ann Surg.* 2004;240(2):389-390.
16. Cummings DE, Weigle DS, Frayo RS, et al. Plasma ghrelin levels after diet-induced weight loss or gastric bypass surgery. *N Engl J Med.* 2002;346(21);1623-1630.
17. Holdstock C, Engstrom BE, Ohrvall M, Lind L, Sundbom M, Karlsson FA. Ghrelin and adipose tissue regulatory peptides: effect of gastric bypass surgery in obese humans. *J Clin Endocrinol Metab.* 2003;88(7):3177-3183.
18. Proceedings of the American College of Endocrinology Task Force on Inpatient Diabetes and Metabolic Control Consensus Conference. Washington, DC, USA, December 2003. *Endocr Pract.* 2004;10(suppl 2):3-108.
19. Clinical guidelines on the identification, evaluation, and treatment of overweight and obesity in adults—the evidence report. National Institutes of Health. *Obes Res.* 1998;6(suppl 2):51S-209S.
20. MacMahon S, Cutler J, Brittain E, Higgins M. Obesity and hypertension: epidemiological and clinical issues. *Eur Heart J.* 1987;8(suppl B):57-70.
21. Stevens VJ, Obarzanek E, Cook NR, et al. Long-term weight loss and changes in blood pressure: results of the Trials of Hypertension Prevention, phase II. *Ann Intern Med.* 2001;134(1):1-11.
22. Schauer, PR; Ikramuddin, S; Gourash W, Ramanathan R, Luketich J. Outcomes after laparoscopic Roux-en-Y gastric bypass for morbid obesity. *Ann Surg.* 2000;232(4):515-529.
23. Gokce N, Vita JA, McDonnell M, et al. Effect of medical and surgical weight loss on endothelial vasomotor function in obese patients. *Am J Cardiol.* 2005;95(2):266-268.
24. Snow LL, Weinstein LS, Hannon JK, et al. The effect of Roux-en-Y gastric bypass on prescription drug costs. *Obes Surg.* 2004;14(8):1031-1035.
25. Lim PO, Rodgers P, Cardale K, Watson AD, MacDonald TM. Potentially high prevalence of primary aldosteronism in a primary-care population. *Lancet.* 1999;353(9146):40.

26. Mingrone G, DeGaetano A, Greco AV, et al. Reversibility of insulin resistance in obese diabetic patients: role of plasma lipids. *Diabetologia.* 1997;40(5):599-605.

27. Frantzides CT, Carlson MA, Moore RE, et al. Effect of body mass index on nonalcoholic fatty liver disease in patients undergoing minimally invasive bariatric surgery. *J Gastrointest Surg.* 2004;8(7):849-855.

28. Luyckx FH, Scheen AJ, Desaive C, Thiry A, Lefebvre PJ. Parallel reversibility of biological markers of the metabolic syndrome and liver steatosis after gastroplasty-induced weight loss in severe obesity. *J Clin Endocrinol Metab.* 1999;84(11):4293.

29. Dixon JB, Bhathal PS, Hughes NR, O'Brien PE. Nonalcoholic fatty liver disease: improvement in liver histological analysis with weight loss. *Hepatology.* 2004;39(6):1647-1654.

30. Luyckx FH, Desaive C, Thiry A, et al. Liver abnormalities in severely obese subjects: effect of drastic weight loss after gastroplasty. *Int J Obes Relat Metab Disord.* 1998;22(3):222-226.

31. Silverman EM, Sapala JA, Appelman HD. Regression of hepatic steatosis in morbidly obese persons after gastric bypass. *Am J Clin Pathol.* 1995;104(1):23-31.

32. Scheuller M, Weider D. Bariatric surgery for treatment of sleep apnea syndrome in 15 morbidly obese patients: long-term results. *Otolaryngol Head Neck Surg.* 2001;125(4):299-302.

33. Pillar G, Peled R, Lavie P. Recurrence of sleep apnea without concomitant weight increase 7.5 years after weight reduction surgery. *Chest.* 1994;106(6):1702-1704.

34. Huerta S, DeShields S, Shipner R, et al. Safety and efficacy of postoperative continuous positive airway pressure to prevent pulmonary complications after Roux-en-Y gastric bypass. *J Gastrointest Surg.* 2002;6(3):354-358.

35. Gastrointestinal surgery for severe obesity. National Institutes of Health consensus development conference statement, March 1991. *Am J Clin Nutr.* 1992;55:615S-619S.

36. Institute of Medicine, National Academy of Sciences: *Nutrition During Pregnancy. Part I, Weight Gain; Part II, Nutrient Supplements.* National Academy Press, 1990.

37. Pratt JS, Blackburn GL. Surgical approaches to the treatment of obesity: a practical guide for the covering physician. In: Bray GA, ed. *Office Management of Obesity.* Philadelphia, Pa: W.B. Saunders; 2004:275-298.

38. Carvajal SH, Mulvihill SJ. Postgastrectomy syndromes: dumping and diarrhea. *Gastroenterol Clin North Am.* 1994;23(2):261-279.

39. MacLean, LD, Rhode BM, Sampalis J, Forse RA. Results of the surgical treatment of obesity. *Am J Surg.* 1993;165(1):155-160.

40. Huang CS, Forse RA, Jacobson BC, Farraye FA. Endoscopic findings and their clinical correlations in patients with symptoms after gastric bypass surgery. *Gastrointest Endosc.* 2003;58(6):859-866.

41. Creutzfeldt W. The incretin concept today. *Diabetologia.* 1979;16(2):75-85.

42. Kellum JM, Kuemmerle JF, O'Dorisio TM, et al. Gastrointestinal hormone responses to meals before and after gastric bypass and vertical banded gastroplasty. *Ann Surg.* 1990;211(6):763-770.

43. Clements RH, Gonzalez QH, Long CI, Wittert G, Laws HL. Hormonal changes after Roux-en-Y gastric bypass for morbid obesity and the control of type-II diabetes mellitus. *Am Surg.* 2004;70(1):1-4.

44. Gudmand-Hoyer E, Asp NG, Skovbjerg H, Andersen B. Lactose malabsorption after bypass operation for obesity. *Scand J Gastroenterol.* 1978;13(6):641-647.

45. Bouhnik Y, Alain S, Attar A, et al. Bacterial populations contaminating the upper gut in patients with small intestinal bacterial overgrowth syndrome. *Am J Gastroenterol.* 1999:94(5):1327-1331.

46. Bengmark S. Ecological control of the gastrointestinal tract. The role of probiotic flora. *Gut.* 1998;42(1):2-7.

47. Skroubis G, Sakellaropoulos G, Pouggouras K, Mead N, Nikiforidis G, Kalfarentzos F. Comparison of nutritional deficiencies after Roux-en-Y gastric bypass and after biliopancreatic diversion with Roux-en-Y gastric bypass. *Obes Surg.* 2002;12(4):551-558.

48. Brolin RE, Leung M. Survey of vitamin and mineral supplementation after gastric bypass and biliopancreatic diversion for morbid obesity. *Obes Surg.* 1999;9(2):150-154.

49. Brolin RE, Gorman JH, Gorman RC, et al. Prophylactic iron supplementation after Roux-en-Y gastric bypass: a prospective, double-blind, randomized study. *Arch Surg.* 1998;133(7):740-744.

50. Ortega J, Escudero MD, Mora F, et al. Outcome of esophageal function and 24-hour esophageal pH monitoring after vertical banded gastroplasty and Roux-en-Y gastric bypass. *Obes Surg.* 2004;14(8):1086-1094.

51. Chang CG, Adams-Huet B, Provost DA. Acute post-gastric reduction surgery (APGARS) neuropathy. *Obes Surg.* 2004;14(2):182-189.

52. Vinik AI, Mehrabyan A. Diabetic neuropathies. *Med Clin North Am.* 2004;88(4): 947-999.

53. Kennedy C. The spectrum of inflammatory skin disease following jejuno-ileal bypass for morbid obesity. *Br J Dermatol.* 1981;105(4):425-435.

54. Slater GH, Kerlin P, Georghiou PR, Fielding GA. Bowel-associated dermatosis-arthritix syndrome after biliopancreatic diversion. *Obes Surg.* 2004;14(1):133-135.

55. Dicken CH. Bowel-associated dermatosis-arthritis syndrome: bowel bypass syndrome without bowel bypass. *J Am Acad Dermatol.* 1986;14(5, Pt 1):792-796.

56. Stein HB, Schlappner OL, Boyko W, Gourlay RH, Reeve CE. The intestinal bypass: arthritis-dermatitis syndrome. *Arthritis Rheum.* 1981;24(5):684-690.

57. Ely PH. The bowel bypass syndrome: a response to bacterial peptidoglycans. *J Am Acad Dermatol.* 1980;2(6):473-487.

58. Bolognia JL, Braverman IM. Skin manifestations of internal disease. In: Braunwald E, ed. *Harrison's Principles of Internal Medicine.* 15th ed. New York, NY: McGraw Hill; 2001:315-330.

59. Brolin RE, Gorman JH, Gorman RC, et al. Are vitamin B12 and folate deficiency clinically important after Roux-en-Y gastric bypass? *J Gastrointest Surg.* 1998;2(5):436-442.

60. Adachi S, Kawamoto T, Otsuka M, Todoroki T, Fukao K. Enteral vitamin B12 supplements reverse post-gastrectomy B12 deficiency. *Ann Surg.* 2000;232(2):199-201.

61. Kalarchian MA, Marcus MD, Wilson GT, Labouvie EW, Brolin RE, LaMarca LB. Binge eating among gastric bypass patients at long-term follow-up. *Obes Surg.* 2002;12(2) 270-275.

62. Busetto L, Segato G, De Marchi F, et al. Postoperative management of laparoscopic gastric banding. *Obes Surg.* 2003;13(1):121-127.

63. Garza E Jr, Kuhn J, Arnold D, Nicholson W, Reddy S, McCarty T. Internal hernias after laparoscopic Roux-en-Y gastric bypass. *Am J Surg.* 2004;188(6):796-800.

64. Shaker JL, Norton AJ, Woods MF, Fallon MD, Findling JW. Secondary hyperparathyroidism and osteopenia in women following gastric exclusion surgery for obesity. *Osteoporos Int.* 1991;1(3):177-181.

65. Goode LR, Brolin RE, Hasina A. Bone and gastric bypass surgery: effects of dietary calcium and vitamin D. *Obes Res.* 2004;12:40-46.

66. Slater GH, Ren DJ, Siegel N, et al. Serum fat-soluble vitamin deficiency and abnormal calcium metabolism after malabsorptive bariatric surgery. *J Gastrointest Surg.* 2004;8:48-55.

67. Newbury L, Dolan K, Hatzifotis M, Low N, Fielding G. Calcium and vitamin D depletion and elevated parathyroid hormone following biliopancreatic diversion. *Obes Surg.* 2003;13(6):893-895.

68. Malabanan A, Veronikis IE, Holick MF. Redefining vitamin D insufficiency. *Lancet.* 1998;351(9105):805-806.

69. Grace DM. Patient selection for obesity surgery. *Gastroenterol Clin North Am.* 1987;16(3):399-413.

70. About Us resource page. Longitudinal Assessment of Bariatric Surgery (LABS) web site. Available at: http://www.edc.gsph.pitt.edu/labs/public/. Accessed February 27, 2005.

10

Endoscopy After Bariatric Surgery

Christopher S. Huang, MD and Francis A. Farraye, MD, MSc

Introduction

Performing upper endoscopic procedures in patients after bariatric surgery can be a challenging task because of the anatomic alterations created during surgery, as well as the unique postoperative complications that can arise. This is particularly true when dealing with patients post Roux-en-Y gastric-bypass (RYGB) surgery, in which the bypassed segments of stomach and small intestine are present *in situ* and yet are not readily accessible using standard endoscopic techniques. The keys to performing endoscopy after bariatric surgery include: (1) understanding the indications and contraindications for endoscopy, (2) being familiar with the expected postsurgical anatomy and endoscopic appearance after bariatric surgery, and (3) anticipating the common structural complications. This chapter will address these issues as well as discuss various aspects of performing therapeutic endoscopy in the bariatric surgical patient.

General Principles and Guidelines for Performing Endoscopy After Bariatric Surgery

Prior to performing upper endoscopy in the bariatric surgical patient, the endoscopist should observe the following basic principles, modified from Stellato et al[1]:

1. Whenever possible, discuss the specific operation with the patient's bariatric surgeon to best understand the altered anatomy. (Be aware that modifications to the standard operations are not uncommon.)
2. Review the operative report and pertinent perioperative records, as well as all available postoperative abdominal imaging studies.
3. Select the most appropriate type of endoscope and accessories based on the indication for the procedure and information gathered from the above investigations. Obtain any specially designed accessories that may be necessary before starting the procedure.

Selection of Endoscopic Equipment

For most RYGB patients, a standard diagnostic gastroscope is the most appropriate type of endoscope for evaluating the esophagus, gastric pouch, gastrojejunal anastomosis, and proximal portion of the Roux limb. A pediatric colonoscope or enteroscope may be required to examine the jejunojejunal anastomosis, particularly in patients with a long-limb RYGB.

Peroral retrograde evaluation of the bypassed stomach and biliopancreatic limb is difficult, but it can be accomplished using a pediatric colonoscope or enteroscope of sufficient length to traverse the Roux-en-Y.[2,3] A long-limb RYGB or acute angulation at the jejunojejunostomy often precludes successful evaluation of the bypassed segments, for which intraoperative enteroscopy or antegrade examination via percutaneous gastrostomy may be required.[4-6]

Indications and Contraindications

Indications

Endoscopy after bariatric surgery is indicated for the evaluation of persistent or unexplained upper gastrointestinal (UGI) symptoms, such as nausea, vomiting, abdominal pain, dysphagia, and hemorrhage. Weight regain, or failure to lose weight, should also prompt an endoscopic examination. In our experience, the most common symptoms reported by patients referred for endoscopy were epigastric abdominal pain (53%), nausea/vomiting (35%), and dysphagia (16%).[7] These symptoms are often multifactorial in etiology; dumping syndrome, inappropriate eating habits, and poor food selection frequently contribute, but upper endoscopy should be performed to exclude structural abnormalities in the surgically altered gastrointestinal (GI) tract.

Upper GI hemorrhage is a relatively uncommon complication after bariatric surgery.[8-10] Studies have demonstrated that hemorrhage during the early postoperative period usually arises from the staple lines of the gastrojejunostomy, gastric remnant, or jejunojejunostomy.[10] Late GI hemorrhage is commonly from a marginal ulcer at the gastrojejunostomy, but bleeding from the bypassed stomach and duodenum should be considered when no apparent source is identified.[9]

The failure to lose weight or the presence of weight regain after gastric bypass or gastroplasty may indicate the development of a staple-line dehiscence. An excessively wide stoma at the gastrojejunal anastomosis can also present as weight gain, presumably due to reduced restriction of food intake. Weight gain after vertical banded gastroplasty (VBG) or laparoscopic adjustable gastric banding (LAGB) also commonly occurs with band erosion into the gastric lumen, which is best diagnosed endoscopically. In many cases, infection at the access-port site (following LAGB) is the first sign of band erosion.[11] Therefore, band erosion should be excluded by endoscopy at the first sign of port infection.

Heartburn has been reported to be a common complication of gastric banding,[12-14] but the actual effect of this procedure on gastroesophageal reflux is controversial.[15,16] Reflux appears to be worsened when a large gastric pouch is present but improved when the band is placed at or just below the gastroesophageal junction, thereby augmenting the effect of the lower esophageal sphincter.[17] Endoscopists should be aware that heartburn after LAGB may be due to an excessively tight band, and there may be an increased risk

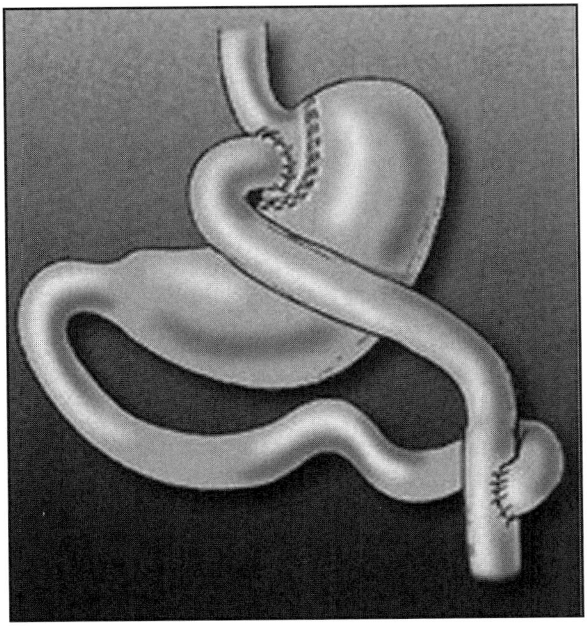

Figure 10-1. Illustration of the RYGB. (Courtesy of the American Society for Bariatric Surgery [ASBS]; Gainesville, FL.) *For a full-color version, see page CA-V of the Color Atlas.*

of endoscopy-related perforation in this setting.[17] A barium contrast study should be performed first to assess the degree of constriction and the position of the band. Endoscopy should be performed if heartburn persists after band deflation.

Contraindications

Upper endoscopy is generally contraindicated when the risks to patient health or life are judged to outweigh the most favorable benefits of the procedure, when adequate patient cooperation or consent cannot be obtained, or when a perforated viscus is known or suspected.[18] It is also advisable to defer endoscopic procedures during the immediate postoperative period to avoid the risk of disrupting the fresh anastomoses.

Postsurgical Anatomy and Expected Endoscopic Appearance

The major types of bariatric procedures that endoscopists may encounter are discussed here. It is critical to have a basic understanding of the anatomical changes after bariatric surgery before endoscopy is performed. A more thorough discussion of the various bariatric operations is covered in Chapter 3.

Gastric Bypass

The RYGB is currently the most commonly performed bariatric operation in the United States (Figure 10-1).[19] Although there are several modifications of the RYGB, in the standard procedure, a small gastric pouch (typically <30 ml) is created along the lesser curve and transected from the remainder of the stomach. The pouch is anastomosed to a Roux

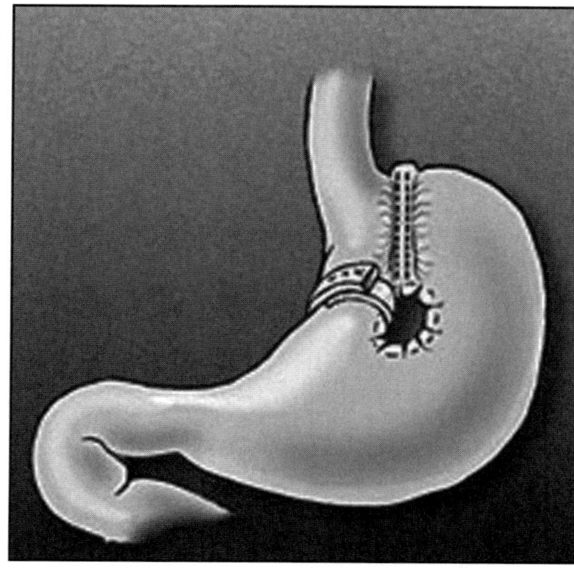

Figure 10-2. Illustration of the VBG. (Courtesy of the ASBS; Gainesville, FL.) *For a full-color version, see page CA-V of the Color Atlas.*

limb in an end-to-side fashion, creating a gastrojejunostomy with a stomal diameter of approximately 10 to 12 mm. The length of the Roux limb is typically 60 to 75 cm but varies, depending on the degree of malabsorption that is desired, and can be as long as 150 cm in the long-limb RYGB. The original gastric bypass was fashioned with a loop gastrojejunostomy,[20] which was subsequently abandoned because of problems with alkaline reflux into the pouch.

Endoscopically, the esophagus and gastroesophageal junction should have a normal, unaltered appearance following RYGB. The normal gastric pouch is small, so minimal amounts of air should be insufflated. Special attention should be paid to the gastrojejunostomy, which, being an end-to-side anastomosis, typically has a short, blind limb of jejunum in addition to the Roux limb, which drains the pouch. The Roux limb should be of normal caliber and generally free of food residue or fluid.

Vertical Banded Gastroplasty

The VBG is a purely restrictive operation and is generally comparable to RYGB in terms of long-term excess weight loss.[21] The key components of this operation include a vertically-oriented 15-ml gastric channel (pouch) and an outlet (stoma) from the channel into the remainder of the stomach (Figure 10-2). The stoma is reinforced by a polypropylene mesh collar or a silastic ring to prevent stomal dilation. The remainder of the stomach and small intestine are unaltered in VBG.

Endoscopy following VBG is relatively straightforward. The vertical lesser-curvature channel permits easy endoscopic visualization. The stoma is located at the lower end of the channel, typically 7 to 8 cm distal to the gastroesophageal junction. The stoma should be approximately 10 to 12 mm wide and endoscopically may appear similar to the pylorus or the diaphragmatic narrowing of a hiatal hernia. After the endoscope passes beyond the stoma, complete examination of the unaltered antrum, pylorus, and duodenum can be performed without difficulty.

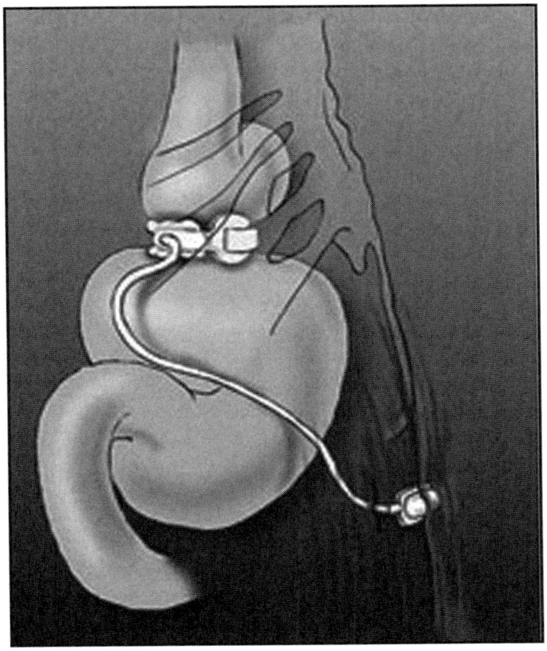

Figure 10-3. Illustration of the LAGB. (Courtesy of the ASBS; Gainesville, FL.) *For a full-color version, see page CA-VI of the Color Atlas.*

Gastric Banding

Gastric banding is another purely restrictive procedure in which a constricting prosthetic band is placed around the proximal stomach, creating a small proximal pouch and a large remnant in an "hour-glass" configuration.[22] An adjustable band, which is lined by an inflatable balloon that is connected to a subcutaneous saline port, allows for changes in the degree of constriction.[23] This procedure is typically performed laparoscopically—the so-called LAGB operation (Figure 10-3).[24]

Biliopancreatic Diversion and Duodenal Switch

Biliopancreatic diversion (BPD) is primarily a malabsorptive procedure with 2 key components: a distal gastrectomy, which results in mild restriction of oral intake, and construction of a long-limb Roux-en-Y anastomosis with a short common alimentary channel (Figure 10-4).[25,26] A modification of the BPD is the "duodenal switch" (BPD/DS), which utilizes a sleeve gastrectomy rather than distal gastrectomy and an anastomosis of the jejunal limb end-to-end with the proximal duodenum (Figure 10-5).[27,28] These procedures are performed infrequently in the United States.

Common Endoscopic Abnormalities

Among symptomatic patients following RYGB, the most common endoscopic abnormalities are marginal (anastomotic) ulcer, stomal stenosis, and staple-line dehiscence.[7]

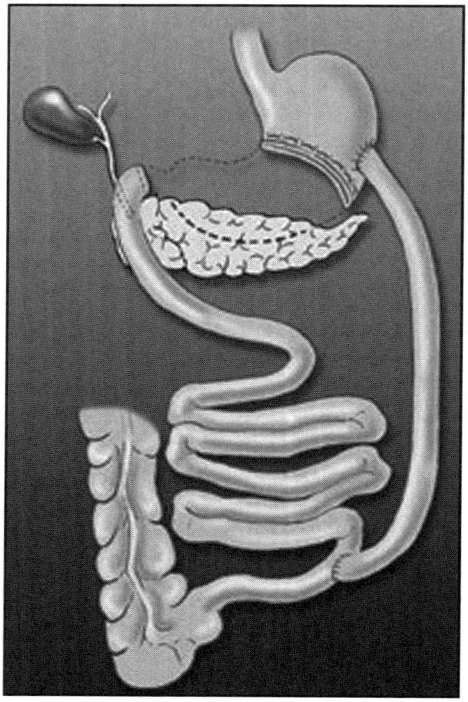

Figure 10-4. Illustration of the BPD. (Courtesy of the ASBS; Gainesville, FL.) *For a full-color version, see page CA-VI of the Color Atlas.*

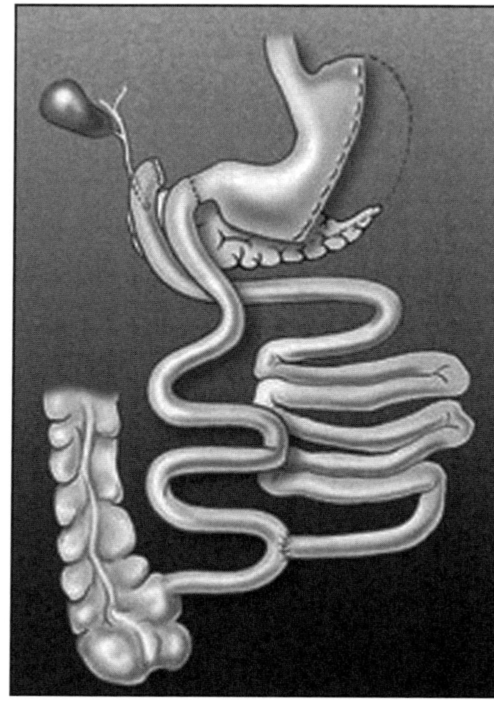

Figure 10-5. Illustration of the BPD/DS. (Courtesy of the ASBS; Gainesville, FL.) *For a full-color version, see page CA-VI of the Color Atlas.*

Marginal Ulcer

Marginal ulcers, or ulcers at the gastrojejunal anastomosis, occur in up to 16% of patients who have had RYGB (Figure 10-6).[29-32] Their etiology remains unclear, but potential contributory factors include gastric acidity (especially in the presence of a staple-line dehiscence and gastrogastric fistula), nonsteroidal anti-inflammatory drug use, *Helicobacter pylori (H. pylori)* infection, and local ischemia and tension at the anastomosis.[31,33-36] Marginal ulcers are frequently located on the jejunal side of the anastomosis, so special attention should be paid to this area during endoscopy. The detection of a marginal ulcer should prompt biopsies for *H. pylori* and a careful search for a gastrogastric fistula, both of which have been implicated in the formation of marginal ulcers.[31,35]

Stomal Stenosis

Stomal stenosis is another important complication of bariatric surgery. It occurs in approximately 3% to 12% of patients following RYGB, with reported rates as high as 27% following laparoscopic RYGB.[32,37-42] In our experience, nearly 20% of symptomatic patients after RYGB had some degree of stomal stenosis. Significant stomal stenosis is readily identified during endoscopy as a pinhole orifice in the distal pouch, precluding passage of the endoscope beyond the gastrojejunal anastomosis (Figure 10-7). Other indicators of stomal stenosis include gastric-pouch dilatation, undigested food in the pouch, or foreign material (eg, phytobezoar) obstructing the stoma.

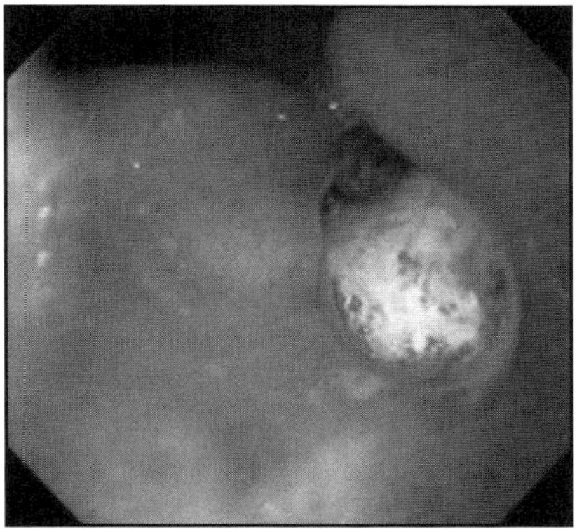

Figure 10-6. Endoscopic appearance of a marginal ulcer following RYGB. *For a full-color version, see page CA-VII of the Color Atlas.*

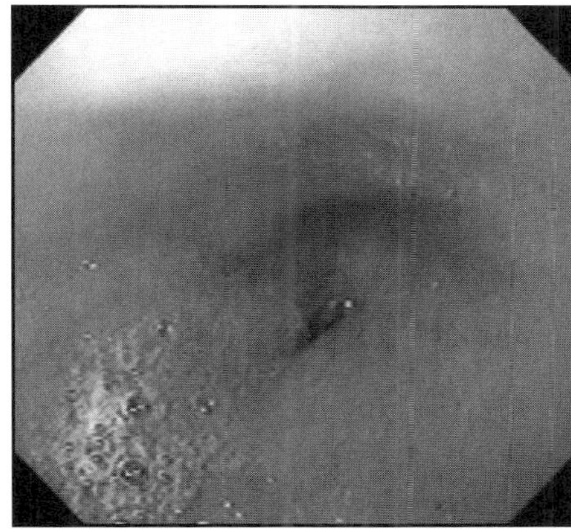

Figure 10-7. Endoscopic appearance of stomal stenosis, characterized by a pinhole orifice in the distal pouch. *For a full-color version, see page CA-VII of the Color Atlas.*

Staple-Line Dehiscence

Staple-line dehiscence with gastrogastric fistula following RYGB can be complicated by weight gain and marginal-ulcer formation. The incidence of staple-line dehiscence following gastric bypass appears to be highly dependent on surgical technique, with rates as high as 20% when the pouch and bypassed stomach are stapled in continuity, compared to 1% when the segments are completely transected.[30] Dehiscences may be small and easily overlooked, having an endoscopic appearance similar to that of a diverticulum (Figure 10-8). Barium studies are particularly helpful in identifying small dehiscences (Chapter 11). In contrast, large dehiscences are easily identified and may permit passage of the endoscope into the bypassed stomach and duodenum.

Other Endoscopic Abnormalities

Band Erosion

Band erosion is a relatively uncommon complication of VBG and LAGB, occurring in approximately 1% to 2% of VBG patients and 1% to 11% of LAGB patients.[11,43,44] In VBG patients, band erosion may cause pain but more often presents with weight gain and reduced restriction to food intake. Band erosion is a potentially serious complication after LAGB and can result in pain, vomiting, bleeding, intra-abdominal abscess, or fistula formation.[45] As in VBG patients, sudden weight gain can occur with band erosion after LAGB; in many cases, the first sign of band erosion is infection at the access port site via the connecting tube.[11] Endoscopic removal of an eroded band has been described,[46,47] but surgical removal is generally recommended as patients will typically require a redo bariatric operation.

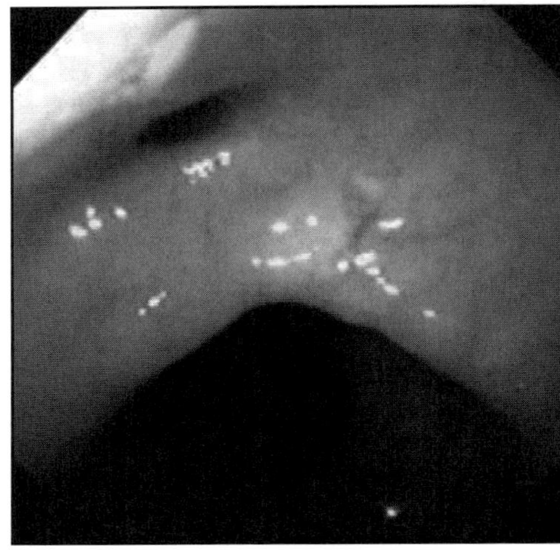

Figure 10-8. Endoscopic appearance of a small staple-line dehiscence within the gastric pouch following RYGB. *For a full-color version, see page CA-VII of the Color Atlas.*

Pathology in the Bypassed Segments

Few studies have investigated the endoscopic findings in the bypassed stomach and duodenum following RYGB.[3,48] One study shows a high prevalence of bile-associated gastritis in the bypassed stomach.[3] Intestinal metaplasia was also detected on histologic examination in a small percentage of patients. Isolated case reports of gastric carcinoma arising within the bypassed stomach have been published, but it is not yet known whether the incidence of carcinoma in this setting is actually increased.[49-51]

Therapeutic Endoscopy in the Bariatric Surgical Patient

Endoscopic Dilation of Stomal Stenosis

Endoscopic dilation of stomal stenosis after bariatric surgery is safe and effective and can be performed using a variety of methods, including balloon dilation, passage of dilators over a guidewire (Eder-Puestow, Savary-Guilliard), and endoscopic electrosurgical incision.[32,37-40,52-58]

The optimal technique for dilation of stomal stenosis is not yet known. The goal stomal diameter after dilation is 10 to 12 mm to a maximum of approximately 15 mm.[45] In a recent series using through-the-scope (TTS) balloons, nearly 60% of patients had complete symptomatic resolution after a single dilation session with a 15-mm balloon, which suggests that this should be the initial target diameter.[37] Very tight stenoses should be gradually dilated over several sessions using progressively larger balloons to reduce the risk of perforation. The incidence of perforation was 3% in a recent study in which the mean initial and final balloon sizes were 13 mm and 16 mm, respectively.[58] Overaggressive dilation should be avoided, not only to reduce the perforation risk but also to reduce the risk of exacerbating dumping symptoms or inducing weight regain. Although there are reports

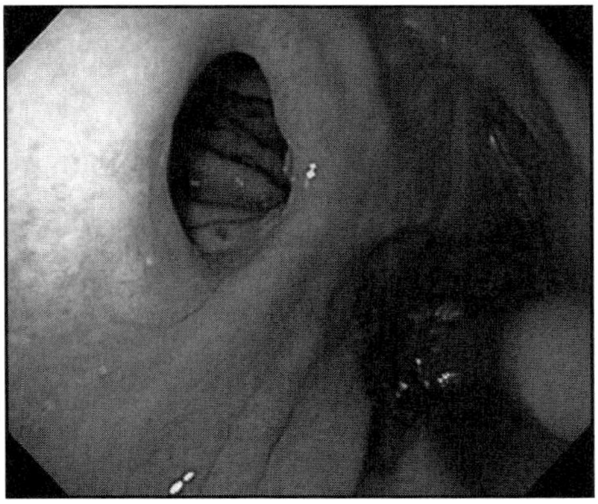

Figure 10-9A. Endoscopic appearance of staple-line dehiscence prior to closure. (Courtesy of Christopher Thompson, MD; Boston, MA.) *For a full-color version, see page CA-VIII of the Color Atlas.*

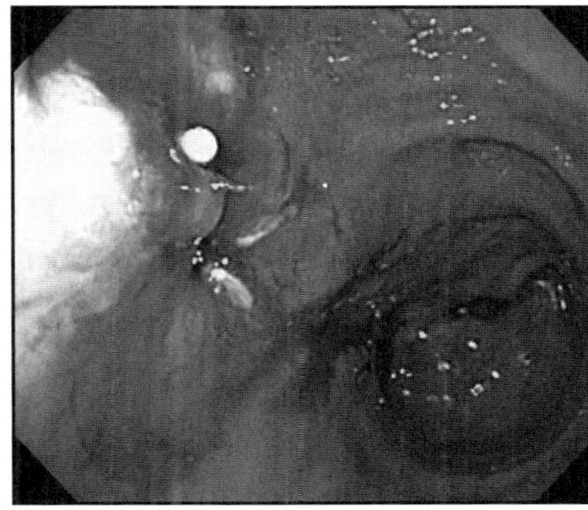

Figure 10-9B. Staple-line dehiscence successfully closed using combination of endoscopic suturing, argon plasma coagulation, and endoscopic clips. (Courtesy of Christopher Thompson, MD: Boston, MA.) *For a full-color version, see page CA-VIII of the Color Atlas.*

of successful dilation to 18 to 20 mm without resulting reoperation for weight regain,[37,53] it is our recommendation to perform serial dilations up to a maximum of 15 mm using TTS balloons. Endoscopists should exercise caution when passing TTS-balloon catheters through a tightly strictured stoma, recognizing that there is a short blind loop of jejunum beyond the gastrojejunostomy. In such situations, a wire-guided balloon should be passed under fluoroscopic visualization.

Endoscopic Management of Staple-Line Dehiscence and Excessive Stomal Dilation

Staple-line dehiscence resulting in weight regain following RYGB and VBG traditionally requires surgical revision, and experience with endoscopic closure is limited. In a small series of VBG patients, local injection of sodium morrhuate surrounding the area of dehiscence was ineffective.[59] A more promising, but technically difficult, technique involves a combination of endoscopic suturing, hemoclip application, and argon-plasma coagulation. In a preliminary study, Thompson et al achieved complete staple-line closure in 6 of 8 RYGB patients by using this method, with a resulting reduction in symptoms and cessation of weight gain (Figures 10-9A and B).[60] Additional experience and clinical trials with long-term follow-up are necessary before endoscopic closure of staple-line dehiscence can be routinely recommended.

An excessively dilated stoma that results in weight gain after gastric bypass can be managed endoscopically with sodium-morrhuate injection in 4 quadrants surrounding the stoma. In one small series, presented in abstract form, this technique resulted in a decrease in stomal size (to 12 mm or less) and resumption of weight loss in 5 of 8 (63%) gastric-bypass patients.[59] Dilated stomas can also be plicated using an endoscopic suturing device, which in a recently published series of 4 patients resulted in reduction of stomal diameter (from >2 cm preprocedurally to <15 mm postprocedurally) and in successful resumption of weight loss.[61]

Endoscopic Retrograde Cholangiopancreatography

Performing endoscopic retrograde cholangiopancreatography (ERCP) in RYGB patients is very challenging but can be successfully accomplished by a variety of methods.[62] Elton et al reported an 84% success rate using an enteroscope or pediatric colonoscope in patients who had undergone a long-limb surgical bypass, including 3 RYGB patients.[63] However, there were several disadvantages with this technique, including the lack of ERCP accessories compatible with the enteroscope, the lack of an elevator, and the limitations of forward-viewing endoscopes in performing biliopancreatic therapy. Wright et al described successful ERCP in 6 of 11 (55%) RYGB patients, with advancement of the duodenoscope over a stiff guidewire previously placed into the bypassed stomach with a forward-viewing endoscope or with "pulling up" the duodenoscope by means of a wire-guided biliary balloon anchored at the pylorus.[64]

An alternative technique involves establishing percutaneous access to the bypassed stomach via a percutaneous gastrostomy, through which the duodenoscope is then passed.[64-66] This method allows for rapid, reliable access to the duodenum and visualization of the papilla in the usual anatomic orientation for ERCP.

Endoscopic Therapy for Acute Gastrointestinal Bleeding

The management of acute GI bleeding in the early postoperative period is often challenging because of the inaccessibility of the excluded stomach and duodenum, as well as the risks associated with early postoperative endoscopy. Some authorities have advised against the use of therapeutic endoscopy in this setting, given the risk of perforation at the surgical anastomoses.[10] There are, however, isolated reports of safe and effective therapeutic endoscopy in the treatment of early GI bleeding after RYGB.[67,68] In general, early reoperation with intraoperative endoscopy (or laparoscopy-assisted enteroscopy) is considered the preferred management approach in these patients who fail conservative therapy.[10,69]

Late GI bleeding is most commonly due to marginal ulcers and can be managed endoscopically using standard hemostatic interventions such as injection and thermal and mechanical therapy.

Summary

Endoscopy after bariatric surgery poses a new challenge for gastroenterologists because of the anatomic alterations created during surgery, as well as the unique postoperative complications that can occur. Special equipment and innovative techniques may be required to perform endoscopy in this patient population. Endoscopy (in conjunction with radiologic studies) is a critical diagnostic modality for evaluating patients with UGI symptoms after bariatric surgery. Therapeutic endoscopy in bariatric surgical patients is evolving and may eventually enable endoscopic correction of structural complications.

References

1. Stellato TA, Crouse C, Hallowell PT. Bariatric surgery: creating new challenges for the endoscopist. *Gastrointest Endosc.* 2003;57:86-94.
2. Flickinger EG, Sinar DR, Pories WJ, Sloss RR, Park HK, Gibson JH. The bypassed stomach. *Am J Surg.* 1985;149:151-156.
3. Sinar DR, Flickinger EG, Park HK, Sloss RR. Retrograde endoscopy of the bypassed stomach segment after gastric bypass surgery: unexpected lesions. *South Med J.* 1985;78:255-258.
4. Sundbom M, Nyman R, Hedenstrom H, Gustavsson S. Investigation of the excluded stomach after Roux-en-Y gastric bypass. Obes Surg. 2001;11:25-27.
5. Baron TH, Vickers SM. Surgical gastrostomy placement as access for diagnostic and therapeutic ERCP. *Gastrointest Endosc.* 1998;48:640-641.
6. Fobi MA, Chicola K, Lee H. Access to the bypassed stomach after gastric bypass. *Obes Surg.* 1998;8:289-295.
7. Huang CS, Forse RA, Jacobson BC, Farraye FA. Endoscopic findings and their clinical correlations in patients with symptoms after gastric bypass surgery. *Gastrointest Endosc.* 2003;58:859-866.
8. Schauer PR, Ikramuddin S, Gourash W, Ramanathan R, Luketich J. Outcomes after laparoscopic Roux-en-Y gastric bypass for morbid obesity. *Ann Surg.* 2000;232:515-529.
9. Braley SC, Nguyen NT, Wolfe BM. Late gastrointestinal hemorrhage after gastric bypass. *Obes Surg.* 2002;12:404-407.
10. Nguyen NT, Rivers R, Wolfe BM. Early gastrointestinal hemorrhage after laparoscopic gastric bypass. *Obes Surg.* 2003;13:62-65.
11. Abu-Abeid S, Keidar A, Gavert N, Blanc A, Szold A. The clinical spectrum of band erosion following laparoscopic adjustable silicone gastric banding for morbid obesity. *Surg Endosc.* 2003;17:861-863.
12. Ovrebo KK, Hatlebakk JG, Viste A, Bassoe HH, Svanes K. Gastroesophageal reflux in morbidly obese patients treated with gastric banding or vertical banded gastroplasty. *Ann Surg.* 1998;228:51-58.
13. Dixon JB, O'Brien PE. Gastroesophageal reflux in obesity: the effect of lap-band placement. *Obes Surg.* 1999;9:527-531.
14. Morino M, Toppino M, Garrone C. Disappointing long-term results of laparoscopic adjustable silicone gastric banding. *Br J Surg.* 1997;84:868-869.
15. Lundell L, Ruth M, Olbe L. Vertical banded gastroplasty or gastric banding for morbid obesity: effects on gastro-oesophageal reflux. *Eur J Surg.* 1997;163:525-531.
16. Angrisani L, Iovino P, Lorenzo M, et al. Treatment of morbid obesity and gastroesophageal reflux with hiatal hernia by Lap-Band. *Obes Surg.* 1999;9:396-398.
17. de Jong JR, van Ramshorst B, Timmer R, Gooszen HG, Smout AJ. The influence of laparoscopic adjustable gastric banding on gastroesophageal reflux. *Obes Surg.* 2004;14:399-406.
18. Appropriate use of gastrointestinal endoscopy. *Gastrointest Endosc.* 2000;52:831-837.
19. Mun EC, Blackburn GL, Matthews JB. Current status of medical and surgical therapy for obesity. *Gastroenterology.* 2001;120:669-681.
20. Mason EE, Ito C. Gastric bypass in obesity. *Surg Clin North Am.* 1967;47:1345-1351.
21. Buchwald H, Avidor Y, Braunwald E, et al. Bariatric surgery: a systematic review and meta-analysis. *JAMA.* 2004;292:1724-1737.
22. Bo O, Modalsli O. Gastric banding, a surgical method of treating morbid obesity: preliminary report. *Int J Obes.* 1983;7:493-499.
23. Kuzmak LI. A review of seven years' experience with silicone gastric banding. *Obes Surg.* 1991;1:403-408.
24. Cadiere GB, Himpens J, Hainaux B, Gaudissart Q, Favretti S, Segato G. Laparoscopic adjustable gastric banding. *Semin Laparosc Surg.* 2002;9:105-114.

25. Scopinaro N, Gianetta E, Pandolfo N, Anfossi A, Berretti B, Bachi V. [Bilio-pancreatic bypass. Proposal and preliminary experimental study of a new type of operation for the functional surgical treatment of obesity]. *Minerva Chir.* 1976;31:560-566.
26. Scopinaro N, Gianetta E, Civalleri D, Bonalumi U, Bachi V. Bilio-pancreatic bypass for obesity: II. Initial experience in man. *Br J Surg.* 1979;66:618-620.
27. Marceau P, Hould FS, Simard S, et al. Biliopancreatic diversion with duodenal switch. *World J Surg.* 1998;22:947-954.
28. Hess DS, Hess DW. Biliopancreatic diversion with a duodenal switch. *Obes Surg.* 1998;8:267-282.
29. Capella JF, Capella RF. Gastro-gastric fistulas and marginal ulcers in gastric bypass procedures for weight reduction. *Obes Surg.* 1999;9:22-27.
30. Capella JF, Capella RF. Staple disruption and marginal ulceration in gastric bypass procedures for weight reduction. *Obes Surg.* 1996;6:44-49.
31. MacLean LD, Rhode BM, Nohr C, Katz S, McLean AP. Stomal ulcer after gastric bypass. *J Am Coll Surg.* 1997;185:1-7.
32. Sanyal AJ, Sugerman HJ, Kellum JM, Engle KM, Wolfe L. Stomal complications of gastric bypass: incidence and outcome of therapy. *Am J Gastroenterol.* 1992;87:1165-1169.
33. Sapala JA, Wood MH, Sapala MA, Flake TM Jr. Marginal ulcer after gastric bypass: a prospective 3-year study of 173 patients. *Obes Surg.* 1998;8:505-516.
34. Pope GD, Goodney PP, Burchard KW, et al. Peptic ulcer/stricture after gastric bypass: a comparison of technique and acid suppression variables. *Obes Surg.* 2002;12:30-33.
35. Schirmer B, Erenoglu C, Miller A. Flexible endoscopy in the management of patients undergoing Roux-en-Y gastric bypass. *Obes Surg.* 2002;12:634-638.
36. Jordan JH, Hocking MP, Rout WR, Woodward ER. Marginal ulcer following gastric bypass for morbid obesity. *Am Surg.* 1991;57:286-288.
37. Ahmad J, Martin J, Ikramuddin S, Schauer P, Slivka A. Endoscopic balloon dilation of gastroenteric anastomotic stricture after laparoscopic gastric bypass. *Endoscopy.* 2003;35:725-728.
38. Barba CA, Butensky MS, Lorenzo M, Newman R. Endoscopic dilation of gastroesophageal anastomosis stricture after gastric bypass. *Surg Endosc.* 2003;17:416-420.
39. Sataloff DM, Lieber CP, Seinige UL. Strictures following gastric stapling for morbid obesity. Results of endoscopic dilatation. *Am Surg.* 1990;56:167-174.
40. Kretzschmar CS, Hamilton JW, Wissler DW, Yale CE, Morrissey JF. Balloon dilation for the treatment of stomal stenosis complicating gastric surgery for morbid obesity. *Surgery.* 1987;102:443-446.
41. Blachar A, Federle MP. Gastrointestinal complications of laparoscopic roux-en-Y gastric bypass surgery in patients who are morbidly obese: findings on radiography and CT. *AJR Am J Roentgenol.* 2002;179:1437-1442.
42. Matthews BD, Sing RF, DeLegge MH, Ponsky JL, Heniford BT. Initial results with a stapled gastrojejunostomy for the laparoscopic isolated roux-en-Y gastric bypass. *Am J Surg.* 2000;179:476-481.
43. Greve JW. Surgical treatment of morbid obesity: role of the gastroenterologist. *Scand J Gastroenterol Suppl.* 2000:60-64.
44. Westling A, Bjurling K, Ohrvall M, Gustavsson S. Silicone-adjustable gastric banding: disappointing results. *Obes Surg.* 1998;8:467-474.
45. Ukleja A, Stone RL. Medical and gastroenterologic management of the post-bariatric surgery patient. *J Clin Gastroenterol.* 2004;38:312-321.
46. Weiss H, Nehoda H, Labeck B, Peer R, Aigner F. Gastroscopic band removal after intragastric migration of adjustable gastric band: a new minimal invasive technique. *Obes Surg.* 2000;10:167-170.
47. Chaptini L, Bhambri S, Greenbaum D, Elfant A. Successful endoscopic management of band erosion complicating gastric bypass surgery. *J Clin Gastroenterol.* 2004;38:914-915.

48. Strodel WE, Knol JA, Eckhauser FE. Endoscopy of the partitioned stomach. *Ann Surg.* 1984;200:582-586.

49. Khitin L, Roses RE, Birkett DH. Cancer in the gastric remnant after gastric bypass: a case report. *Curr Surg.* 2003;60:521-523.

50. Lord RV, Edwards PD, Coleman MJ. Gastric cancer in the bypassed segment after operation for morbid obesity. *Aust N Z J Surg.* 1997;67:580-582.

51. Raijman I, Strother SV, Donegan WL. Gastric cancer after gastric bypass for obesity. Case report. *J Clin Gastroenterol.* 1991;13:191-194.

52. Lineaweaver W, Ryckman F, Hawkins I, Robertson J, Woodward ER. Endoscopic balloon dilation of outlet stenosis after gastric bypass. *Am Surg.* 1985;51:194-196.

53. Rajdeo H, Bhuta K, Ackerman NB. Endoscopic management of gastric outlet obstruction following surgery for morbid obesity. *Am Surg.* 1989;55:724-727.

54. Al-Halees ZY, Freeman JB, Burchett H, Brazeau-Gravelle P. Nonoperative management of stomal stenosis after gastroplasty for morbid obesity. *Surg Gynecol Obstet.* 1986;162:349-354.

55. Wolper JC, Messmer JM, Turner MA, Sugerman HJ. Endoscopic dilation of late stomal stenosis. Its use following gastric surgery for morbid obesity. *Arch Surg.* 1984;119:836-837.

56. Froyen J, Rosseland AR, Helsingen N. Endoscopic diathermy incision in the treatment of stoma obstruction after gastroplasty for obesity. *Endoscopy.* 1985;17:91-93.

57. Bell RL, Reinhardt KE, Flowers JL. Surgeon-performed endoscopic dilatation of symptomatic gastrojejunal anastomotic strictures following laparoscopic Roux-en-Y gastric bypass. *Obes Surg.* 2003;13:728-733.

58. Go MR, Muscarella P 2nd, Needleman BJ, Cook CH, Melvin WS. Endoscopic management of stomal stenosis after Roux-en-Y gastric bypass. *Surg Endosc.* 2004;18:56-59.

59. Catalano MF, George S, Thomas M, Geenen JE, Chua T. Weight gain following bariatric surgery secondary to staple line disruption and stomal dilation: endotherapy using sodium morrhuate to induce stomal stenosis prevents need for surgical revision [abstract]. *Gastrointest Endosc.* 2004;59(5):AB149.

60. Thompson CC, Carr-Locke DL, Saltzman J, et al. Peroral endoscopic repair of staple-line dehiscence in Roux-en-Y gastric bypass: a less invasive approach [abstract]. *Gastroenterology.* 2004;126(Suppl 2):A-810.

61. Schweitzer M. Endoscopic intraluminal suture plication of the gastric pouch and stoma in postoperative Roux-en-Y gastric bypass patients. *J Laparoendosc Adv Surg Tech A.* 2004;14:223-226.

62. Feitoza AB, Baron TH. Endoscopy and ERCP in the setting of previous upper GI tract surgery. Part I: reconstruction without alteration of pancreaticobiliary anatomy. *Gastrointest Endosc.* 2001;54:743-749.

63. Elton E, Hanson BL, Qaseem T, Howell DA. Diagnostic and therapeutic ERCP using an enteroscope and a pediatric colonoscope in long-limb surgical bypass patients. *Gastrointest Endosc.* 1998;47:62-67.

64. Wright BE, Cass OW, Freeman ML. ERCP in patients with long-limb Roux-en-Y gastrojejunostomy and intact papilla. *Gastrointest Endosc.* 2002;56:225-232.

65. Pimentel RR. Laparoscopy-assisted transgastrostomy ERCP after bariatric surgery: case report of a novel approach. *Gastrointest Endosc.* 2004;59(2):325-328.

66. Peters M, Papasavas PK, Caushaj PF, Kania RJ, Gagne DJ. Laparoscopic transgastric endoscopic retrograde cholangiopancreatography for benign common bile duct stricture after Roux-en-Y gastric bypass. *Surg Endosc.* 2002;16:1106.

67. Moretto M, Mottin CC, Padoin AV, Berleze D, Repetto G. Endoscopic management of bleeding after gastric bypass—a therapeutic alternative. *Obes Surg.* 2004;14:706.

68. Steffen R. Early gastrointestinal hemorrhage after laparoscopic gastric bypass. *Obes Surg.* 2003;13:466; author reply 466-467.

69. Mehran A, Szomstein S, Zundel N, Rosenthal R. Management of acute bleeding after laparoscopic Roux-en-Y gastric bypass. *Obes Surg.* 2003;13:842-847.

11

Imaging of the Gastrointestinal Tract After Bariatric Surgery

Jose C. Varghese, MD; Brian C. Lucey, MD; and Jorge A. Soto, MD

Introduction

Imaging plays a vital role in the prompt and accurate diagnosis of complications arising from bariatric surgery and is helpful in directing patients to life-saving therapeutic interventions.[1] Up to 10% of bariatric patients experience postoperative complications (Chapter 7); therefore, imaging is routinely performed in the immediate postsurgical period—to confirm adequacy of surgery—and in the delayed postoperative period in symptomatic patients—to detect complications and direct treatment.[1-4] While conducted on a variety of individuals, these procedures are particularly indispensable in the bariatric patient, as clinical examination is often inconclusive because of patient size.[4] The effectiveness of imaging is maximized when tests are interpreted with clinical findings and results from other tests, such as upper gastrointestinal endoscopy (Chapter 10).

The barium upper gastrointestinal (UGI) series and the abdominal computed tomography (CT) are the most common imaging tests used to investigate patient problems after bariatric surgery. The UGI series provides functional and intraluminal information about the gastrointestinal (GI) tract, while CT provides extraluminal information of the surrounding structures. The 2 tests are complementary and should be used in conjunction for complete evaluation of the persistently symptomatic patient when a single test has normal results. Other tests, such as ultrasonography and nuclear scintigraphy, are occasionally used to diagnose specific complications (eg, gallbladder disease and gastric motility disorders, respectively).

Surgeons are performing a variety of weight-reduction procedures, most of which fall into the malabsorptive, restrictive, or combination (both malabsorptive and restrictive) classifications (Chapter 3). This chapter's discussion is confined to the 2 most commonly performed bariatric operations in the United States: the Roux-en-Y gastric bypass (RYGB) and the laparoscopic adjustable gastric band (LAGB).

The investigation of postoperative GI complications can be considered in 3 specific groups. The first group—early postoperative (perioperative) complications—includes those that occur in the first 30 days after surgery, most of which are diagnosed in the immediate perioperative period (before the patient is discharged from the hospital).

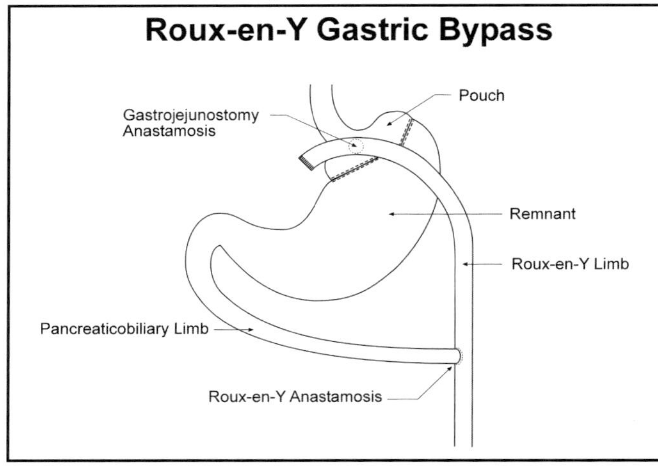

Figure 11-1. Diagram showing normal Roux-en-Y surgical anatomy.

The second group—delayed complications—includes those that occur after the patient's postoperative hospitalization is over and the patient has returned to his or her normal daily activity. The third group consists of the investigation of specific complaints of pain, vomiting, and weight gain that occur after bariatric surgery.

Roux-en-Y Gastric-Bypass Surgery

RYGB is a combination procedure and is currently the most commonly performed weight-reduction surgery in the US (Figure 11-1). It is performed with open and laparoscopic techniques, with the choice depending on the center where it is performed and on the preference and experience of the attending surgeon.

Technique of UGI Series

The UGI series is the mainstay of investigation and is routinely performed in all bariatric patients before they commence oral food intake, usually 1 to 8 days after surgery.[1,5-7] For this diagnostic-imaging test, the patient is placed supine on the fluoroscopy table. A preliminary abdominal radiograph is taken to identify any radio-opaque surgical suture material at the left upper quadrant of the abdomen and to identify any abnormal gas-distended or dilated bowel, which can suggest staple-line dehiscence or bowel obstruction. Most patients have a nasogastric tube transgressing the gastrojejunal anastomosis, which is retracted under fluoroscopic guidance to the lower esophagus. This is done so that an obstruction or leak at the gastrojejunostomy anastomosis is not obscured by the presence of that tube.

Any water-soluble contrast material can be used for the examination. The patient drinks through a straw and swallows 2 to 3 mouthfuls of contrast material while undergoing fluoroscopy. The patient's position is not particularly critical for this examination, although some physicians suggest the left posterior position.[1] Ideally, the patient should be examined in multiple positions to increase the confidence with which a leak is excluded; however, this can be difficult due to patient size, postoperative pain, and attached support lines and tubes. Once the water-soluble contrast study is deemed satisfactory, the patient repeats the swallow with dilute barium. This enables the radiologist to take full advantage of the high-density properties of barium to reveal any small leaks or fistulas that may not be evident with water-soluble contrast material alone.

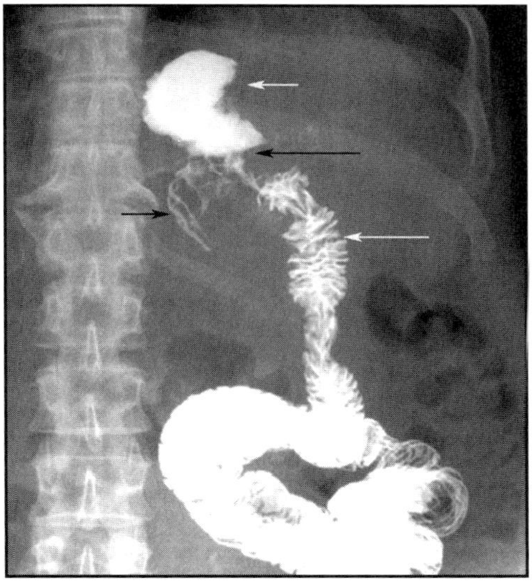

Figure 11-2. Single-contrast barium UGI series showing normal postoperative Roux-en-Y radiological appearance. This shows the gastric pouch (short white arrow), side-to-side gastrojejunostomy anastomosis (long black arrow), blind-ending Roux-loop stump (short black arrow), and Roux-en-Y limb (long white arrow).

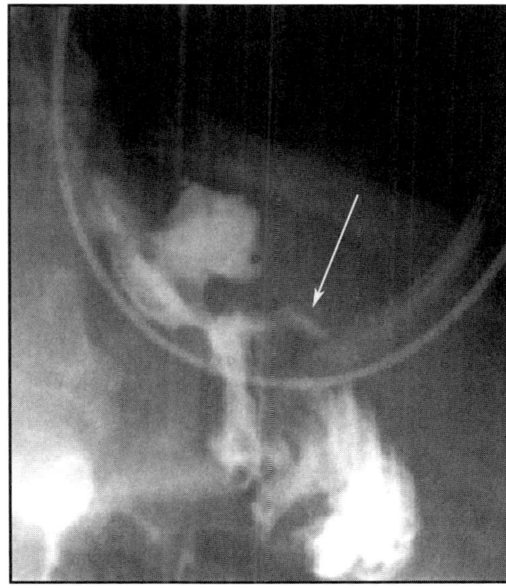

Figure 11-3. Gastrografin UGI series in the immediate postoperative period showing a small localized leak (arrow) from the gastrojejunostomy anastomosis.

Attention to the following details in the technique of performing an UGI series will increase its sensitivity for the detection of complications occurring after bariatric surgery: (1) reduction in pain and discomfort to the patients by not using gas distention; (2) detection of occult leak by intermittent fluoroscopic examination of the left upper quadrant of the abdomen to identify any pooling of contrast material in the subphrenic or perisplenic regions; (3) detection of occult leaks by fluoroscopic examination of any surgical drains present to look for evidence of contrast material within these drains; (4) detection of a staple line dehiscence by the use of intermittent obliqued spot views of the stomach to identify any filling of the gastric remnant; (5) distinguish incomplete from complete obstruction at the gastrojejunostomy anastamosis by obtaining delayed films to look for passage of contrast distally; and (6) exclusion of any complications, such as obstruction or leak, at the Roux-en-Y anastamosis by making sure that contrast material has progressed beyond this point before completion of the examination. A normal early postoperative UGI series is shown in Figure 11-2.

Complications

Early Postoperative Complications

The most dangerous perioperative complications include bowel leaks, bowel obstruction, and staple-line dehiscence. GI hemorrhage into the bowel lumen, the bowel wall, or the peritoneum is a rare but concerning complication that requires immediate investigation and treatment. Less critical complications include temporary hold-up of contrast at the gastrojejunostomy anastomosis and gastroesophageal reflux.

Intra-abdominal infection due to GI leak is the most common cause of perioperative mortality after bariatric surgery (Figure 11-3). The leak usually arises from the gastric

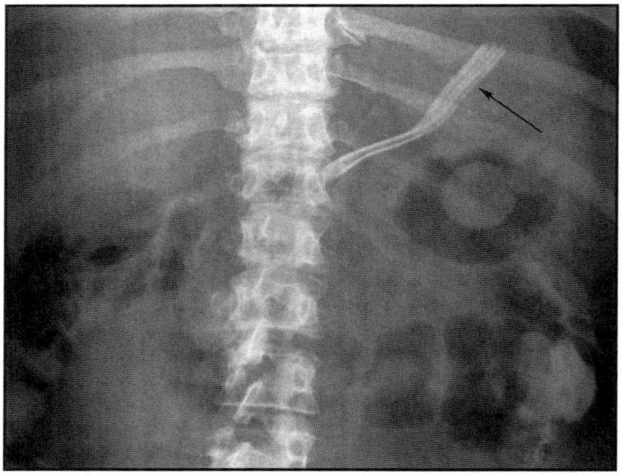

Figure 11-4A. Gastrografin UGI series showing a leak. This preliminary image shows a surgical drain (arrow) in situ.

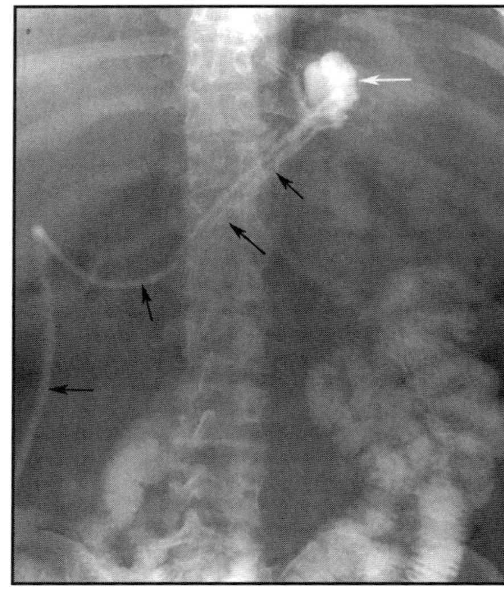

Figure 11-4B. After grastrografin swallow, there is filling of the gastric pouch (white arrow) with immediate contrast opacification of the surgical drain (black arrows) indicative of a leak.

pouch, close to or at the staple line.[1] Less commonly, leaks can arise from the Roux-en-Y anastomotic site. Gastric leaks occur because of devascularization that results from gastric mobilization and stapling, which leads to bowel necrosis and perforation. During an UGI series, contrast extravasates from the stomach into the peritoneal cavity.[8] This may appear as a confined extragastric collection or as a free-flowing peritoneal leak. Occasionally, the only sign of a leak is the occult pooling of contrast in the left subdiaphragmatic space or the presence of contrast material in the surgical drains in situ (Figure 11-4).[6]

CT can also be extremely useful in the diagnosis of a leak.[4] It can show extraluminal gas and contrast material and can occasionally reveal a sealed-off collection that is not detected at UGI study. Patients with a bowel leak usually present with tachycardia, tachypnea, shock, and abdominal pain; however, in many patients, these signs are not present. There should be a low threshold for imaging if the physician has any clinical concern for this diagnosis.[4,9] Treatment includes immediate corrective surgery or percutaneous-catheter drainage in stable patients with localized collections.

Bowel obstruction may occur because of anastomotic stenosis or kinking of the bowel (Figure 11-5). Measures are taken during surgery to ensure anastomotic patency and unimpeded lie of the bowel to prevent bowel kinking. Despite this, bowel kinks leading to obstruction can occasionally occur when patients resume an erect position, with resultant gravity-dependent changes acting on the bowel at the anastomotic sites. In this situation, an UGI study will show persistent non-passage of contrast beyond the point of obstruction, despite changes in patient positioning or use of delayed imaging. This particular complication requires immediate surgery for relief of obstruction.[10]

A more common finding at UGI series is the temporary hold-up of contrast material at the gastrojejunostomy site because of anastomotic edema.[7] The gastrojejunostomy is

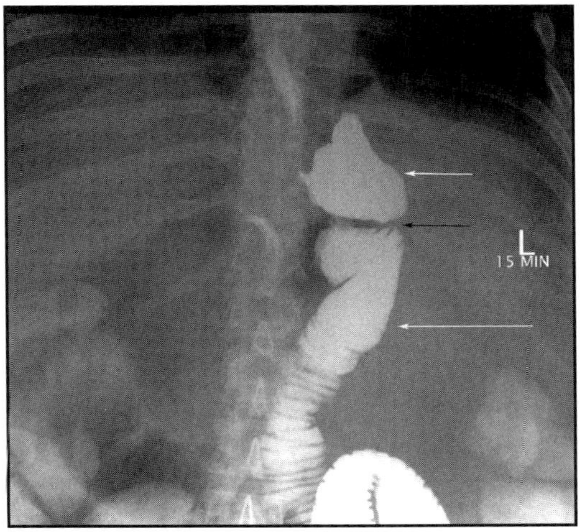

Figure 11-5A. Single contrast barium UGI series showing partial small-bowel obstruction due to stricture at the Roux-en-Y anastomosis. A 15-minute film shows dilatation and hold-up of barium within the gastric pouch (short white arrow), gastrojejunostomy (black arrow), and the Roux-en-Y limb (long white arrow).

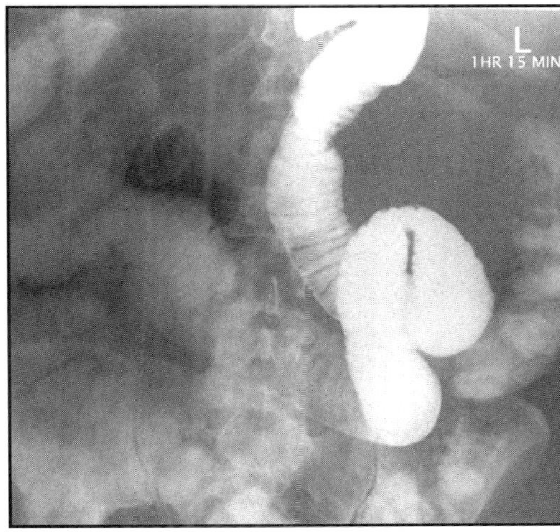

Figure 11-5B. A 75-minute film shows persistent dilatation and opacification of the Roux limb with small amounts of contrast in the distal bowel. A stricture at the Roux-en-Y anastomosis causing partial obstruction was found at surgery.

surgically fashioned to measure 10 to 11 mm in diameter; however, edema in the immediate postoperative period may lead to narrowing of the stoma, which results in temporary hold-up of contrast.[1] In most patients, some contrast material should pass through the ostomy on delayed imaging, which indicates a good prognostic outcome with spontaneous resolution of temporary anastomotic edema. However, if there is complete and persistent obstruction or if the patient becomes symptomatic, endoscopy is required to assess anastomotic patency. Postoperative fibrosis leading to anastomotic stricture, particularly at the gastrojejunostomy site, can occur at a surprisingly early stage. Endoscopy is more sensitive than is UGI series in determining stomal diameter, and endoscopic techniques—such as balloon dilatation—can be used to treat any underlying stricture.[12]

Staple or staple-line dehiscence is an uncommon complication in the immediate postoperative period (Figure 11-6). It occurs because of stress on the staple line, which leads to staple separation. This is diagnosed at UGI series when contrast material enters the gastric remnant from the gastric pouch through a defect in the staple line. There is progressive filling of the isolated stomach remnant and antegrade filling of the duodenal limb. This finding represents a surgical technical failure, and intervention is required to correct the problem. If the staple-line disruption is extensive, revision surgery is required; if the defect is small, repair with endoscopic stapling can be considered. However, long-term data regarding the success of the endoscopic approach is lacking.

Late Complications After Bariatric Surgery

After bariatric surgery, the most commonly encountered late complications are staple dehiscence, marginal ulcers, and bowel obstruction. Investigations are usually triggered when the patient becomes symptomatic.

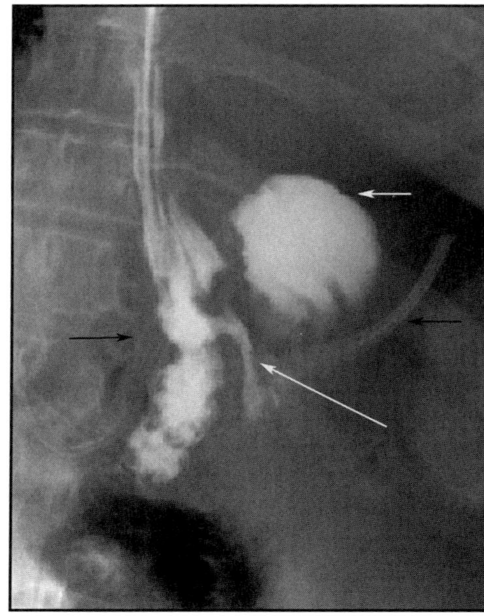

Figure 11-6. Gastrografin UGI series in the early perioperative period showing suture failure with contrast material traversing the suture line (long white arrow) and filling the gastric remnant (short white arrow). Note the surgical drains (black arrows) that are normally present during the perioperative period.

Staple Failure

Staple failure usually presents in the first year after surgery as failure to lose weight, insufficient weight loss, or regaining of weight after initial satisfactory weight loss (Figure 11-7). Staple failure occurs because of many causes, including stress placed on the staple line from overdistension (eating large volumes of food that is not well chewed) and increased pouch pressure from gastrojejunostomy stenosis. The imaging findings and treatment of this condition have been previously discussed.

Marginal Ulcer

A marginal ulcer is most commonly a shallow ulcer near the margin of the gastrojejunostomy anastomosis. Symptoms include abdominal pain, vomiting, and bleeding. The etiology of these ulcers remains unclear, but it has been postulated that they result from overuse of nonsteroidal anti-inflammatory drugs or from local tissue injury related to surgery.[11] There is also a strong association found with staple-line dehiscence. The diagnosis of marginal ulceration is predominantly an endoscopic one, although, when large, these ulcers can be identified at UGI series. An ulcer is recognized as a persistent area of contrast outpouching from the bowel wall, around the anastomotic site (Figure 11-8).[1] In patients undergoing RYGB, peptic disease in the gastric remnant or duodenal limb can be difficult to diagnose and to treat, as these areas remain unseen by endoscopy and contrast studies.

Bowel Obstruction

One of the most common complications after bariatric surgery is bowel obstruction, usually due to anastomotic stricture, adhesions, volvulus, intussusception, or internal

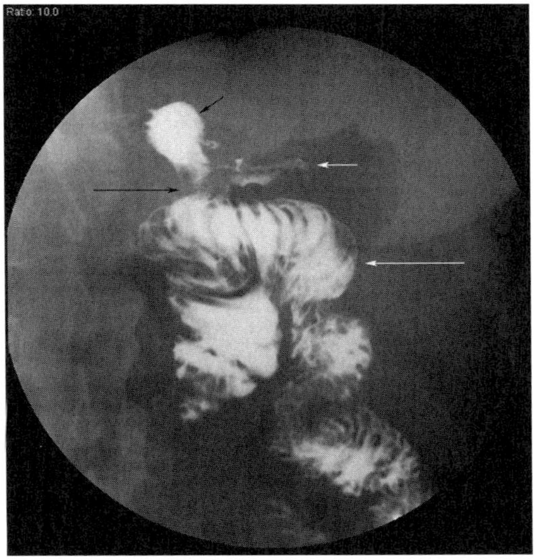

Figure 11-7A. Single-contrast barium UGI series showing delayed staple failure. This shows contrast leak across the suture line (short white arrow). The remainder of the anatomy—including gastric pouch (small black arrow), gastrojejunostomy anastomosis (long black arrow), and the Roux limb (long white arrow)—are shown.

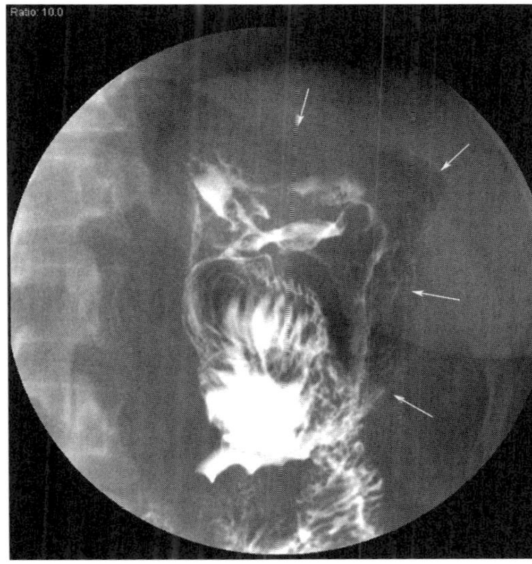

Figure 11-7B. A subsequent film shows progressive filling of the gastric remnant (arrows) with contrast.

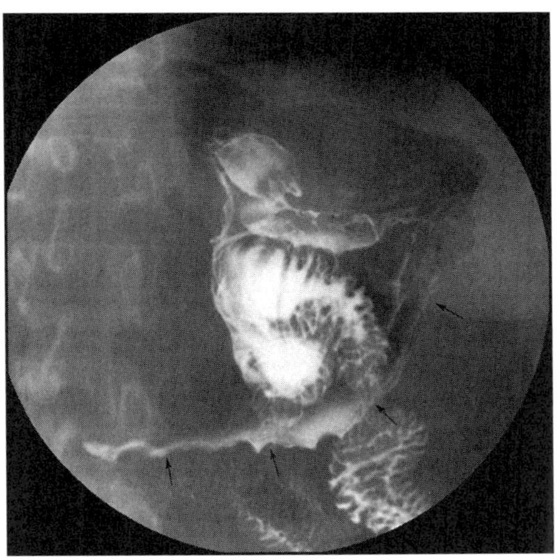

Figure 11-7C. A delayed film shows filling of the gastric antrum (arrows).

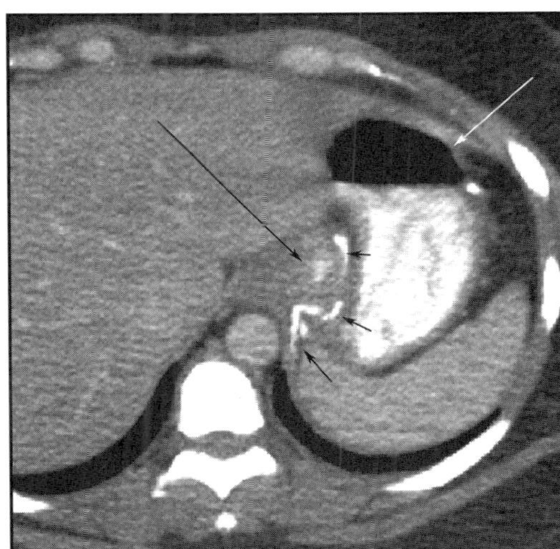

Figure 11-7D. An oral contrast-material–enhanced CT in a different patient shows contrast material within the gastric pouch (long black arrow), as expected, but there is contrast also in the gastric remnant (white arrow), which suggests suture failure. Note the surgical staples (small black arrows) partitioning the gastric pouch from the remnant.

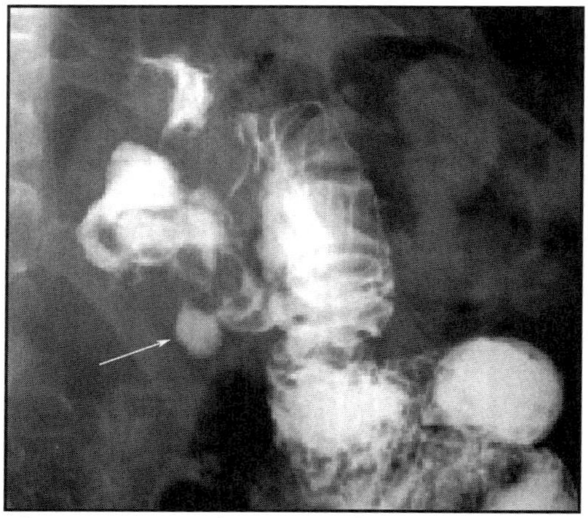

Figure 11-8. Single-contrast barium UGI series showing persistent pooling of contrast (arrow), indicative of an ulcer arising from the Roux limb, close to the gastrojejunostomy site.

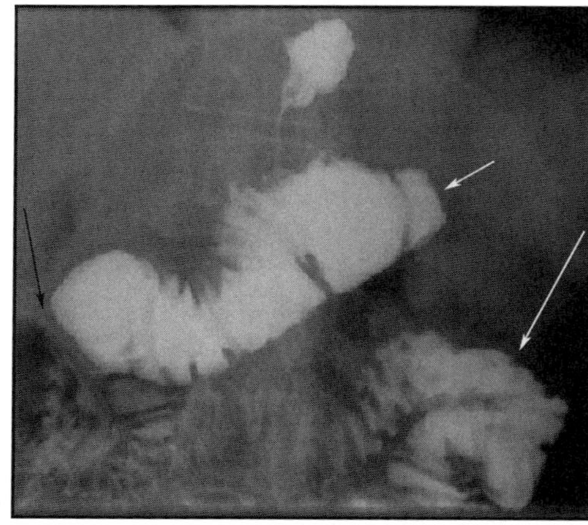

Figure 11-9. Single-contrast barium UGI series showing partial small-bowel obstruction of the Roux limb with persistently dilated, barium-filled proximal bowel (short white arrow); relatively collapsed distal bowel (long white arrow); and site of transition (black arrow)—results of compression from adhesion proved at surgery.

herniation (Figure 11-9).[10,12] As after other surgical procedures, the obstruction can be partial or complete. Patients clinically present with colicky abdominal pain, vomiting, and hypovolemic shock. If untreated, bowel ischemia and death may ensue.

The imaging tests used to diagnose obstruction include the UGI series and CT.[10] Findings on imaging depend primarily on the cause, site, and degree of obstruction. The cardinal finding is that of a transition point with dilated bowel proximal and collapsed bowel distal to the site of obstruction. Imaging is sensitive to the presence and severity of the obstruction but is less accurate in the diagnosis of its cause, unless specific features are present. Intussusception is easily diagnosed when intussusceptum with herniating mesenteric fat is identified within the intussuscipiens (Figure 11-10). However, most obstructions occur because of adhesions or anastomotic stricture where specific diagnostic features are not present. CT is specifically superior to UGI in the diagnosis of closed-loop obstructions such as volvulus or pancreaticoduodenal-limb obstruction, in which segmentally dilated, fluid-filled loops of bowel do not fill with contrast at UGI series.

Imaging of Specific Symptoms

Pain

Pain after bariatric surgery can be due to a variety of causes including rapid, excessive, or improper food ingestion; gastroesophageal reflux; gastric, duodenal, or marginal ulcer; gastric leak; bowel obstruction (pouch or distal); an incisional hernia; or pancreaticobiliary disease.[13] (For more information on postoperative complications, see Chapter 7.)

An UGI series is the initial study of choice to investigate a patient's operative pain because it can detect gastroesophageal reflux and secondary changes of esophagitis that may account for patient symptoms. Gastric-pouch dilatation and stomal widening at UGI may be seen in patients who consume large volumes of food without adequate chewing. These patients require behavioral-modification counseling and training to alleviate their

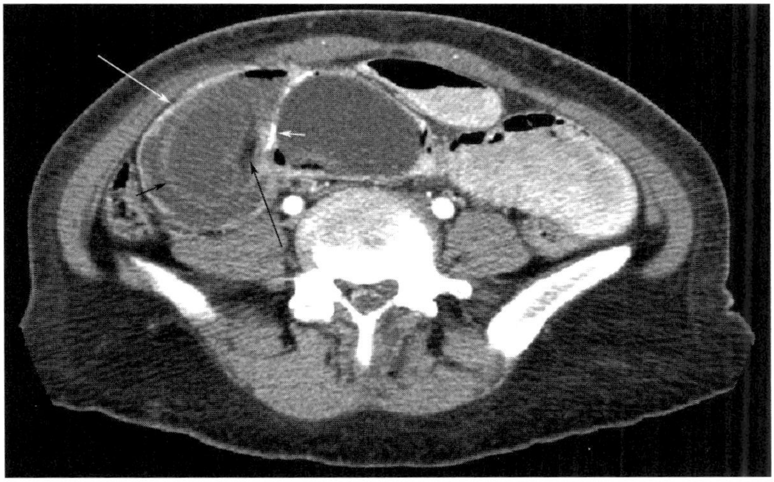

Figure 11-10. CT showing small-bowel obstruction due to intussusception occurring at the Roux-en-Y anastomosis. This shows retrograde migration of distal jejunum (short black arrow) together with its mesentery (long black arrow) intussuscepting through the anastomosis (short white arrow) into the pancreaticobiliary limb (long white arrow).

eating-related pain (Chapter 8). An UGI can show large ulcers; however, marginal ulcers are best diagnosed by endoscopy. Gastric leak is best diagnosed by UGI because free flow of contrast into the peritoneal cavity can be seen.

Detection of a closed-off leak requires CT for the detection of gas or abnormal fluid collections outside the bowel. CT is also useful in the diagnosis of bowel obstruction, particularly one due to closed-loop obstruction.[10] CT also remains the best test for less common causes of postsurgical abdominal pain, such as incisional herniation and fat necrosis.

Various disease of the pancreaticobiliary system can also lead to abdominal pain after bariatric surgery. Not all surgeons perform routine cholecystectomy at the time of weight-reduction surgery, particularly if gallstones are not present; however, these patients are prone to gallstone formation, particularly during the period of rapid weight loss, and they should be monitored closely. Sonography is the most sensitive test for diagnosis of gallstones, while cholescintigraphy is the best test for diagnosis of acute cholecystitis. Pancreatic disease with associated complications—such as acute pancreatitis and pseudocysts—are best shown using CT.

Vomiting

Vomiting, particularly of solid foods, is the most common complaint after bariatric surgery. Postoperative vomiting has a variety of causes, many of which are also sources of postoperative pain: rapid, excessive, or improper food ingestion; gastroesophageal reflux; hiatal hernia; ostomy obstruction by a solid-food particle or bezoar; stomal stenosis or obstruction; Roux limb or distal jejunal obstruction; marginal ulcer; gastric dysmotility; dumping syndrome; biliary disease; or other idiopathic diseases.[11,13]

The UGI series is well suited to evaluate many of the anatomical abnormalities that cause vomiting. The presence of hiatal hernia and gastroesophageal reflux is tested as in normal patients (Figure 11-11). Gross gastroesophageal reflux is recognized by free retrograde flow of contrast material to the cervical esophagus, but intermittent reflux (particularly when small in volume) may require endoscopic methods for diagnosis. Large, undigested food particles or bezoars causing intermittent obstruction can be recognized as filling defects within the gastric pouch on imaging studies.

Gastrojejunostomy stricture is diagnosed at UGI series when narrowing of the anastomosis occurs in conjunction with proximal-pouch or lower-esophageal dilatation and

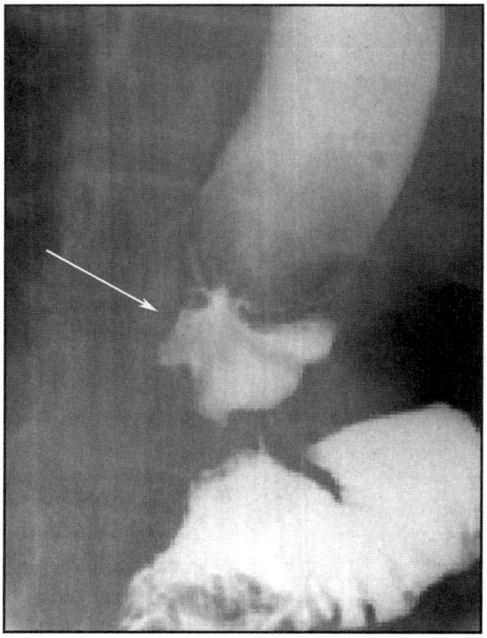

Figure 11-11. Single-contrast barium-swallow study shows the gastric pouch (arrow) situated in the chest with associated free gastroesophageal reflux.

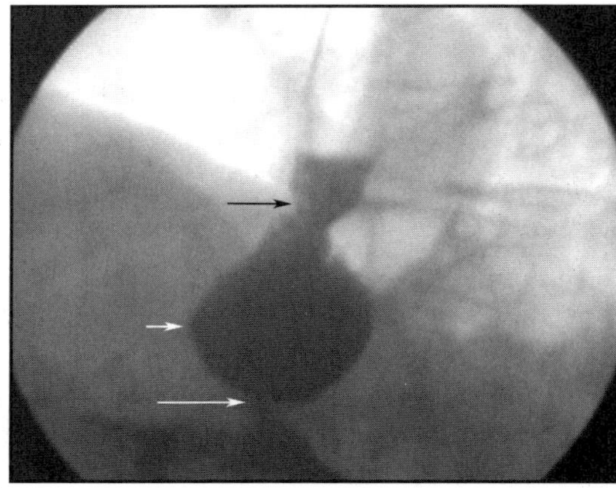

Figure 11-12. Single-contrast barium-swallow study shows a tight gastrojejunostomy stricture (long white arrow) resulting in proximal dilatation of gastric pouch (short white arrow) and esophagus (black arrow) with persistent hold-up of contrast.

delayed gastric emptying (Figure 11-12). This finding is associated with gastroesophageal reflux, pouch dilatation, staple-line dehiscence, and marginal ulcers. Obstruction elsewhere in the bowel, particularly occurring at the Roux-en-Y anastomosis or in the distal small bowel, is diagnosed as in other patients, with impedance to contrast flow and change in bowel caliber at the obstruction.

Physiological causes may also lead to delayed gastric emptying and vomiting. The disruption of intrinsic neuronal integrity during gastric surgery, together with truncal vagotomy, leads to gastric dysmotility. This condition is best diagnosed using a radionuclide solid-phase gastric-emptying study. Gallbladder disease including biliary colic and acute and chronic cholecystitis can present with vomiting. As already mentioned, sonography and cholescintigraphy are the best tests for diagnosis of these biliary conditions. In a few patients, and despite all investigations, there may be no identifiable cause for chronic vomiting, which may cause malnutrition. In such patients, reversal of the weight-reduction surgery may be the only hope for a cure.

Weight Gain

Ideally, a patient should lose weight after bariatric surgery; however, in some rare instances, patients gain weight. The causes of postoperative weight gain include patient's excessive consumption of high-calorific liquid food, enlargement of the surgically reduced gastric pouch, widening of the stoma, or staple-line dehiscence.[11,13]

Ideally, the gastric pouch should measure 15 to 30 ml in volume, and the gastrojejunostomy should measure 10 to 11 mm in diameter to provide sufficient restriction to

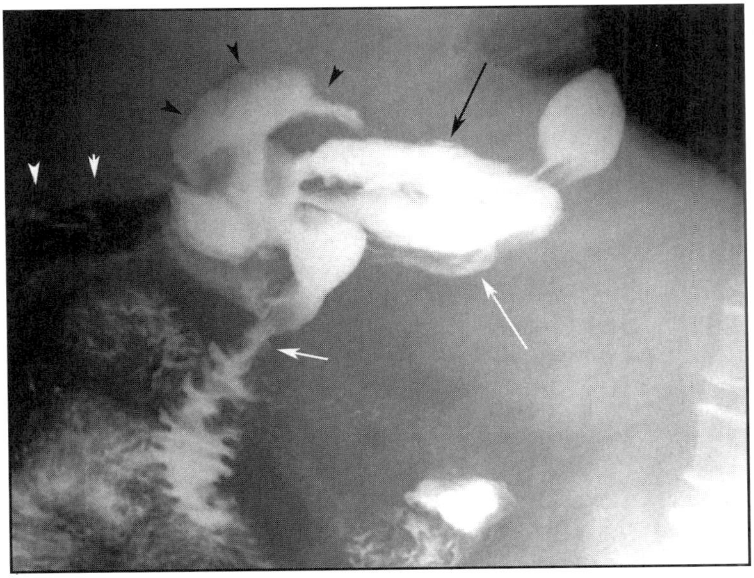

Figure 11-13. Single-contrast barium UGI series showing staple failure associated with a large anastomotic ulcer. This shows contrast in the gastric pouch (long black arrow), but also contrast in the gastric fundus (long white arrow) extending to the antrum (white arrow heads) due to staple failure. There is free flow of contrast through the gastrojejunostomy anastomosis into the Roux-en-Y limb (short white arrow), despite the presence of a large anastomotic ulcer (black arrow heads).

effect weight loss. However, because of surgical technical reasons or overstretching from excessive eating, the pouch or stoma may dilate over time to eventually lose the restrictive effect of the pouch. When this happens, the patient may fail to lose additional weight or may even regain weight. Similar results are evident with staple-line dehiscence, where a loss of the bypass effect results in free communication between the 2 gastric chambers (Figure 11-13). When a patient fails to lose weight or regains lost weight, the health-care provider should investigate and identify the cause.

UGI series is the most sensitive test for evaluating pouch dilatation and detecting staple-line failure. In testing for the latter, the partitioned gastric remnant will progressively fill with contrast material. This test can also expose the site and size of the staple-line defect. Endoscopy best defines the size of gastrojejunostomy anastomosis, although a radiologist can also gauge the ostomy's size during the barium study. When no anatomical cause is identified to account for weight gain, the physician must suspect a behavioral cause—such as excessive intake of high-calorie foods in semi-solid or liquid form—and again educate the patient on necessary behavior modifications.

Laparoscopic Adjustable Gastric Band

LAGB is a restrictive type of weight-reduction surgery that is gaining popularity in the United States (Figure 11-14). The procedure involves the placement of an adjustable silicone band around the upper stomach that constricts the stomach and restricts the amount of food presented for absorption. The band is tightened by saline injection into a subcutaneous port that is attached to the band through a connecting tubing. This surgery is less invasive than is RYGB and is universally performed laparoscopically. Imaging plays a large role in the management of these patients: (1) to evaluate baseline anatomy in the immediate postoperative period; (2) to provide imaging guidance for port access and band adjustment; and (3) to diagnose delayed complications arising from the bariatric surgery.[3,14,15]

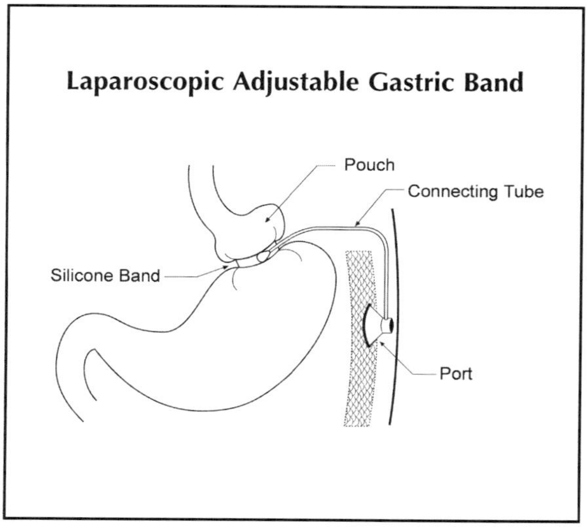

Figure 11-14. Diagram showing normal postoperative LAGB anatomy.

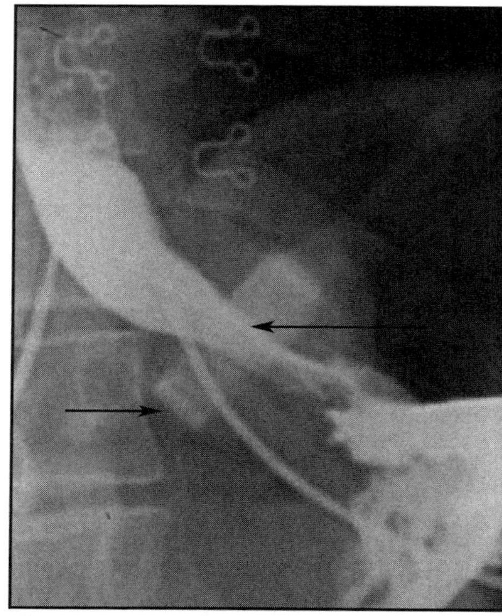

Figure 11-15. Gastrografin swallow showing normal radiologic appearance with adjustable silicone band (short black arrow) causing constriction of the upper stomach (long black arrow). (Courtesy of Scott Shikora, MD; Boston, Mass.)

Assessment of Baseline Anatomy

A dilute-barium UGI study is usually performed in the immediate postoperative period to assess the position of the gastric band and the capacity of the pouch (Figure 11-15).[3] The band should wrap around the stomach just under the gastroesophageal junction to form a small pouch of approximately 15-ml capacity. The band is not inflated for the first 6 to 8 postoperative weeks, when weight loss results from band constriction alone. Unless the band slips or severe postoperative edema occurs, there is usually no obstruction to the contrast flow during the initial barium study.

Guidance for Gastric-Band Adjustment

Usually 6 to 8 weeks after the surgery and periodically thereafter, further weight loss requires inflation of the balloon (attached to the inner surface of the silicone band).[14,15] This necessitates fluoroscopic guidance to locate and access the balloon's port, as is done with the more familiar subcutaneous ports used for chemotherapy. Small volumes of saline are injected through the port to inflate the balloon and increase the constriction on the stomach. To properly tighten the silicone band and achieve the desired constriction of the stomach (ideally a stomal width of 3 to 4 mm) without complete obstruction, the radiologist observes and directs such adjustments under fluoroscopy during the patient's barium swallow.[14,15]

Table 11-1

Primary Causes of Mechanical Gastric Obstruction After Laparoscopic Adjustable Gastric Banding

- Edema around band
- Overtightening of band
- Improper placement of band
- Food bolus impaction
- Band slippage
- Paragastric herniation of distal stomach through band

Adapted from Frigg A, Peterli R, Zynamon A, Lang C, Tondelli P[14] and Roy-Choudhury SH, Nelson WM, El Cast J, et al.[15]

Diagnosis of Postsurgical Complications

The potential complications arising after LABG include persistent nausea and vomiting, band slippage or erosion into the stomach, esophageal and pouch dilatation, persistent gastroesophageal reflux, dysphagia, infection, and mechanical malfunction of prosthetic components. The most common complication—persistent nausea and vomiting—occurs postoperatively in up to 23% to 38% of patients, perhaps because of noncompliance, such as overeating, or mechanical causes resulting in obstruction (Table 11-1). An UGI series will graphically demonstrate pouch obstructions that cause vomiting (ie, causes resulting from band overtightening, slippage, or paragastric herniation).[14,15] In the case of a mechanical obstruction caused by a slipped band, an UGI series will find gastric-pouch dilatation and obstruction to the flow of contrast material (Figure 11-16). When chronic overtightening of the prosthesis causes obstruction, marked esophageal dilatation may be found with loss of the normal stripping peristalsis.

Band erosion into the lumen of the stomach is a rare (1% to 3%) but late complication of LAGB that can be related to overtightening of the gastric band.[16] This circumstance can present with weight gain, gastric fistulation, hematemesis, or (rarely) a leak. The diagnosis is equally made at endoscopy or UGI series. During the latter, the adjustable band is seen as a filling defect lying freely within the stomach, with loss of its restrictive function. The treatment for this is removal of the band and replacement once healing is complete.

Finally, there are a number of technical complications that can affect the port (malalignment, infection), the connecting tube (kinking, detachment), and the band (balloon leakage), many of which can be diagnosed with imaging.[3,15] Specifically, a connecting-tube disruption and band leakage can be diagnosed by observation of a leak of injected water-soluble contrast material under fluoroscopy. Recently, nuclear-scintigraphy techniques were also described where technetium radiopharmaceuticals were injected through the port and the leakage site was identified with a gamma camera.[17]

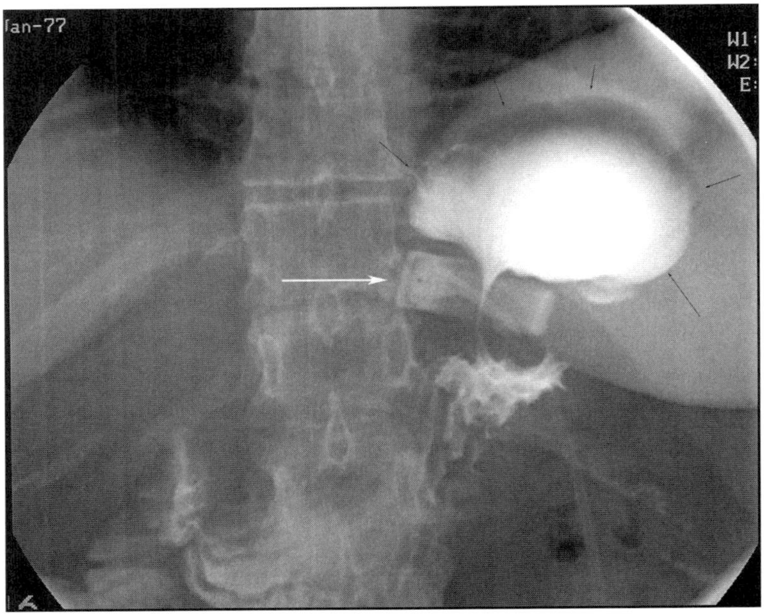

Figure 11-16. Gastrografin UGI series showing distal slip of the adjustable gastric band (white arrow) to constrict the gastric body, resulting in gastric obstruction and pouch dilatation (black arrows). (Courtesy of Scott Shikora, MD; Boston, Mass.)

Summary

Imaging is used in bariatric patients to evaluate the technical success of surgery, document baseline anatomy, and diagnose postoperative complications. The UGI series and CT are the most common investigations used. They are complementary, and together, they provide functional, dynamic, and cross-sectional information that is sufficient to diagnose most complications that occur after bariatric surgery. Physicians should consider performing imaging in symptomatic patients, even when symptoms seem minimal, as early diagnosis can lead to lifesaving therapy. The radiologists performing these tests should be experienced and knowledgeable in the normal postoperative anatomy, as findings of potential complications can be subtle and easily missed.[7] The value of imaging is maximized when interpreted in the context of clinical findings and with the results of other tests, such as upper gastrointestinal endoscopy.

References

1. Monteduro F, Cappello I, Mazzoni G, et al. Radiological contrast studies after vertical banded gastroplasty (VBG) and Roux-en-Y gastric bypass (RYGBP) in patients with morbid obesity. Study of the complications. *Radiol Med (Torino)*. 2004;107(5-6):515-523.
2. Livingston EH. Procedure incidence and in-hospital complication rates of bariatric surgery in the United States. *Am J Surg*. 2004;188(2):105-110.
3. Hainaux B, Coppens E, Sattari A, Vertruyen M, Hubloux G, Cadiere GB. Laparoscopic adjustable silicone gastric banding: radiological appearances of a new surgical treatment for morbid obesity. *Abdom Imaging*. 1999;24(6):533-537.
4. Lyass S, Khalili TM, Cunneen S, et al. Radiological studies after laparoscopic Roux-en-Y gastric bypass: routine or elective? *Am Surg*. 2004;70(10):918-921.
5. Ganci-Cerrud G, Herrera MF. Role of radiologic contrast studies in the early postoperative period after bariatric surgery. *Obes Surg*. 1999;9(6):532-534.
6. Serafini F, Anderson W, Ghassemi P, Poklepovic J, Murr MM. The utility of contrast studies and drains in the management of patients after Roux-en-Y gastric bypass. *Obes Surg*. 2002;12(1):34-38.
7. Toppino M, Cesarani F, Comba A, et al. The role of early radiological studies after gastric bariatric surgery. *Obes Surg*. 2001;11(4):447-454.
8. Moffat RE, Peltier GL, Jewell WR. The radiological spectrum of gastric bypass complications. *Radiology*. 1979;132(1):33-36.
9. Gonzalez R, Nelson LG, Gallagher SF, Murr MM. Anastomotic leaks after laparoscopic gastric bypass. *Obes Surg*. 2004;14(10):1299-1307.
10. Srikanth MS, Keskey T, Fox SR, Oh KH, Fox ER, Fox KM. Computed tomography patterns in small bowel obstruction after open distal gastric bypass. *Obes Surg*. 2004;14(6):811-822.
11. Ukleja A, Stone RL. Medical and gastroenterologic management of the post-bariatric surgery patient. *J Clin Gasteroenterol*. 2004;38(4):312-321.
12. MacGregor AM. Small bowel obstruction following gastric bypass. *Obes Surg*. 1992;2(4):333-339.
13. Knol JA. Management of the problem patient after bariatric surgery. *Gastroenterol Clinic North Am*. 1994;23(2):345-369.
14. Frigg A, Peterli R, Zynamon A, Lang C, Tondelli P. Radiologic and endoscopic evaluation for laparoscopic adjustable gastric banding: preoperative and follow-up. *Obes Surg*. 2001;11(5):594-599.
15. Roy-Choudhury SH, Nelson WM, El Cast J, et al. Technical aspects and complications of laparoscopic banding for morbid obesity—a radiological perspective. *Clin Radiol*. 2004;59(3):227-236.
16. Hainaux B, Agneessens E, Rubesova E, et al. Intragastric band erosion after laparoscopic adjustable gastric banding for morbid obesity: imaging characteristics of an underreported complication. *AJR Am J Roentgenol*. 2005;184(1):109-112.
17. Mittermair RP, Weiss HG, Nehoda H, et al. Band leakage after laparoscopic adjustable gastric banding. *Obes Surg*. 2003;13(6):913-917.

Selected Readings

Balchar A, Federle MP, Pealer KM, Abu Abeid S, Graif M. Radiographic manifestations of normal postoperative anatomy and gastrointestinal complications of bariatric surgery, with emphasis on CT imaging findings. *Semin Ultrasound CT MR*. 2004;25(3):239-251.

Fielding GA, Ren CJ. Laparoscopic adjustable gastric band. *Surg Clin North Am*. 2005;85(1):129-140.

Martin LF. Managing postoperative complications after bariatric surgery. In: Martin LF, ed. *Obesity Surgery*. New York, NY: McGraw-Hill; 2004:259-274.

12

Psychological Issues and the Bariatric-Surgery Patient

Linda Lin, PhD and Frank Perna, PhD, EdD

Introduction

In the study of obesity surgery, understandably, much attention has been paid to the surgery's effects on physical health. However, the psychological aspects of obesity surgery significantly impact the individual as well, playing a major role in the patient's experience of and success with the surgery. Health professionals specializing in obesity surgery can improve patient preparedness for surgery and care by examining the psychological correlates of obesity and obesity surgery. This is particularly important because mental health professionals are being utilized more frequently to assess individuals' psychological appropriateness for obesity surgery. Although the research on the psychological factors related to obesity surgery is still in its infancy, the existing research sheds light on how to best assess and treat patients seeking obesity surgery and provides future direction for the field.

Psychological Issues Within the Morbidly Obese Population

Studies suggest that individuals with morbid obesity experience different psychosocial stressors than do nonobese individuals. Prejudice and discrimination are prevalent in society and negatively impact individuals with obesity. Although bariatric surgery corrects a biological predisposition to weight gain, it does not necessarily address the psychosocial issues and self-beliefs that patients may have formed and that may remain or influence the patient postsurgically. For this reason, it is important to understand the psychological context of the patient with obesity.

Prejudice and Discrimination

In societies that greatly value thinness, individuals with obesity suffer from prejudice and discrimination. The negative attitudes that American society has against individuals with obesity have been called the "last safe prejudice" in the United States. Although there is growing recognition of the biological and genetic factors that affect weight, research shows that American society continues to view weight as a controllable characteristic.[1] The assumption that weight is dependent on will power leads to the common belief that obesity is the result of character defects within the individual who is obese.[2,3] For instance, studies have shown that individuals with obesity are perceived as lazy, slow, dirty, stupid, ugly, sloppy, and as having poor willpower.[4] These studies show that these negative stereotypes are prevalent in children as young as 6 years old.[5] These negative stereotypes are held despite the fact that there are few differences in personality characteristics between obese and nonobese individuals.[6]

These negative attitudes often translate into discriminatory behaviors. The discrimination faced by individuals with obesity has measurable effects on major life events. One long-term study of females with obesity found that they are paid less money, receive fewer years of education, and are less likely to be married than are nonobese females.[7] Another study found discriminatory treatment in the workplace in employee selection, placement, salary, promotion, and discharge.[8] Unfortunately, individuals with obesity suffer from societal prejudice and discrimination that nonobese individuals do not encounter.

Because individuals with obesity are subject to greater psychosocial stressors, one would suspect that these individuals experience greater psychological distress than do nonobese individuals. Research has examined both subclinical psychological distress and gross psychopathology. Although most research suggests that individuals with obesity do not inherently suffer from greater rates of gross psychopathology than do nonobese individuals, findings suggest that individuals with obesity experience higher rates of subclinical distress. Moreover, these patients' distress levels and dissatisfaction with themselves are most likely to occur when they attempt to diet—when, presumably, self-to-others comparisons are heightened.[9,10] This point is salient in that a negative affect accompanies an attempt at behavior change, as opposed to having affect reinforce an attempted behavior change.

Psychopathology

It has been commonly assumed that there are greater levels of clinical distress among individuals with obesity than are among nonobese individuals. Although this assumption has been widely held, research suggests that there are no greater levels of psychopathology among individuals with obesity than in their nonobese counterparts. In fact, psychological distress such as depression and anxiety, which were once widely considered a cause of obesity, are now considered by some to be consequences of obesity.[11] Although individuals with obesity who are within the general population do not experience greater rates of clinical distress, research does suggest greater rates of clinical distress among individuals seeking obesity treatment. In addition, some researchers have hypothesized that there may be specific subgroups of individuals with obesity that are particularly at risk for developing psychopathology, such as females and individuals with binge-eating disorder.

General Population Studies

One way to determine whether individuals with obesity suffer from greater rates of clinical distress is to compare the psychopathology rates of obese and nonobese individuals from the general population. Research comparing pathology rates of these individuals suggests that there is no greater incidence of pathology among individuals with obesity than among the nonobese.[12-16]

Although there is consensus that individuals with obesity do not display greater rates of clinical distress, some researchers suggest that definitive conclusions cannot be drawn because of inconsistencies and methodological problems within the literature (eg, lack of uniform definitions of psychopathology and obesity and small, unrepresentative samples). Friedman and Brownell suggest that these inconsistencies reflect the heterogeneity of the obese population and that a second generation of studies must examine specific subsets of the obese population to determine whether specific characteristic (eg, gender, age, degree of obesity) place certain individuals with obesity at increased risk for developing future problems.[17]

The few studies that have examined the existence of psychopathology within obese subgroups found greater incidence of depression in females with obesity than in males with obesity, which mirrors gender differences in depression in the general population. One such study of over 40,000 adults concluded that the relationship between obesity and depression varied by gender: in females, the greater the body mass index (BMI), the greater the incidence of major depression and suicidal ideation, whereas the opposite was found in males.[18] Another study similarly reported that females with higher BMIs reported higher rates of depression than did those with lower BMIs.[19] These results suggest that, although obesity itself may not inherently be associated with higher rates of clinical distress, there may be specific subgroups within the general obese population, such as females and those with greater degrees of obesity, that are at risk for developing psychopathology.

Clinical Population Studies

Researchers have also examined the incidence of psychopathology among individuals seeking general obesity treatment. Perhaps because of greater dissatisfaction with their weight and its impact on their quality of life, individuals seeking obesity treatment are likely to be a specific subset within the greater obese population because they are motivated to seek treatment. Of individuals with obesity who are seeking bariatric surgery, studies have found rates of psychopathology that range from 27.3% to 44.8% for Axis I disorders[20,21] and 22% to 24% for Axis II (personality) disorders.[22-24] These results suggest that individuals seeking treatment suffer from higher rates of psychopathology, but they do not include adequate control groups for comparison. One study with adequate control groups found similar results when comparing individuals with obesity who were seeking treatment, individuals with obesity who were not seeking treatment, and nonobese individuals on a variety of psychosocial measures. The study found that the patients with obesity who were seeking treatment had higher rates of psychopathology and binge eating.[25]

Studies examining rates of psychopathology among individuals specifically seeking obesity surgery have found similar results. One study compared the scores of 118 females with morbid obesity who were seeking Roux-en-Y gastric bypass (RYGB) with age-matched controls on measures of psychosocial adjustment. Participants with obesity scored significantly higher on phobic anxiety, somatization, depression, and hostility.[26]

Another study compared 88 individuals with obesity seeking RYGB with age and gender-matched controls on a psychological assessment interview. Individuals with obesity had significantly higher rates of mood and anxiety disorders and bulimia.[27] Although research has not shown that individuals with obesity suffer from a greater incidence of gross psychopathology than do nonobese individuals, these studies suggest that those seeking obesity treatment experience a higher incidence of pathology than those not seeking obesity treatments.

Binge Eating

The term "binge eating" is widely, but incorrectly, used to describe any overeating or form of emotion-linked eating. While binge eating has entered the common vernacular and is also used by professionals, binge-eating episodes have distinct qualities that are important to differentiate from emotion-linked eating and simple overeating. The latter 2 may commonly occur; however, binge-eating episodes meeting clinical criteria, as opposed to emotion-linked eating, may be less frequent. This distinction is important because many individuals with obesity will report "binging" unless they are specifically probed regarding clinical criteria. Binge-eating disorder is characterized by recurrent episodes (twice a week for at least 6 months) of uncontrollably eating large amounts of food within a brief period. Binge-eating episodes are different from overeating in that the amount of food consumed tends to be considerably greater and eaten at a faster rate, individuals feel a loss of control of their eating, and they are markedly distressed after the episode. Binge-eating–disorder rates among the general population are less than 5% in community samples[28]; however, among individuals with obesity who are seeking obesity treatment, the rates of binge-eating episodes are estimated to be over 40%.[29,30] The psychological comorbidity and outcome differs markedly between patients with and without clinical binge-eating disorder.

Binge-eating disorder appears to be an indicator for comorbid psychopathology. Studies comparing psychopathology rates among patients with morbid obesity show a higher prevalence of clinical distress among individuals with binge-eating disorder. In particular, studies have found that individuals with obesity who are suffering from binge-eating disorder display greater levels of personality and mood disorders and lower self-esteem.[31-33] One comparison of psychopathology rates of 25 individuals with obesity and binge-eating disorder and 25 without the disorder found that 60% of those with the disorder had a comorbid psychiatric disorder versus 28% of those without binge-eating disorder.[34]

Subclinical Distress

Poor Body Image

Body-image dissatisfaction refers to the degree to which an individual's perception or evaluation of his or her body shape and size is positive or negative. Studies that have compared the body-image dissatisfaction of obese and nonobese individuals have shown that individuals with obesity are consistently less satisfied with their body shapes and sizes and have more negative evaluations of their bodies than do nonobese individuals.[35,36] Negative body image has been found, not only in adults with obesity, but also in adolescents[37-39] and children.[40,41] Another measure of body image is how an individual perceives his or her body shape and size.

Body-image distortion refers to the degree to which an individual perceives his or her body as larger than its actual size. Studies examining body-image distortion typically ask each participant to chose a silhouette size from a range of differently sized silhouettes or adjust the width of a video image of a body so that it best reflects his or her own actual body size. These studies have found that individuals with obesity overestimate the size of their bodies more than nonobese individuals do.[36,42-44] Body image may vary among different ethnicities and races, depending on cultural expectations and norms for body size. For example, studies have found that non-Hispanic black females' ideal body size is larger than non-Hispanic white females' ideal body size[45] and that they are more likely to want to gain weight than are white females.[46]

Poor Self-Esteem

Research examining self-esteem suggests that individuals with obesity suffer from lower self-esteem than do nonobese individuals. A majority of the research conducted on self-esteem and obesity has been with child and adolescent samples. The research on childhood self-esteem is equivocal, with studies finding lower self-esteem[47] or no differences in self-esteem[40] in children with overweight compared with that of nonobese children. Results are more consistent within obese adolescent and adult populations, showing that they suffer from lower self-esteem than do nonobese adolescents and adults.[48-50] This research suggests that adolescents and adults with obesity tend to suffer from lower self-esteem, but the same may not necessarily be true for children with overweight.

Summary

Research suggests that individuals with obesity suffer from greater psychosocial stressors in the form of prejudice and discrimination. They are at greater risk for having poorer body image and lower self-esteem than are nonobese individuals. Although it was widely assumed that individuals with obesity suffer from greater psychopathology than do nonobese individuals, research suggests that individuals with obesity, as a group, do not experience more clinically significant psychological disturbance than do nonobese individuals. However, specific subgroups within the obese population may be at greater risk for clinically significant disturbance. For example, individuals who seek obesity treatment, including surgery, do experience a higher rate of clinical disturbance. In addition, it has been suggested that females with obesity and individuals with a higher degree of obesity are at greater risk for diagnosable psychopathology.

Preoperative Psychosocial Factors That Predict Postoperative Outcomes

Obesity surgery requires numerous changes in eating and lifestyle habits. Postoperative diets are incredibly restrictive. Individuals who elect to have the surgery must reduce their portion sizes; eat at a slower rate; avoid high-sugar, high-fat foods; and avoid drinking beverages with meals (Chapter 8). While weight loss is significant and rapid in the first postsurgical year, studies have shown that a significant number of individuals who undergo obesity surgery regain weight within 18 months to 2 years after their surgery.[51] Weight regain may be due, in part, to a lack of psychological and behavioral readiness. For example, individuals who do not have good coping mechanisms in place to help manage the stress related to major lifestyle changes may have more difficulty complying with the diet and may experience greater amounts of psychological distress postoperatively. Identifying psychological and behavioral variables that predict postoperative success is useful. In addition, evaluation may help medical professionals identify individuals who may benefit from preoperative interventions designed to increase surgery readiness.

Psychopathology

Contrary to popular belief, the presence of psychopathology does not appear to be associated with poor postoperative weight loss. A majority of studies suggest that preoperative levels of clinical distress do not predict less postoperative weight loss. A study of 65 individuals undergoing RYGB who underwent semi-structured psychiatric interviews before surgery and 16 months after surgery found that psychiatric status was not related to postoperative weight loss.[52] Another study grouped individuals undergoing vertical banded gastroplasty (VBG) into 3 categories with regard to psychological disturbance: no psychiatric abnormality, minor psychiatric disorders, and major psychiatric disturbance. Findings showed no differences in postoperative weight loss among the 3 groups at a mean follow-up period of 33 months.[53] A study of 131 RYGB found no relationship between preoperative psychiatric diagnosis and postoperative weight loss after a follow-up period of more than 5 years.

In fact, some studies have suggested that greater clinical distress predicts greater weight loss. One assessment of depression levels of RYGB patients found that greater depression scores predict greater weight loss at 1-year follow-up.[54] Another study found that those who experienced depression preoperatively experienced greater weight loss postoperatively at the over 2–year follow-up.[55] In contrast, a study of 89 patients undergoing VBG divided subjects into three groups, according to severity of psychological and behavioral dysfunction, and found no differences in weight loss at 1-year follow-up.[56]

Although a majority of studies found that preoperative psychopathology does not predict poorer outcomes postoperatively, a few studies suggest otherwise. One study of 103 patients assessed before undergoing horizontal gastric-banding surgery found that individuals with diagnosed personality disorders prior to surgery were less likely to have lost sufficient weight at the 3-year follow-up.[24] Patients who were more likely to seek preoperative psychiatric counseling were more likely to experience negative psychosocial outcomes, although counseling rates did not correlate with weight loss. A study of 57 patients with horizontally reinforced gastric surgery found history of psychiatric inpatient hospitalization to be linked to postoperative medical and psychiatric complications, although not to weight loss.[57] Some anxiety disorders (generalized anxiety disorder and phobia) are negatively related with weight loss 1 year after surgery according to a study of 71 patients undergoing RYGB.[58] Another study, which included 20 RYGB patients, did not find a relationship between anxiety and postoperative weight loss at 2-year follow-up.[59]

It is suggested that individuals who suffer from severe or chronic psychopathology may not experience as great a success after bariatric surgery as do individuals with milder forms of the disorder. A review of 29 studies—both prospective and retrospective—with a follow-up of 1 year examined psychosocial predictors of weight loss and mental health after obesity surgery. The conclusion suggests that it is not the mere presence or absence of psychopathology that predicts poorer outcomes but the severity of the disorder. For example, individuals with a prior history of inpatient hospitalization or chronic disorder, such as personality disorders, may experience less weight loss and worse psychosocial outcomes than do individuals suffering from milder forms of mood and anxiety disorders.[60] Little research has been conducted on the severely mentally ill who have had obesity surgery, perhaps because of the typical screening procedures involved in receiving surgery. Many patients are referred by their primary-care physician and must receive a psychological evaluation prior to being approved for the surgery. Individuals with severe and chronic mental illness are often screened out of the process prior to the surgery, which artificially restricts the range of psychopathology and hence the ability of psychological function to correlate with surgical outcomes. Therefore, less is known about the effects of serious mental illness on weight loss and psychosocial outcomes. The results of the current research reflect a higher functioning subgroup.

Individuals who suffer from preoperative psychopathology may benefit from psychological intervention prior to surgery, according to a study of 141 bariatric patients who were screened for clinical disorder (eg, substance abuse, depression, anxiety) and then referred for treatment as a prerequisite for surgery. Compared with bariatric patients who had no preoperative clinical disorders, study participants who successfully completed preoperative treatment lost more weight at 2 postoperative years than did those with no preoperative disorder.[61] Although this study is limited by a small follow-up sample size, reliance on self-report weight, and a limited range of disorders, it suggests that individuals with preoperative psychopathology have postoperative weight loss with treatment prior to surgery.

Subclinical Distress

Two studies that examined history of sexual abuse show equivocal results. Of 243 individuals seeking RYGB, 28% reported a history of sexual abuse; those individuals had lost significantly less weight 1 year after surgery than had those who did not report a history of sexual abuse.[62] This is contrasted by another study of females undergoing RYGB: subjects with histories of sexual abuse had greater levels of postoperative depression at the 5- to 9-month follow-up but no differences in postoperative weight loss and depression levels at the 1-year follow-up.[63] A patient's history of sexual abuse in itself may not be a predictor of postoperative outcomes; however, the degree of psychological distress experienced as a result of the abuse may predict an outcome.

Studies suggest that preoperative stress levels do not predict poorer postoperative outcomes. A study of 131 individuals undergoing RYGB in high- and low-psychosocial stress groups did not differ in physical and psychological well-being 1 year after surgery.[64] Surprisingly, 1 study suggests that individuals with greater life stress lose more weight 1 to 2 years postoperatively than do individuals with less life stress.[62]

Eating Behaviors

Binge Eating

Research examining preoperative binge-eating disorder in 191 patients undergoing RYGB[65] and 80 individuals undergoing adjustable silicone gastric banding (ASGB)[66] suggests that this eating behavior does not predict poorer weight loss in the first year after surgery. These studies did find, however, that individuals with binge-eating disorder had significantly higher vomiting frequency postoperatively, although it did not appear to affect weight loss. Latner et al[52] found that higher levels of binge eating were predictive of greater weight loss by the patient at 16-month follow-up.

Although most studies have not shown binge-eating disorder to be predictive of less postoperative weight loss after 1 year, studies with longer follow-up periods suggest that preoperative binge eating may predict poorer weight loss and psychosocial adjustment long-term. One study of 27 individuals undergoing VBG compared weight-loss results of individuals with and without preoperative binge-eating disorder and found no difference in weight loss 1 year after surgery; however, after 5 years, individuals with binge-eating disorder had regained significantly more weight than had those without the disorder.[67] A cross-sectional study of 99 individuals who had RYGB 2 to 7 years earlier found that 46% reported postoperative binge-eating episodes and weight regain.[68] Powers et al examined the eating disordered pathology in 116 individuals undergoing gastric-restrictive surgeries and 5 years after the surgery. They found no difference in postoperative weight; however, 79% of patients reported occasional vomiting and 33% were vomiting weekly, which suggested failed attempts to overeat.[69] These studies suggest that individuals with binge-eating problems prior to surgery may see a sharp reduction of binge-eating problems within the first few years after the surgery but a recurrence of problems long-term.

General Eating Habits

Researchers have examined what preoperative eating habits are linked to postoperative success. Studies suggest that infrequent snacking and eating triggered by pleasant emotions are associated with better outcomes. According to a study of eating triggers for 33 patients undergoing RYGB, individuals who eat in response to positive emotions (eg, pleasant feelings, a sense of accomplishment) have greater weight loss postoperatively than do those whose eating is triggered by negative emotions (eg, stress).[20] Brolin et al examined preoperative eating habits of individuals undergoing horizontal gastroplasty and found that frequent snacking prior to surgery is associated with poor postoperative weight loss.[70]

Studies have compared individuals who eat sweets with those who do not and suggest that there is no difference between the groups. Investigators examining the preoperative sugar intake of 375 individuals undergoing VBG found that sugar intake was not linked to postoperative weight at 2-year follow-up.[71] A retrospective study of 200 individuals undergoing laparoscopic adjustable gastric banding (LAGB) had similar findings.[72] An examination of 260 patients undergoing restrictive LAGB found that those who did not eat sugary foods preoperatively experienced greater weight gain by the 3-year follow-up.[73] The type of gastric surgery may affect this outcome, according to findings of Sugerman and colleagues. "Sweets eaters" (ingest >300 cal/day of sweets or ≥3 sweet beverages a week) and "non-sweets eaters" were randomly assigned to either VBG or RYGB. Weight loss at 1 year between the two RYGB groups did not differ; however, there were significant differences in weight loss with VBG. "Non-sweets eaters" lost significantly more weight with VGB at the 1-year follow-up than did "sweets eaters."[74]

Limitations to Predicting Surgical Outcome from Psychological Assessment

Although a number of studies have examined whether clinical distress, binge eating, and general eating behavior predict postoperative weight loss and other outcomes, the research on postoperative outcomes is still in its early stages, and inconsistencies still exist. Some discrepancy in results may result from differences in measures, research design, and follow-up periods across studies. Many studies used retrospective and observational designs without consistent measures, omitted appropriate control groups, and did not have follow-up periods longer than 2 years, when some gains made after surgery begin to reverse. There has also been a lack of attention to assessment of factors positively associated with postsurgical weight loss. Regardless of the confusion in the field, preoperative psychological assessment is recommended as a means of identifying contraindications to obesity surgery and giving patients realistic expectations of surgery and its outcomes.[75,76]

Summary

Research does not suggest that the mere presence of preoperative psychopathology predicts poorer weight loss postsurgically. However, the sample groups studied have been limited to higher functioning individuals, and it has been suggested that individuals with more severe psychopathology may have problems adjusting postoperatively. A patient's history of sexual abuse does not clearly suggest poor outcomes, although poor outcomes may be linked to the level of unresolved distress experienced after the surgery. Stress levels, in general, have not been linked to postoperative weight loss; in fact, 1 study suggests that greater preoperative stress was linked to greater weight loss. In terms of eating behaviors, preoperative binge eating has not been linked to poorer weight loss in the first 2 years following surgery, although problems with weight regain and adjustment have been found long-term. Studies also suggest that infrequent snacking and eating triggered by positive emotions have been linked to better outcomes. Eating sweets preoperatively does not appear linked to a patient's postsurgical weight loss, although this may depend on the type of procedure done.

Psychological Assessment for Obesity Surgery

Psychological evaluation has been widely recommended for bariatric-surgery candidates.[77] Some programs require a brief assessment interview with a mental health professional, while others require multiple visits and may employ a variety of data gathering approaches including chart review, patient clinical and family interview, psychological-test administration, and behavioral observation. While assessment program requirements vary, they share many common and recommended questions about psychosocial functioning that patients should anticipate. As with all assessment, it is helpful to prepare the patient for the interview, as there is often considerable anxiety about the psychological evaluation. Psychosocial evaluation should occur toward the end of a comprehensive assessment, which allows time for patients to try a presurgical diet.

Patient Preparation

Patients must be informed that psychological evaluations are routine and that, just as they see other medical specialists prior to surgery, all bariatric patients undergo mental and emotional evaluation as part of the preoperative process. Patients should know that a standard protocol is routinely administered as a means of normalizing their experience (ie, "We have a set series of questions that we ask everyone."). Patients also need to understand the purpose of the evaluation—to see how they are coping emotionally and to discuss lifestyle changes that will be necessary to accommodate the procedure. Patients are usually reassured when they hear that it is common to feel stress or anxiety as they wait for the procedure. Mental health professionals should communicate that their role is to evaluate how the patient is coping with the anticipated surgery and other events that may be occurring in his or her life. Data and experience indicate that surgery should not be delayed or denied because a patient is experiencing emotional distress, even distress that rises to the level of clinical significance. Rather, the patient should be assured that mental health care is available and acceptable to address distress, depression, anxiety, or other psychopathology in order to ensure that appropriate psychiatric supports are in place to facilitate the best possible outcome. Part of this discussion should also address the degree to which the patient sees emotional distress as an influence on self-regulatory behavior.

Common Assessment Areas

A variety of topics should be discussed with patients before bariatric surgery. While these assessments may not be part of a program's formal evaluation process, addressing them can prepare the patient, thus ensuring that he or she understands the implications of his or her decision, decreasing the patient's pre- and postsurgical stressors and equipping mental health professionals with information specific to each patient that can help with future care, if necessary.

Rationale for and Expectations of Surgery

The majority of patients typically report improved health as their primary rationale for undergoing bariatric surgery. Many also mention desiring improved quality of life resulting from health-related changes after surgery. However, some patients report a primary desire for improved body appearance or are largely motivated to pursue surgery in order to maintain, regain, or initiate romantic relationships. Patient motivation is related to patient outcome: those seeking surgery primarily for health-related reasons have significantly greater weight loss postsurgically than do patients motivated by social reasons.[62] Asking a patient how he or she heard of surgery frequently leads to a discussion of the individual's rationale and provides the evaluator with an idea of how much forethought the patient put into the decision (ie, how many sources of information were used) and of his or her expectations.

Understanding of Surgical Procedure and Recovery

Beyond an assessment of competence, patients are often queried regarding their level of understanding regarding the procedure, time required to recuperate from surgery, work arrangements, and plans for self and assisted care. Patients do not always remember that different surgical procedures and their own medical characteristics may influence recovery time, and they may not have considered the extent to which they may need help to care for their dependent children or dependent parents.

Level of Social Support

The degree of tangible and emotional support is commonly assessed. Tangible support includes the degree to which others may perform tasks or otherwise help the patient during the recovery period. Emotional support entails the degree to which patients feel others will provide understanding and empathy as well as participate in lifestyle changes that the patient may have to make during the pre- and postsurgical periods.

Knowledge of Pre- and Postsurgery Diet

While the dietician's note covers this area, reassessment is helpful and provides an indication of the patient's level of understanding, motivation, and judgment regarding the importance and difficulty of making lifestyle changes. Specifically, the patient must know dietary stages, size of stomach postsurgically, amount of food he or she can eat, pacing of eating and drinking, and if the patient has been prescribed and attempted any dietary changes. Data are then compared with the dietician's note. The patient should also be able to identify commonly prohibited foods and possible consequences of dietary nonadherence, specifically dumping syndrome. Using a trans-theoretical model framework, the patient is then classified according to his or her stage of change (eg, precontemplation, contemplation, preparation, action, or maintenance).

Participation in Exercise

The patients should be questioned regarding the extent of his or her physical activity. Using a trans-theoretical model framework, the patient is then classified according to stage of change (eg, precontemplation, contemplation, preparation, action, or maintenance).

Psychosocial Factors Influencing Eating Behavior

Evaluation usually includes a determination of mood influences, both positive and negative, to eating, environmental factors (ie, cue-related eating, such as relative availability of high calorie snack foods in home or at work), and social influences related to eating. Assessment may entail use of a structured interview, validated questionnaire,[78] or a combination of both methods.

Psychopathology

As discussed in prior sections of this chapter, assessment of psychopathology typically involves, at minimum, a mental status exam and, where appropriate, a more thorough assessment of Axis I diagnostic criteria for depression and anxiety states via structured interview or standardized testing. Assessment of substance use (including caffeine and tobacco) and disordered eating and history of pathogenic weight-control behavior and psychosocial stressors (such as trauma history) are also routinely conducted. As mentioned, the presence of a clinical disorder or clinical history is not in itself sufficient to deny or delay surgery. However, assessment should determine if treatment was provided, if it was relatively successful, if appropriate psychiatric supports exists, and the degree to which the patient's history suggests that he or she will seek help should distress increase. Lastly, patients may be asked the degree to which they have discussed bariatric surgery with their mental-health provider and the provider's opinion regarding the appropriateness of surgery at this time.

Typical Bariatric-Surgery Preparation Programs

In addition to counseling by a dietician, pre- and postoperative counseling may, but not necessarily, be available to patients. Currently, no standard-of-care approach to counseling exists for the preparation of bariatric-surgery patients. Programs fall along a continuum with respect to which psychological preparation simply entails assessment and treatment recommendation to full-fledged surgical-preparation counseling. Similarly, counseling may be individual, group-based, or some combination of both. In programs that do provide counseling, it is typically related to lifestyle-adherence counseling in conjunction with dietician recommendations, addresses psychosocial factors related to emotion-food relationships, and may entail stress management to prepare patients for surgery and post-surgical life. Programs may also involve other patients in psychoeducational groups involving pre-surgical candidates and patients at various post-surgical stages. Patients may also be directed toward online sources for information and support. Internet-based sources can help patients, but, as with any online sources, providers should view website content prior to making a referral. Many programs do not provide treatment for primary diagnoses of depression, anxiety, substance use, or post-traumatic stress, but most make provision for referral and provide counseling related to eating disorders. As is apparent, the availability, approach, and extent of counseling vary greatly.

Psychosocial Outcomes of Obesity Surgery

In the study of obesity surgery, much attention has been paid to the surgery's effects on physical health; however, obesity surgery has a significant impact on psychological health and social well-being as well. Although the surgery's effects on physical health have been well documented, research of the effects on psychological health is still in its infancy.

PSYCHOPATHOLOGY

It has been a commonly held assumption that the stress and lifestyle changes associated with obesity surgery would cause preexisting distress to increase after surgery; contrary to popular belief, studies do not support this. In fact, studies show that most individuals experience either no change or reductions in levels of distress postoperatively. Gentry et al assessed psychopathology of 33 individuals preoperatively and found a history of affective disorder in 4 individuals. At the 2-year follow-up, they found no change in psychiatric status.[20] Using the Minnesota Multiphasic Personality Inventory (MMPI)-2, Maddi et al[79] measured psychopathology in 52 individuals undergoing bariatric surgery. At 1-year follow-up, individuals showed significant decreases in 7 of the 10 clinical scales, and the number of individuals showing clinical levels of distress prior to surgery had declined below the test's norms after surgery. One study reported that half of the 41% of individuals who met criteria for an Axis I disorder prior to surgery had reported postoperative mental-health improvements.[23]

Although it appears that psychopathology improves after surgery, studies suggest that psychological gains made postoperatively dissipate approximately 2 years after the surgery. Waters et al examined the mental health of 157 individuals undergoing Greenville gastric-bypass surgery and found that significant improvements in mental health were achieved at 6- and 12-month follow-ups; however, these gains disappeared by 2 years, suggesting that longer-term follow-up may show variations in clinical course.[80] A study of 90 individuals found differences in reduction rates depending on the type of disorder: at the 3-year follow-up, half of the 41% who preoperatively met criteria for an Axis I disorder no longer met criteria, whereas the numbers were relatively stable for the 22% who met criteria for an Axis II (personality) disorder prior to surgery.[24]

Few studies have followed postoperative psychosocial adjustment long term. One study examined 20 individuals 25 years after they had received a jejunoileal bypass (JIB). Of the 6 individuals who had reported depression and anxiety problems prior to surgery, only 2 reported current distress, suggesting that reductions in clinical distress levels maintained long-term. However, this study was limited by a small sample size and estimated preoperative psychological-distress scores from chart review rather than use of a consistent, validated measure of distress.[81] More studies need to be conducted with follow-up periods longer than 2 years to determine the long-term course of obesity surgery on preoperative distress.

Subclinical Distress

Studies conducted on subclinical distress suggest that the surgery does not cause increases in distress. Several studies have compared preoperative and postoperative distress using the MMPI and found the surgery had no effect.[82-84] Interestingly, several did find reductions in subclinical distress after surgery: 2 studies report that intestinal-bypass patients evaluated with the MMPI preoperatively and 1 year postoperatively had significant decreases in the Depression and Hysteria Scales.[85,86]

Binge Eating and Vomiting

Preoperative binge-eating rates have been estimated to be over 40% among bariatric patients.[29,30] Studies conducted on the occurrence of binge eating postoperatively suggest that the frequency of this disorder decreases dramatically immediately after surgery. A study of 50 individuals before and after RYGB found that 100% of the binge eating had discontinued at the 4-month follow-up,[87] and a study of eating pathology in 40 RYGB patients showed resolution of the disorder in 100% of the patients at the 6-month follow-up.[88] Malone and Alger-Mayer measured binge eating in 109 RYGB patients and found that binge-eating behaviors declined significantly at the 1-year follow-up.[65]

Although incidence of binge eating decreases dramatically immediately after the surgery, there is evidence to suggest that this improvement may deteriorate after 2 years. Kalarchian et al conducted a cross-sectional study of 99 individuals who had undergone RYGB between 2 and 7 years prior. They found that 46% reported postoperative binge-eating episodes and weight regain.[68] Perhaps individuals with binge-eating problems prior to surgery may see a sharp reduction of binge-eating problems within the first few years after the surgery but a recurrence of problems long-term.

In a comprehensive review, Herpertz et al examined 40 studies on the psychosocial outcomes of obesity surgery and found that eating pathology postoperatively differed depending on the type of surgery. Their review suggests that individuals who underwent restrictive procedures and RYGB experienced a decrease in postoperative binge eating, although they had an increase in vomiting. Individuals who underwent a biliopancreatic diversion (also called a BPD/DS) also had improvements in binge eating but did not increase vomiting.[60]

However, specific studies have noted the development of postoperative vomiting. A study of disordered eating pathology in 116 individuals undergoing gastric-restrictive surgeries showed no difference in postoperative weight after 5 postoperative years, but 79% of patients reported occasional vomiting and 33% were vomiting weekly. Patients reported purposely overeating knowing that they might vomit. Despite a sharp reduction in patients' binge-eating behavior after surgery, frequent vomiting after the surgery may be a consequence of a binge-eating attempt. Although frequent intentional vomiting is associated with bulimia, all but 1 of the participants reported that the vomiting was unintentional.[69] Future studies should examine the role of vomiting in postsurgical adjustment.

Quality of Life

Individuals with obesity have increased health risks and experience greater medical problems and social stigmatization than do nonobese individuals. The subjective emotional, social, and physical well-being of an individual who suffers from obesity is significantly poorer than that of a nonobese individual.[89] In particular, it has been shown that individuals with morbid obesity who are seeking bariatric surgery suffer from poorer quality of life than do individuals with obesity who are not seeking surgery.[90]

Although one would imagine intuitively that obesity surgery would have a great impact on quality of life, few studies had examined this until recently. The few studies examining the quality of life in RYGB patients have found that quality of life dramatically improves following surgery. Several cross-sectional studies have been conducted examining differences in quality of life between surgical candidates and individuals after surgery. One cross-sectional study examined health-related quality of life in 20 individuals 25 years after they had undergone JIB. The comparison group of individuals with morbid obesity reported having poor quality of life, whereas individuals who had received the surgery had significantly improved on all measured areas of quality of life including physical functioning, bodily pain, general health, vitality, and social functioning. Moreover, those who had the surgery 25 years prior had similar ratings of quality of life as the comparison group of nonobese individuals.[81] Other cross-sectional studies have found similar differences in quality of life between pre- and postoperative groups.[91-94]

Studies using prospective designs have shown similar changes in quality of life. Mathus-Vliegen et al examined quality of life in 50 individuals undergoing VBG prior to surgery and at 1 postoperative year. One year after surgery, the patients' quality of life improved significantly, as did general well-being, health distress, depression, self-esteem, physical activity, and social activity.[95] Freys et al examined the changes in quality of life of 188 VBG patients and found significant changes between 6 months and 2 years after surgery.[96] A study comparing quality of life outcomes of individuals undergoing VBG and RYGB found no differences between surgery groups in quality of life improvements; all had improved equally.[97]

Marital Adjustment and Sexual Functioning

A majority of studies that have examined the impact of obesity surgery on marriage and sexual functioning have found that, although many individuals report improved sex life following surgery, this does not necessarily correspond with improved marital adjustment. Several studies have found improvement in both marital adjustment and sexual functioning. One study reported that, after an average follow-up of 21 months, 59% of the 160 VBG patients participating reported an improvement in the quality of their relationships and 45% reported an increase in sexual functioning; only 2% and 4% respectively reported declines.[98] Similarly, a study of 54 bariatric patients with follow-ups at 1 and 3 postoperative years reported that, at the 1-year follow-up, 52% experienced marital improvement and 61% testified to improvements in sex life. At the 3-year follow-up, 87% reported their marriages to be good, which did not differ from the normal-weight control group. Interestingly, the divorce rate was higher among couples experiencing greater problems preoperatively.[99]

To the contrary, several studies report postoperative decrease in either marital adjustment or sexual functioning. A study of 12 females who had undergone JIB reported that at 3-year follow-up, patients had improved sex lives but increased strain in their marriages related to lifestyle changes.[83] Crisp et al found that only 2 of 10 patients reported improvements in their marriages, although 46% of married and 18% of unmarried subjects reported increased sexual interest.[100] Hafner examined 69 females and their husbands 1 year after gastric-restriction surgery and found that females rated themselves as significantly more attractive and sociable and their husbands as less sociable and interesting.[101] In another study, 12 of 14 participating couples reported declines in marital adjustment and increases in spousal jealousy and anxiety postoperatively; however, 9 of the 14 couples reported increased interest in sexual fantasies and intercourse.[102]

Rand et al suggest that differences in marital adjustment are related to the level of preoperative marital discord: marriages with high levels of adjustment preoperatively do better after surgery, whereas marriages with low levels of preoperative adjustment do worse.[99]

Summary

Studies do not show that obesity surgery increases preexisting psychopathology. In fact, studies have shown that most individuals experience either no change or reductions in levels of distress postoperatively. Similar results have been found for subclinical distress levels. Incidence of binge eating decreases dramatically in the first 2 years after the surgery, although evidence suggests that disordered eating may return long-term and includes increases in vomiting. Studies show that quality of life dramatically improves following surgery. A majority of studies that have examined the impact of obesity surgery on marriage and sexual functioning have found that, although many individuals report improved sex life following surgery, this does not necessarily correspond with improved marital adjustment.

Conclusion

Health care professionals working with individuals undergoing obesity surgery improve patient care by understanding the psychological issues relevant to their patients. Although research of psychological factors related to bariatric surgery is still in its infancy, existing research sheds light onto how to best assess and treat patients seeking obesity surgery and provides direction for the field. Individuals with morbid obesity who are seeking surgery have psychological concerns that are different from those of the general population. Understanding these concerns allows health professionals to tailor preoperative programs to the specific needs of their patients as well as anticipate any special needs the patients may have. In addition, the surgery itself has a significant impact on patients' psychological and social well-being. A better understanding of the effects of the surgery on psychosocial well-being helps health professionals to better prepare the patient for these changes and address any issues that arise after surgery.

References

1. Klaczynski PA, Goold KW, Mudry JJ. Culture, obesity stereotypes, self-esteem, and the "thin ideal": a social identity perspective. *J Youth Adolesc.* 2004;33(4):307-317.
2. Bocchieri LE, Meana M, Fisher BL. A review of psychosocial outcomes of surgery for morbid obesity. *J Psychosom Res.* 2002;52(3):155-165.
3. Fabricatore AN, Wadden TA. Psychological aspects of obesity. *Clin Dermatol.* 2004 Jul-Aug;22(4):332-337.
4. Ryckman RM, Robbins MA, Kaczor LM, Gold JA. Male and female raters' stereotyping of male and female physiques. *Pers Soc Psychol Bull.* 1989;15(2):244-251.
5. Staffieri JR. A study of social stereotype of body image in children. *J Pers Soc Psychol.* 1967;7(1):101-104.
6. Poston WS 2nd, Ericsson M, Linder J, Nilsson T, Goodrick GK, Foreyt JP. Personality and the predication for weight loss and relapse in the treatment of obesity. *Int J Eat Disord.* 1999;25(3):301-309.

7. Gortmaker SL, Must A, Perrin JM, Sobol AM, Dietz WH. Social and economic consequences of overweight in adolescence and young adulthood. *N Engl J Med.* 19930;329(14):1008-1012.
8. Roehlin MV. Weight-based discrimination in employment: psychological and legal aspects. *Pers Soc Psychol Bull.* 1999;29:28-38.
9. Perna F, Bryner R, Donley D, et al. The effect of diet and exercise on quality of life and fitness parameters among obese individuals. *J Exer Physiol.* 1999;2(1). Available at: http://www.css.edu/users/tboone2/asep/.april998.htm. Accessed January 23, 2005.
10. Ross CE. Overweight and depression. *J Health Soc Behav.* 1994;35:63-78.
11. Wooley SC, Wooley OW, Dyrenforth SR. Theoretical, practical, and social issues in behavioral treatments of obesity. *J Appl Behav Anal.* 1979;12(1):3-25.
12. Faubel M. Body image and depression in women with early and late onset obesity. *J Psychol.* 1989;123(4):385-395.
13. O'Neil PM, Jarrell MP. Psychological aspects of obesity and very-low-calorie diets. *Am J Clin Nutr.* 1992;56(1 Suppl):185S-189S.
14. Rodin J, Schank D, Striegel-Moore R. Psychological features of obesity. *Med Clin North Am.* 1989;73:47-66.
15. Stewart AL, Brook RH. Effects of being overweight. *Am J Public Health.* 1983;73(2):171-8.
16. Stunkard AJ, Wadden TA. Psychological aspects of severe obesity. *Am J Clin Nutr.* 1992;55(2 Suppl):524S-532S.
17. Friedman MA, Brownell KD. Psychological correlates of obesity: moving to the next research generation. *Psychol Bull.* 1995;117(1):3-20.
18. Carpenter KM, Hasin DS, Allison DB, Faith MS. Relationships between obesity and DSM-IV major depressive disorder, suicide ideation, and suicide attempts: results from a general population study. *Am J Public Health.* 2000;90(2):251-257.
19. Istvan J, Zavela K, Weidner G. Body weight and psychological distress in NHANES. *Int J Obes Relat Metab Disord.* 1992;16(12):999-1003.
20. Gentry K, Halverson JD, Heisler S. Psychological assessment of morbidly obese patients undergoing gastric bypass: a comparison of preoperative and postoperative adjustment. *Surgery.* 1984;95(2):215-220.
21. Gertler R, Ramsey-Stewart G. Pre-operative psychiatric assessment of patients presenting for gastric bariatric surgery (surgical control of morbid obesity). *Aust N Z J Surg.* 1986;56(2):157-161.
22. Powers PS, Boyd F, Blair CR, Stevens B, Rosemurgy A. Psychiatric issues in bariatric surgery. *Obes Surg.* 1992;2(4):315-325.
23. Powers PS, Rosemurgy A, Boyd F, Perez A. Outcome of gastric restriction procedures: weight, psychiatric diagnoses, and satisfaction. *Obes Surg.* 1997;7(6):471-477.
24. Larsen F. Psychosocial function before and after gastric banding surgery for morbid obesity: a prospective psychiatric study. Acta Psychiatr *Scand Suppl.* 1990;359:1-57.
25. Fitzgibbon ML, Stolley MR, Kirschenbaum DS. Obese people who seek treatment have different characteristics than those who do not seek treatment. *Health Psychol.* 1993;12(5):342-345.
26. Hafner RJ, Watts JM, Rogers J. Psychological status of morbidly obese women before gastric restriction surgery. *J Psychosom Res.* 1987;31(5):607-612.
27. Black DW, Goldstein RB, Mason EE. Prevalence of mental disorder in 88 morbidly obese bariatric clinic patients. *Am J Psychiatry.* 1992;149(2):227-234.
28. Stunkard AJ. Binge-eating disorder and night-eating syndrome. In: Wadden TA, Stunkard AJ, eds. *Handbook of Obesity Treatment.* New York: NY; 2002:107-118.
29. Adami GF, Gandolfo P, Bauer B, Scopinaro N. Binge eating in massively obese patients undergoing bariatric surgery. *Int J Eat Disord.* 1995;17(1):45-50.
30. Hsu LK, Sullivan SP, Benotti PN. Eating disturbances and outcome of gastric bypass surgery: a pilot study. *Int J Eat Disord.* 1997;21(4):385-390.
31. Specker S, de Zwaan M, Raymond N, Mitchell J. Psychopathology in subgroups of obese women with and without binge eating disorder. *Compr Psychiatry.* 1995;35(3):185-190.
32. Mitchell JE, Mussell MP. Comorbidity and binge eating disorder. *Addict Behav.* 1995;20(6);725-732.

33. van Hanswijcke de Jonge P, Van Furth EF, Lacey JH, Waller G. The prevalence of DSM-IV personality pathology among individuals with bulimia nervosa, binge eating disorder and obesity. *Psychol Med.* 2003;33(7):1311-1317.

34. Marcus MD, Wing RR, Ewing L, Kern E, Gooding W, McDermott M. Psychiatric disorders among obese binge eaters. *Int J Eat Disord.* 1990;9:69-77.

35. Brodie DA, Slade PD. The relationship between body-image and body-fat in adult women. *Psychol Med.* 1988;18(3):623-631.

36. Pearlson GD, Flournoy LH, Simonson M, Slavney PR. Body image in obese adults. *Psychol Med.* 1981;11(1):147-154.

37. Wadden TA, Foster GD, Stunkard AJ, Linowitz JR. Dissatisfaction with weight and figure in obese girls: discontent but not depression. *Int J Obes.* 1989;13(1):89-97.

38. Cash TF, Counts B, Huffine CE. Current and vestigial effects of overweight among women: fear of fat, attitudinal body image, and eating behaviors. *J Psychopathol Behav Assess.* 1990;12:157-167.

39. Cash TF, Green GK. Body weight and body image among college women: perception, cognition, and affect. *J Pers Assess.* 1986;50:290-301.

40. Klesges RC, Haddock CK, Stein RJ, Klesges LM, Eck LH, Hanson CL. Relationship between psychosocial functioning and body fat in preschool children: a longitudinal investigation. *J Consult Clin Psychol.* 1992;60(5):793-796.

41. Mendelson BK, White DR. Relation between body-esteem and self-esteem of obese and normal children. *Percept Mot Skills.* 1982;54(3):899-905.

42. Gardner RM, Martinez R, Espinoza T, Gallegos V. Distortion of body image in the obese: a sensory phenomenon. *Psychol Med.* 1988;18(3):633-641.

43. Schonbu SS, Chell RE. Judgments of body appearance by fat and skinny male college students. *Percept Mot Skills.* 1967;24(3):999-1002.

44. Cappon D, Banks R. Distorted body perception in obesity. *J Nerv Ment Dis.* 1968;146(6):465-467.

45. Rucker CE, Cash TF. Body images, body-size, perceptions, and eating behaviors among African-American and white college women. *Int J Eat Disord.* 1992;12:291-300.

46. Rosen JC, Gross J. Prevalence of weight reducing and weight gaining in adolescents girls and boys. *Health Psychol.* 1987;6(2):131-147.

47. Kaplan KM, Wadden TA. Childhood obesity and self-esteem. *J Pediatr.* 1986;109(2): 367-370.

48. Kim O, Kim K. Comparisons of body mass index, perception of body weight, body shape satisfaction, and self-esteem among Korean adolescents. *Percept Mot Skills.* 2003;97(3, Pt 3):1339-1346.

49. Stein RF. Comparison of self-concept of nonobese and obese university junior female nursing students. *Adolescence.* 1987;22(85):77-90.

50. Davis JM, Wheeler RW, Willy E. Cognitive correlates of obesity in a nonclinical population. *Psychol Rep.* 1987;60(3, Pt 2):1151-1156.

51. Powers PS, Rosemurgy A, Boyd F, Perez A. Outcome of gastric restriction procedures: weight, psychiatric diagnoses, and satisfaction. *Obes Surg.* 1997;7(6):471-477.

52. Latner JD, Wetzler S, Goodman ER, Glinski J. Gastric bypass in a low-income, inner-city population: eating disturbances and weight loss. *Obes Res.* 2004;12(6):956-961.

53. Davidson T, Rohde P, Wastell C. Psychological profile and outcome in patients undergoing gastroplasty for morbid obesity. *Obes Surg.* 1991;1(2):177-180.

54. Averbukh Y, Heshka S, El-Shoreya H, et al. Depression score predicts weight loss following Roux-en-Y gastric bypass. *Obes Surg.* 2003;13(6):833-836.

55. Dubovsky SL, Haddenhorst A, Murphy J, Liechty RD, Coyle DA. A preliminary study of the relationship between preoperative depression and weight loss following surgery for morbid obesity. *Int J Psychiatry Med.* 1985-86;15(2):185-196.

56. Vallis TM, Butler GS, Percy B, et al. The role of psychological functioning in morbid obesity and its treatment with gastroplasty. *Obes Surg.* 2001;11(6):716-725.

57. Valley V, Grace DM. Psychosocial risk factors in gastric surgery for obesity: identifying guidelines for screening. *Int J Obes.* 1987;11(2):105-113.

58. Hafner RJ, Watts JM, Rogers J. Quality of life after gastric bypass for morbid obesity. *Int J Obes.* 1991;15(8):555-560.

59. Delin CR, Watts JM, Bassett DL. An exploration of the outcomes of gastric bypass surgery for morbid obesity: patient characteristics and indices of success. *Obes Surg.* 1995;5(2):159-170.

60. Herpertz S, Kielmann R, Wolf AM, Langkafel M, Senf W, Hebebrand J. Does obesity surgery improve psychosocial functioning? A systematic review. *Int J Obes Relat Metab Disord.* 2003;27(11):1300-1314.

61. Clark MM, Balsiger BM, Sletten CD, et al. Psychosocial factors and 2-year outcome following bariatric surgery for weight loss. *Obes Surg.* 2003;13(5):739-745.

62. Ray E, Nickels MW, Sayeed S, Sax HC. Predicting success after gastric bypass: the role of psychosocial and behavioral factors. *Surgery.* 2003;134(4):555-564.

63. Buser A, Dymek-Valentine M, Hilburger J, Alverdy J. Outcome following gastric bypass surgery: impact of past sexual abuse. *Obes Surg.* 2004;14(2):170-174.

64. Buddeberg-Fischer B, Klaghofer R, Sigrist S, Buddeberg C. Impact of psychosocial stress and symptoms on indication for bariatric surgery and outcome in morbidly obese patients. *Obes Surg.* 2004;14(3):361-9.

65. Malone M, Alger-Mayer S. Binge status and quality of life after gastric bypass surgery: a one-year study. *Obes Surg.* 2004;12(3):473-481.

66. Busetto L, Valente P, Pisent C, et al. Eating pattern in the first year following adjustable silicone gastric banding (ASGB) for morbid obesity. *Int J Obes Relat Metab Disord.* 1996;20(6):539-546.

67. Pekkarinen T, Koskela K, Huikuri K, Mustajoki P. Long-term results of gastroplasty for morbid obesity: binge-eating as a predictor of poor outcome. *Obes Surg.* 1994;4(3):248-255.

68. Kalarchian MA, Marcus MD, Wilson GT, Labouvie EW, Brolin RE, LaMarca LB. Binge eating among gastric bypass patients at long-term follow-up. *Obes Surg.* 2002;12(2):270-275.

69. Powers PS, Perez A, Boyd F, Rosemurgy A. Eating pathology before and after bariatric surgery: a prospective study. *Int J Eat Disord.* 1999;25(3):293-300.

70. Brolin RE, Clemow LP, Kasnetz KA, Fynan TM, Silva EM, Greenfield DP. Outcome predictors after gastroplasty for morbid obesity. *Nutr Int.* 1986;2:322-326.

71. Lindroos AK, Lissner L, Sjostrom L. Weight change in relation to intake of sugar and sweet foods before and after weight reducing gastric surgery. *Int J Obes Relat Metab Disord.* 1996;20(7):634-643.

72. Hudson SM, Dixon JB, O'Brien PE. Sweet eating is not a predictor of outcome after Lap-Band placement. Can we finally bury the myth? *Obes Surg.* 2002;12(6):789-794.

73. Busetto L, Segato G, De Marchi F, et al. Outcome predictors in morbidly obese recipients of an adjustable gastric band. *Obes Surg.* 2002;12(1):83-92.

74. Sugerman HJ, Starkey JV, Birkenhauer R. A randomized prospective trial of gastric bypass versus vertical banded gastroplasty for morbid obesity and their effects on sweets versus non-sweets eaters. *Ann Surg.* 1987;205(6):613-624.

75. Wadden TA, Brownell KD, Foster GD. Obesity: responding to the global epidemic. *J Consult Clin Psychol.* 2002;70(3):510-525.

76. Hunter SM, Larrieu JA, Ayad FM, et al. Roles of mental health professionals in multidisciplinary medically supervised treatment programs for obesity. *South Med J.* 1997;90(6):578-586.

77. Greenberg I, Perna F, Kaplan M, Sullivan MA. Behavioral and psychological factors in the assessment and treatment of obesity surgery patients. *Obes Surg.* 2005;13(2):244-249.

78. Schlundt DG, Zimering RT. The dieter's inventory of eating temptations: a measure of weight control competence. *Addict Behav.* 1988;13(2):151-164.

79. Maddi SR, Fox SR, Khoshaba DM, Harvey RH, Lu JL, Persico M. Reduction in psychopathology following bariatric surgery for morbid obesity. *Obes Surg.* 2001;11(6):680-685.

80. Waters GS, Pories WJ, Swanson MS, Meelheim HD, Flickinger EG. May HJ. Long-term studies of mental health after the Greenville gastric bypass operation for morbid obesity. *Am J Surg* 1991;161(1) 154-157.

81. Vage V, Solhaug JH, Viste A, Bergsholm P, Wahl AK. Anxiety, depression and health-related quality of life after jejunoileal bypass: a 25-year follow-up study of 20 female patients. *Obes Surg.* 2003;13(5):706-713.

82. Bull RH, Engels WD, Engelsmann F, Bloom L. Behavioural changes following gastric surgery for morbid obesity: a prospective, controlled study. *J Psychosom Res.* 1983;27(6):457-467.

83. Castelnuovo-Tedesco P, Schiebel D. Studies of superobesity: II. Psychiatric appraisal of jejuno-ileal bypass surgery. *Am J Psychiatry.* 1976;133(1),:26-31.

84. Castelnuovo-Tedesco P, Weinberg J, Buchanan DC, Scott HW Jr. Long-term outcome of jejuno-ileal bypass surgery for superobesity: a psychiatric assessment. *Am J Psychiatry.* 1982;139(10):1248-1252.

85. Leon GR, Eckert ED, Teed D, Buchwald H. Changes in body image and other psychological factors after intestinal bypass surgery for massive obesity. *J Behav Med.* 1979;2(1):39-55.

86. Wampler RS, Lauer JB, Lantz JB. Psychological effects of intestinal bypass surgery. *J Counsel Psychol.* 1980;27(5):492-499.

87. Kalarchian MA, Wilson GT, Brolin RE, Bradley L. Effects of bariatric surgery on binge eating and related psychopathology. *Eat Weight Disord.* 1999;4(1):1-5.

88. Boan J, Kolotkin RL, Westman EC, McMahon RL, Grant JP. Binge eating, quality of life and physical activity improve after Roux-en-Y gastric bypass for morbid obesity. *Obes Surg.* 2004;14(3):341-348.

89. Hassan MK, Joshi AV, Madhavan SS, Amonkar MM. Obesity and health-related quality of life: a cross-sectional analysis of the US population. *Int J Obes Relat Metab Disord.* 2003;27(10):1227-1232.

90. Kolotkin RL, Crosby RD, Pendleton R, Strong M, Gress RE, Adams T. Health-related quality of life in patients seeking gastric bypass surgery vs non-treatment-seeking controls. *Obes Surg.* 2003;13(3):371-377.

91. De Zwaan M, Lancaster KL, Mitchell JE, et al. Health-related quality of life in morbidly obese patients: effect of gastric bypass surgery. *Obes Surg.* 2002;12(6):773-780.

92. Larsen JK, Geenen R, van Ramshorst, B, et al. Psychosocial functioning before and after laparoscopic adjustable gastric banding: a cross-sectional study. *Obes Surg.* 2003;13(4):629-636.

93. Tolonen P, Victorzon M. Quality of life following laparoscopic adjustable gastric banding—the Swedish band and the Moorehead-Ardelt questionnaire. *Obes Surg.* 2003;13(3):424-426.

94. Dymek MP, Le Grange D, Neven K, Alverdy J. Quality of life after gastric bypass surgery: a cross-sectional study. *Obes Res.* 2002;10(11):1135-1142.

95. Mathus-Vliegen EM, de Weerd S, de Wit LT. Health-related quality-of-life in patients with morbid obesity after gastric banding for surgically induced weight loss. *Surgery.* 2004;135(5):489-497.

96. Freys SM, Tigges H, Heimbucher J, Fuchs KH, Fein M, Thiede A. Quality of life following laparoscopic gastric banding in patients with morbid obesity. *J Gastrointest Surg.* 2001;5(4):401-407.

97. Arcila D, Velazquez D, Gamino R, et al. Quality of life in bariatric surgery. *Obes Surg.* 2002;12(5);661-665.

98. Kinzl JF, Traweger C, Trefalt E, Biebl W. Psychosocial consequences of weight loss following gastric banding for morbid obesity. *Obes Surg.* 2003;13(1):105-110.

99. Rand CS, Kuldau JM, Robbins L. Surgery for obesity and marriage quality. *JAMA.* 1982;247(10):1419-1422.

100. Crisp AH, Kalucy RS, Pilkington TR, Gazet JC. Some psychosocial consequences of ileojejunal bypass surgery. *Am J Clin Nutr.* 1977;30(1):109-120.

101. Hafner RJ. Morbid obesity: effects on the marital system of weight loss after gastric restriction. *Psychother Psychosom.* 1991;56(3):162-166.

102. Neill JR, Marshall JR, Yale CE. Marital changes after intestinal bypass surgery. *JAMA.* 1978:240(5):447-458.

Appendix: Bariatric-Related Abbreviations

25(OH)D	25 hydroxy vitamin D
ABG	arterial blood gas
ABW	adjusted body weight
APGARS	acute post-gastric reduction surgery
ASBS	American Society of Bariatric Surgeons
ASGB	adjustable silicone gastric banding
BADAS	bowel-associated dermatosis-arthritis syndrome
BEE	basal energy expendature
BID	twice a day
BMI	body mass index
BMR	basal metabolic rate
BPD	biliopancreatic diversion
BPD/DS	biliopancreative diversion with duodenal switch
CAD	coronary artery disease
CHF	congestive heart failure
CPK	creatinine phosphokinase
CT	computed tomography
DM	diabetes mellitus
DRI	daily reference intake
DVT	deep vein thrombosis
EBW	excess body weight
ECG	electrocardiogram
ERCP	endoscopic retrograde cholangiopancreatography
FRC	functional residual capacity
GERD	gastroesophageal reflux disease
GI	gastrointestinal
GIP	glucose-dependent insulinotropic peptide
GLP-1	glucagon-like peptide-1
G-tube	gastrostomy tube
HTN	hypertension
IAP	intra-abdominal pressure
IBW	ideal body weight
ICU	intensive care unit
JIB	jejunoileal bypass
LAGB	laparoscopic adjustable gastric banding
LCD	low-calorie diets
MAO	monoamine oxidase [inhibitors]

NG nasogastric
NHANES National Health and Nutrition Examination Surveys
NPO "nothing by mouth"

OHS obesity hypoventilation syndrome
OSA obstructive sleep apnea

PAC pulmonary-artery catheter
PAL physical activity level
PCOS polycystic ovary syndrome
PCP primary-care provider
PE pulmonary embolism
PEEP positive end expiratory pressure
PEM protein energy malnutrition
PPI proton pump inhibitor

QD once a day

RYGB Roux-en-Y gastric bypass

TEE total energy expenditure
TID three times a day
TPN parenteral (total parenteral nutrition)
TTS through-the-scope (TTS) (balloons)

UGI upper gastrointestinal

VBG vertical banded gastroplasty
VLCD very-low–calorie diets
VTE venous thromboembolism

INDEX

WAIT ...There's More!

SLACK Incorporated's Professional Book Division offers a wide selection of products in the field of Gastroenterology. We are dedicated to providing important works that educate, inform and improve the knowledge of our customers. Don't miss out on our other informative titles that will enhance your collection.

Handbook of Digestive Diseases
Anil Minocha, MD, FACP, FACG
448 pp., Soft Cover, 2004,
ISBN 1-55642-665-8, Order #76658, **$35.95**

Handbook of Digestive Diseases provides clinical information essential to the management of various digestive disorders in a handy, quick reference format. This concise, yet complete resource offers practical tips for treatment, as well as common errors to avoid, based on digestive complaints and symptoms.

Bariatric Surgery: A Primer for Your Medical Practice
Francis A Farraye, MD, MSc and R. Armour Forse, MD, PhD
300 pp., Soft Cover, 2006,
ISBN 1-55642-736-0, Order #77360, **$59.95**

Bariatric Surgery: A Primer for Your Medical Practice is a user-friendly, practical reference text that provides all the necessary information that the health care professional will need to assist in patient selection and preoperative assessment, as well as recommendations in dealing with complex postoperative care of the bariatric patient.

The Clinician's Guide to Inflammatory Bowel Disease
Gary R Lichtenstein, MD
336 pp., Soft Cover, 2003,
ISBN 1-55642-554-6 Order #75546, **$46.95**

The Clinician's Guide to Gastrointestinal Oncology
Michael Kochman, MD
440 pp., Soft Cover, 2005,
ISBN 1-55642-682-8, Order #76828, $59.95

The Clinician's Guide to Pancreaticobiliary Disorders
Gregory Ginsberg, MD and Nuzhat Ahmad, MD
336 pp., Soft Cover, 2006,
ISBN 1-55642-694-1, Order #76941, **$59.95**

The Clinician's Guide to Liver Disease
K. Rajender Reddy, MD and Thomas Faust, MD
336 pp., Soft Cover, 2006,
ISBN 1-55642-675-5, Order #76755, **$59.95**

The Clinician's Guide to Acid/Peptic Disorders and Motility Disorders of the Gastrointestinal Tract
Henry Parkman, MD and Robert S. Fisher, MD
400 pp., Soft Cover, 2006,
ISBN 1-55642-716-6, Order #77166, **$59.95**

Please visit

www.slackbooks.com

to order any of these titles!

24 Hours a Day...7 Days a Week!

Attention Industry Partners!

Whether you are interested in buying multiple copies of a book, chapter reprints, or looking for something new and different — we are able to accommodate your needs.

Multiple Copies

At attractive discounts starting for purchases as low as 25 copies for a single title, SLACK Incorporated will be able to meet all your of your needs.

Chapter Reprints

SLACK Incorporated is able to offer the chapters you want in a format that will lead to success. Bound with an attractive cover, use the chapters that are a fit specifically for your company. Available for quantities of 100 or more.

Customize

SLACK Incorporated is able to create a specialized custom version of any of our products specifically for your company.

Please contact the Marketing Manager of the Professional Book Division for further details on multiple copy purchases, chapter reprints or custom printing at 1-800-257-8290 or 1-856-848-1000.

**Please note all conditions are subject to change.*

CODE: 328

SLACK INCORPORATED

SLACK Incorporated • Professional Book Division

6900 Grove Road • Thorofare, NJ 08086

1-800-257-8290 or 1-856-848-1000

Fax: 1-856-853-5991 • E-mail: orders@slackinc.com • Visit www.slackbooks.com